JULIAN'S
MATERIA MEDICA
OF
NOSODES
WITH
REPERTORY

TREATISE ON
DYNAMISED MICRO-IMMUNOTHERAPY

Part I
ISOPATHIC CONCRETOLOGY
Part II
MATERIA MEDICA OF BIOTHERAPIC NOSODES
Part III
REPERTORY

Translated from the original French

by

RAJKUMAR MUKHERJI, M.A., L.H.M.S.

B. JAIN PUBLISHERS (P) LTD.
An ISO 9001 : 2000 Certified Company
USA — EUROPE — INDIA

First Indian edition, 1980

By arrangement with Dr. O.A. Julian, France
Second revised edition, 1985
Reprint 1988, 1995, 1996 1997, 1999, 2000, 2003, 2005
© Copyright with the Publishers

Reprint Edition: 2007

Published by

KULDEEP JAIN

for

B. Jain Publishers (P) Ltd.
1921, Chuna Mandi, St. 10th, Paharganj,
New Delhi-110 055
Ph.: 2358 0800, 2358 1100, 2358 1300, 2358 3100
Fax: 011-2358 0471
Website: www.bjainbooks.com, Email: bjain@vsnl.com

Printed in India by
J.J. Offset Printers
522, FIE, Patpar Ganj, Delhi-110 092

BOOK CODE / ISBN 978-81-319-0075-8

DR. O.A. JULIAN
A Biographical Note

Born on the 18th June, 1910, Dr. O.A. Julian did all his studies on medicine at Strassbourg. He was profited by the teachings of masters like professors Ambard, Merklen and Leriche etc.

While quite young during a replacement at Saverne, he met Dr. Pfister, who practised Homoeopathy. He became immediately interested in Homoeopathy. On the 1st April, 1935, he installed himself at Normandy, at Beaumesnil, in Eure.

He practised a complete medicine with a small surgery, a delivery section and a section for labour accidents, open day and night.

In this village having 500 inhabitants, he was himself a propharmacist, having the help of Mme Julian, who administered the stock of medicine.

Advised by Maurice Delpeche, he began Homoeopathy, which he soon adopted totally.

The world war began. He was engaged as a volunteer. He actively participated in the defence. Being warned of being arrested, he was finally arrested on the 13th November, 1942, was interned at Casseneuil near Agen. He came out of his arrestation thanks to the intervention of his superior, a colonel under whom he worked in the hospital of Agen as a biologist.

He was soon sent to take refuge in Switzerland with his family. Interned from the 6th December, 1942 to May 1943, he organised medical service of refugee camps at Morgins, Presles, Espaligne etc. Always active, he got the possibility of doing researches in the cancer laboratory of the hospital of Lausanne.

He returned to France in May 1945. He found his house completely devastated and his clientele dispersed. He began again his medical activities as well as those of a pro-pharmacist, always helped by Mme Julian. He learnt acupuncture and vertebrotherapy. Soon his fame passed beyond the boundaries of Normandy and from far away patients were coming to him. He was forced to stop visits and accouchement.

iii

In 1956, he founded the Societe Homoeopathique of Normandy which united the homoeopaths of that region: Drs. H. Vannier, Flamen, Poisson, Dadu, Bernard, Amoyal and others, and soon he began to publish the Revue des Archives Homoeopathiques de Normandy, and was the editor of this review for 10 years.

In 1959, he transferred his chamber to Paris, on the 1st May.

He participated always in national and international congresses. He desired also more friendly meetings. Thus from the year 1962 began the meetings in his house at 11, Avenue Carnot, where most able homoeopaths used to meet, who desired to exchange their experiences. Young students of medicine, veterinary doctors, pharmacists and even artists, painters, writers, philosophers whom he liked to meet gathered in his house.

His mind was always open to new ideas and he was full of energy. He met at Strassbourg Dr. Pol Henry who helped him to learn his Gemmotherapy.

He organised seminar on Electro-acupuncture together with its founder Dr. Voll in 1971, 1972, 1973. He also organised seminars on Auriculotherapy with Dr. Bourdiol.

In 1963 he founded the Societe Medicale de Biotherapie. It is he who created the term Biotherapy, a symbol of his open mind. He associated with Homoeopathy some other therapeutics: Acupuncture, Anthroposophotherapy, Vertebrotherapy.

He published in 1964 the Revue des Cahiers de Biotherapie which gradually became successful.

In 1972, wishing to assure a teaching, he established the foundation of the Institut de Hecherches d'Enseignement de la Societe Medicale de Biotherapie (S.M.B.).

Soon began the seminaries of teaching which continued for three years.

He began under the guidance of Professor Henri Baruk and Dr. J. Dannay homoeopathic experiments on rats and cobayes, with substances like Rauwolfia, and Cicuta virosa, in l'Ecole pratique des Hauses etudes in the experimental school of psycho-pharmacology.

Above all a physician, an endowed teacher, a fervent researcher, he was also a writer. He has published many books. In January 1984, a little before his death, he published his last book "Homoeopathie et terrain" (Homoeopathy and ground) in collaboration with Mac Haffen.

After having struggled during his life in many fields he died on the 14th March, 1984.

CONTENTS

CONTENTS
PART I
ISOPATHIC CONCRETOLOGY

PART II

MATERIA MEDICA OF BIOTHERAPICS (EX-NOSODES)

x

PART III
REPERTORY OF NOSODES

PART I

ISOPATHIC CONCRETOLOGY

CHAPTER 1

INTRODUCTION

Short Epistemology of Homoeopathic Concretology

I. GENERAL INTRODUCTION

The peculiar characteristic of humanity is never to stop progressing by a stubborn fight for the conquest of scientific knowledge by discovering the laws of nature and trying to transform them. It is for this reason "dogmatism and conformism are the terrible powers of immobility," said Rene Leriche.

In order to understand the progress of medicine which goes from the doctor to the patient, in order to apprehend the pathology and to make a deduction for the treatment, it is useful, even necessary to have a comprehension of the whole of the human biopathology and the harmony of a renovated Homoeopathology.

II. METHODOLOGICAL AND PHILOSOPHICAL CONSIDERATION ON MEDICINE

We have, as our modest part, made the choice of a philosophical conception of medicine which we are going to designate by the term **Contradictional Monist Concretology** (CMC).

Concretology : It indicates the real expressing itself by the help of matter, which is conceived as movement and change.

Man the concrete is a whole by his possibilities, as well as by the relations of his "Being", caught in the whole of his manifestations and in his milieu. It is his existence which determines the conscience and in its turn the consciousness influences the existence as well on the sphere of anthropology, as on the sociological sphere.

Contradictional indicates the dialectic process which implies the contradiction in the unity of things. "It is the science of general laws of movement, of the exterior world, as well as of the human thought" (Fr. Engels, Ludwig Feurbach—Ed. Sociales).

The contradictional concretology conception proceeds from the study of the processus, normal or pathological, of its internal content and of its relation to other processus. It is the internal contradiction which is in the **origin** of the development of the processus and the **external causes** constitute the condition of the change, and act by the intermediary of the internal causes.

The *contradiction* is the basis of simple and complex forms of movement and the characteristic of life shows precisely that a being is at every moment the same but however an other.

The *contradiction* presents a **double** aspect, that of the universality and that of the *specific*.

The character of the universality is found in all the stages of the development of symptoms or processus and penetrates each force from the start to finish.

The appearance of a new pathologic process means that the old unity and the contraries that constitute it yields its place to a new unity, to some new contrary symptoms ; the old processus is complete, the new appears and begins in its turn its own history of contradictional clinic.

The **specific** indicates the infinite differenciation of things in the Nature and Society. The pathologic specificity indicates the diversity of biochemical phenomena and their infinite variability.

To **consider unilaterally a pathological process** leads to an impass (unicism according to Kent in Homoeopathy) because it blocks the process of the knowledge of contradiction, therefore the unfolding of the pathological process in time and space.

In the whole pathological process there are different stages and one should try to recognise and differentiate the **principal fundamental contradiction** having the general character and the particular contradiction which is secondary.

The contradictional relation between the principal and the secondary symptom and symptoms, forces us, considering the disease in its totality, to prescribe some remedies analogous to the symptoms present, according to the stages of the pathological processus in course.

But, and this is primordial, not statically, but dynamically because the 'General' exists only in the 'Particular'. In the development of the morbid phenomena what is universal in such a context may become particular in another.

Thus in a given patient, such symptomatology will dominate in the unfolding of the clinical phenomenon, in order to yield place to a secondary contradiction which has *suddenly* become, by the interpretation of the qualitative change, principal contradiction by the fact even of the interpretation and displacement of contradiction.

There is every reason to note that a pathological process which is complex, has many contradictions and it will be necessary to find out the principal contradiction at a given moment of this development.

The disease should then never be considered only its static condition but as a dynamic process having pluri contradictional character and will require a pluri analogic treatment.

What is that which distinguishes the principal contradiction from the secondary one ?

It is the inequality of development in the given pathological process of contradictional forces. To say otherwise the dominating expression of a symptom or a symptomatic complex —the characteristic triade—in the general symptomatologic picture.

The study of the different pathological stages of inequality in the contradictions, of the principal contradiction and the secondary contradiction will determine the clinico-therapeutic line in view of the re-establishment of the health, the new state in the place of the old of which the name only remains the same.

Finally the contradictional concretology or that dialectic materialistic conception is monist.

Monist indicates the unity of things and of phenomena as the state of quantitative change, *i.e.*, to say the passage of a pathological processus to another.

The knowledge is the division of the unity and it characterises the thought which apprehends the "thing itself". The monistic medical knowledge thus apprehends Health in the **unity** of the being.

(a) Methodology of Contradictional Monistic Concretology

The clinical practice of a contradictional monistic concretology implies a **methodological**.

This methodology will be two dimensional : 1. Structural and 2. Cybernetic.

1. *Structural* because of the fact that the pathological elements have not any meaning and existence but in relation to the whole.

That structure, according to Jean Piaget includes three essential characteristics : totality of a pathological process, its internal biological **transformation** and its pathological or normal physiological **auto regulation.**

2. *Cybernatic* because concrete by the fact that there is constant interaction between different biochemical metabolities and that interaction by the intermediary of the process of feed back modifies the lymphoid system bound to the whole of the lymphatic and blood circulation.

Since then it is necessary **not to isolate a symptom of a morbid** process in evolution but to study it in the context of the whole and of the interactions that exist (To think : localised morbid process as manifestation of a general pathological movement).

In this morbid process it is necessary to study the manner in which the modifications obtained following a particular medical intervention, will entail a modification of symptoms by the feed-back reaction of the other changes and so on (Therapeutic action).

The particular character of this successive modifications unfolds itself not according to a mechanical lineary tracing but according to a dialectic undulation, because the successive physiopathological modifications are inseparable from the new and sudden qualitative transformations, which in their turn are originally new contradictions (It is the meaning of meta-stasis and morbid alternance).

(*b*) **Theory of a Knowledge of Contradictional Monistic Concretology**

The C.M.C. conceives the existence of the universe as an existence *by itself* and *for itself,* implying no intervention foreign to its existence and alone the laws of matter will determine the evolution.

It results that some natural phenomena have nothing mysterious or even miraculous even if in a certain stage of our knowledges of the present day sciences there exist some non-resolved problems.

The C.M.C. considers that is the **matter** which is the primordial fact of the reality of the world.

What is that Matter ?

The matter is a philosophical category which means an objective reality. It is not only a simple image (image in the mirror) as Mr. J. Monod understands wrongly, but it is the **concrete real which is given to us a reflex action in the form of a reflexion which is active through the senses.**

The nature of the matter remains in the field of scientific knowledge and for the moment it is understood provisorily in the form of a mass and of energy, corpuscular and undulatory state. Mass, energy are the dialectic and dynamic entities ; the matter being understood as "condensed energy" in the atomic neucleus and H. Laborit will say that our means of apprehension are still limited to the **quantum** as far as the mass is concerned.

In its space-time becoming, that matter is formed in a helicoidal movement, its own development, its own becoming and gives birth to new qualities.

There is why, thought, intelligence, memory are the new manifestations of that particular moment of development of the matter in a given historic phase of its evolution. The development characteristics, a progressive growth and complexification of the structures.

The **concepts** are some specific and complex manifestations of the cortico-endocrino-somatic activity of the organism as the highest product in the complexifying evolution of the matter.

The matter, reached at ʳa very high degree of organisation will give a new aspect, unusual for its existence by the phenomenon of life.

III. CONSIDERATIONS ON GENERAL BIOLOGY AND MEDICAL BIOLOGY

(a) General Biology

The life is a mode existence of the matter characteristing itself by the incessent and contradictory renewal of each of its co-ordinated parts which compose the living matter, by assimilation and disassimilation of materials less ordered in the exterior milieu.

The *Life* is inseparable from this coordinated and contradictory movements, it is this movement itself.

The *Death* is the contradictional aspect of the life as much as a biological manifestation where the functional activities of the matter change the symptom, the coordination to an inverse qualitative change ending in a **process of degradation** which remains open. A dead body is the result of the life which cannot create by itself.

The death is not a nothingness, the absolute rest, but it is a *movement of the negation of the matter*, in a constant process having movement and change.

The phenomenon of life and death are then some manifestations in the particular development and to a high degree of its evolutivity of that matter in incessant movement and change.

(b) Consideration on General Bio-pathology

Normal life and pathological life, health and disease are the contradictional aspects of the same state of the **matter**, of a material phenomenon to a superior degree in the waning of the evolutivity of the latter.

The human body is an unity of contraries, it is more than the same total of its constituents. Its different parts are related to one another, they are in opposition and at the same time interdependence they are bound to each other and the ones act on the others. The body is a process of health in itself.

The **individuality** includes at the same time the molar individual, global and total and the molecular individuality, singular, parcellary, peculiar with its specific characteristics.

The human individuality is thus a **totality** integrated in its milieu sustaining there the laws of matter.

It follows that the external purturbations constitute the condition of the change but that these are the internal purturbations which are its basis and the external causes operate by the intermediary of internal causes.

It is then impossible to treat an organ without knowing that it receives without stop from the whole of the organism some neuro-chemio-hormonal in-flows and that it sends to the whole organism some nervous reflex messages or some biochemic and hormonal modifications which pass in the blood.

Let us mention here that the difference between Spagyric medicine of Paracelsus and the Homoeopathic medicine of Hahnemann lie in this. Paracelsus recommends to treat the organ which is ill while having the recourse to the law of analogy by the intermediary of the "signature".

Hahnemann after experiments of dynamised pharmacology on human body takes the help of the law of analogy to treat the individual who is ill, in his totality. It is for this reason Hahnemann has always refused to see his doctrine referred to the doctrine of Paracelsus.

Thus we can understand :

1. The **pathological phenomenology** which includes the integrality of the individual and disease of the patient in its biological becoming.

2. *The pathological condition* is not considered as an isolated moment of a perspective of a **chemical history of oscillation** between life and death, between health and illness, between the normal and the physiopathological.

The Pathological condition is dialectical. It is characterised by some contradictions in its morbid process, which are and which are not all at the same time and out of these contradictions appear the essential energy of the dynamic therapeutic which, without it, would be mechanical.

3. The *disease is then understood* as a concept. Molar and Global at the same time qualitative and quantitative in a processus where an organism on a determined ground and in a determined milieu meets with some conditions of excitations and inhibitions entailing a pathological retro-action having variable quality and different intensity.

We must understand that the bio-normal *is the state of equilibrium more or less stable of the organism conditioned by its-milieu.*

But that idea of biological equilibrium should not be envisaged as a fixed static and inhert state, because in fact it realises a living concreity, contradictional being characterised by a double process, *viz* :

(*a*) *An internal process*, bio-micro-chemic of anabolism and catabolism.

(*b*) *An external process*, consequences of continual modifications of the environment.

Biological equilibrium is therefore in the last resort a concreity, moving, changing, relative.

The pathological, it is the rupture for disequilibriating retroaction, following a deteriorisation of the liasons, either with the environment, with the organism or with both at the same time or alternately.

A pathological modification in any part of the body may affect the organs in other parts or even the organism as a whole in its turn a new condition of the body in its totality may act on the local pathological modifications.

Thus even in the essence of the pathological phenomenon there is reason to consider the contradictional aspect in all its aspects and to regularise later on the relations between the parts and the whole, taking into account the principal and the secondary contradictions, unique or multiple.

The whole medical art, the whole clinical ingenuity play a part at that moment.

IV. HOMOEOPATHIC CONCRETOLOGY OR HOMOEOPATHY

The honour is due to Samuel Hahnemann (1755-1843) to have given, there is a century and half, the lecture about the comprehension of the totality of a diseased individual, and to have elevated it to the rank of a doctrine and of a praxis.

Under the generic name of Homoeopathy, one should understand according to us at present :

(a) Homoeopathology which is a structural, phenomeno-logical concreity of homoeopathic medicine.

It is the original work of Samuel Hahnemann who formulated theoretical and practical expression about what is understood by Homoeopathy.

It may be summarised by formulating **theoretical and methodological** exigency by the **law of analogy** and the exigency of the praxis by the dynamised attenuations of the pharmacological substances that are to be administered to the patient.

There is therefore every ground to study that law of analogy and let our Master speak first. In his fundamental work 'Organon' of the art of cure (6th ed. fr. tr. by P. Schmidt, 1952, Paris) one reads as follows :

Para 22. The therapeutic properties of medicines reside exclusively in their power to provoke some pathological symptoms in healthy man and to make them disappear in the patient.

Para 24. Consequently there remains no other therapeutic really salutary to apply medicines to the diseases, but that which is based on the principles of similars.

This therapy aims at finding among all medicines (of which the pharmacodynamic action on healthy man is well established) that which has the power to produce the artificial disease the most resembling to the natural disease which is in view. This medicine is directed against the totality symptoms of a given patient, taking into account the cause, if it is known, and concomittent circumstances of the affections of which he suffers."

These definitions taken together may be summarised by the famous phrase :

Similia - Similibus - Curentur

We will frame in the scientific language of our time that **definition** in the following manner :

Homoeotherapy is defined as the therapeutic art which tries stimulate the reactional mode of the patient by the intermediary of a remedy analogous in potentised microdose, which has been determined by a cortico-visceral-pharmadynamic research in sub-toxic dose having provoked some morbid phenomena in a normo-physiologic individual.

What signifies that, that analogy presents itself as an Iso-morphism of relations between some elements qualitatively different : bears upon a system of relations and reciprocal actions and encompasses, in its totality, the singularity of the illness of the patient.

The experimental photogenesis of that research allows to build the constitutional physiognomy of the medicine which is called a pathogenesis or according to us a cartico-visceral pharmacodynamic experimental protocol.

What is Meant by Analogy ?

Analogy (O.A. Julian – Recherches theoriques et pratiques en Homoeopathy, t. 2, pp. 27-36) enters into the philosophical vocabulary with an allusion in the **temaeus** of Plato and is according to Aristotle the idea of equality of relation in mathematical sense.

From the relation one goes to the reason of the relation, which is, according to the relation, Analogy.

Then one passes from the quantitative sense of the Analogy to the qualitative sense of a resemblance of the relation which will give a wider meaning to the term to designate some resemblances of functions. It appears then that the word analogy acquires the quality of a **movement of the thought** which, from the similitude of functions ends in a new idea. It becomes a means of reasoning and Alfred Binet will say "the foundation of all reasoning is the recognition of similitude (M. Dorolle - Le raisonnement par analogie P.U.F., 1949, Paris).

Dorolle specifies that "Reasoning by analogy, it is to take the starting point either on the resemblance of two relations in order to deduce from it a certain resemblance or even an identity, or on the resemblance (superficial) of two relations, for deducing from the two, the nature of - one of the two and the nature of the other."

Analogy is consequently made out of dissimilars which makes every object autonomous and of a dissimilarity which designates their common terms.

Let us add that the existence of the object is never isolated, it is "relation". The analogical methodology suggests some properties which are possible but does not prove it ; it will be there, the necessity of experimental verification.

The analogical reasoning denotes a forward movement which confers to it a great value in the scientific research and "it is the dialectic which is to day formed of idea the most important for the natural science, because it alone can offer the element of analogy and as a result, the method of explanation for the evolution of the whole, for the passage of a field of research into another" (Fr. Engels-Anti-Duhring, p. 445, Ed. Sociale, Paris).

K. Marx has already said that there is a dialectic of the rational and of the experimental and it is to the phenomenon one should attach oneself for the sensible perception and consequently to have taken recourse to analogy (Difference of the philosophy of Democritus and Epicurus) (Oeuvres philosophiques, t.l., p. 24, Ed. Coste, Paris) (K.M. was not then a Marxist, but a young neo-Hegelian).

Thus Analogy appears at the sametime as a static idea of relation of critical value in the Kantian sense of the word and dynamic, contradictional, dialectic, because the similar is a moment of affirmation in a relation and the latter negates itself as much as an idea non-unique and non-equivocal. This determines its own frontiers and is evaluated by the verification in practice.

The essence even of the analogical reasoning requires that the analogous symptoms the latter establishes between the comparative phenomena should be **essential** and not accidental and should come out of the relations of phenomena.

S. Hahnemann made a type of experiment conditioned by a relation of analogy. He has not invented it, having had, here and there some predecessors but, **he has raised it to the rank of a systematised experimental method.**

By giving to a normo-physiologic individual a given medicinal substance, and noting later on the appearance of patho-physiological symptoms and bringing this experimental protocol to the symptomatic picture of a precise and analogous morbid condition, he took the help of the method of analogical reasoning.

But continuing on the movement of the thought of analogy he proceeds a real dialectic bound. to the passage of analogy be induction such as : Two isomorphic states, the one having the pharmaco-dynamic quality, the other having the pathologic quality should coincide, to creat, to invent a therapentic action which becomes Homoeotherapy.

Homoeotherapy is therefore **a moment** in the chain of analogical **reasoning**. There is the necessity of induc ive thought. to end by a **quantitative start** to a practical invention of therapeutic character.

In the first step of our research we may conclude :

There is reason for prescribing a homoeopathic remedy in a given morbid condition by the analogical reasoning. This is what Hahnemann says in para 273 of his Organon.

"In course of the treatment aiming at cure, it is not in that case necessary, and from this fact it is inadmissible, to use in a patient more than a single substance and simple at the same time."

But, we do not stop to repeat that, everything that lives, dies, perish, change to renew itself in an uninterrupted cycle.

The experience of life, of the daily clinical practice caused towards 1816-1817 in Hahnemann an intellectual restlessness which ended in a real thunderbolt from a blue sky in 1828-1830.

Hahnemann did not hesitate to turn upside down his world, and the daily practice of Homoeopathic doctors.

It is the question of a real *fracture* **in the old order formulated in the 1st ed. of 1810 of the Organon with the publication (1828) of the work"** *Doctrine and Homoeopathic Treatment of Chronic Disease* **(Tr. by A.J. L. Jourdan) Ed. Baillere, Paris, 1832.**

What Characterises this Fracture ?

It is the work of a verification and above all the verification of a failure.

Here it is :

"The ills that seemed cured already, came to reappear, the means that one found at the first time was successful much less completely and when it is reiterated a third time, it was crowned with still less success (p. 5) and further on "Some new symptoms of the disease come forth, that one could cure only partially by the help of the most homoeopathic means (p. 6) and still further" the relapses, the frequent relapses of the disease ended in rendering the medicines thought upto that time to be the most homoeopathic and given in the most appropriate dose, still less efficacious when they are repeated.

A time comes when they can hardly cause an amelioration (p. 5-6).

Thus the absoluteness of the Law of Analogy and the unique remedy a severe blow of reprimand.

To the field of the action of a homoeopathic remedy, a **limit**, a frontier was found.

But it is still more serious, it is the absoluteness of the law of Analogy which **put to the cause because** its strict application is proved to be a failure.

Why ?

"To find the cause which makes that all the medicines know to Homoeopathy do not bring a real cure in these diseases, and to arrive, if it is possible, to some more exact views on the true nature of the thousands of diseases which resist to the treatment inspite of the unshakable truths of the Homoeopathic law, such is the problem with which I am occupied day and night since the years 1816 and 1917 (p. 7-8), will say Hahnemann.

Face to face with this failure Hahnemann concluded :

"......that one has before his eyes only a portion of the primitive disease deeply seated" and "that consequently it is necessary to know the entire field of all the diseases and symptoms proper to the unknown primitive disease." (p. 9-10)

These are the three important morbid processes, three miasms, which Hahnemann describes as follows :

The *Sycosis*, the *Syphilis* and the more important of all that thousand headed hydra *psora*. The real nature of the disease and origin of failure resides there. The result is a clinical description of these processus or "miasms" and for each of them there is at first a specific remedy : *Thuya* for *Sycosis*, *Mercury* for *Syphilis* and *Sulphur* for *Psora*.

The individualisation of the analogical remedy falls back, face to face with the advent of the specific remedy of the miasmatic disease.

It is there where one goes beyond the deep significance of which many homoeopaths witness still to-day a certain incomprehension.

It widens the narrowness of the analogical reasoning covering the "Homoeopathic" remedy and helps at the same time to have a new comprehension of the disease of the individual according to another dimension, another height, those of dialectic clinic.

After a period of unvariability comes the period of a drastic revision. The clinical fact and its therapeutic failure is there.

The greatness of S. Hahnemann is to recognise this fact to analyse it to describe later on some variable specific morbid entities of which the etiology is determined and the specific therapeutic is indicated.

But, and this is the dark side of the picture, he proclaims beyond the practical truth which he himself has just denounced the perenneity and the absolutism on an *imaginary* truth that of non-transgression and that of the absoluteness of the law of analogy in the narrow sense of the word.

This intransigence hides in reality a *strategic* retreat, because Hahnemann was conscious that with his work on chronic diseases he opened a new era, but met equally a strong opposition from his own disciples.

There he adds a new idea.

"It is necessary to know the entire extension of all the illnesses and symptoms proper to the unknown primitive disease" which implies a historico-etiologic inquiry of the pathologic syndrome, of the "Chronic disease." In fact it is the narrowness of the comprehension of the definition of the term "analogous" which caused in him the trouble.

Because, unconsciously Hahnemann enlarged the sense of reasoning by *Analogical specification* of a morbid process of which he made an *entity separately* and the *analogical relation* which represents the *remedy*.

There lies the going beyond from *particular* to the *general*.

It is to be regretted that he was not in a position to discern that diatetical mutation. The clinical enquiry which is revealed by the research of causality and the total etiology leads us towards that therapeutic discipline which is the great object of this book.

Isopathy and Isotherapics

We have more particularly insisted on the specific analogy of Homoeopathy by the elaboration of the experimental analytical model of the medicine and analogical symptomatic model of the patient, which totally forms *homoeopathic analogouse*.

But also, looking closely, one sees that the analogical reasoning and the model, the analogical situation, are different.

One will understand it by reading this book.

There remains to explain briefly what is Biotherapy.

Biotherapy means clinico-therapeutic practice hierarchised on its structure and of which Homoeopathy is *one* of its primordial constituents.

These two terms will represent for us, instead of Homoeopathy, *the homoeopathic concretology*, which means : Logic of the Homoeopathic concreity, medicine of our time.

The concept of the typo-pathological totality apprehends the concreity of the cortico-somatic and cortico-visceral functional direction as far as the processus in a given individual conditioned by his ground, his bio-type and his biological perturbation acquired or hereditary, in time and space. The diagnosis will then be a reasoned action.

This is the ground of establishing a nosologic diagnosis according to the methodology, the investigations taught by the universities, a bio-typologic diagnosis (ground, constitution, temperament...) an immunological diagnosis (the diathesis or morbid processes), the allergy (Psora), chronic mesenchymatosis (Sycosis), luetosis toxoplasminosis, the tuberculinosis, the cancerinosis, and to interprete in the practice these informations the therapeutic diagnosis.

In the sphere of our conception of contradictional monist concretology, the pathological personality should therefore be the object of clinical study on many levels as for example :

(*a*) As a typological, morphological and temperamental personality.

(*b*) As aggressologic structuration in the becoming as for example :

Internal aggression on molecular level, then tissular, organic, by the perturbations caused by intoxination by microbes or chemicals, by perturbations of environmental pollution.

External aggression by the traumas of different nature having cortico-somatic reflex.

A reasoned therapeutic action should then proceed to the structurisation by levels, taking into account the principal contradiction and the secondary contradictions.

The therapeutic action contributed to the perishing of the pathological structure by an antagosistic action and on the restructurisation of normo-physiology by a non-antagonistic action.

This return to the normo-physiology is placed on another level of the helicoidal process because it persists, according to the bio-molecular comprehension a reaction of the functional or lesional memory which is cortico-somatic, which introduces a modification of behaviour with which there is ground to take into account the hysteriographic clinic of the individual.

BIOTHERAPIC GEOTAXY

We will define by this term the plan of a tactic and bio-therapic strategy.

We will prescribe on three levels :

(*a*) The level of lifting the barrage or the reactional blockage.

2 F

(*b*) The level of cleansing or drainage.

(*c*) The level of setting aright the entire biological space.

Let us study closely these three levels.

The individual is a biological space closed by his form and his function integrating himself in his environment.

A pathological processus, by the diversity of metabolic perturbations causes some structural modification of the morphology.

Deblocking a patho-morpho type may be considered by taking into account the following categories of biotherapy :

1. Articular manipulation.

2. Neurotherapy.

3. Acupuncturotherapy :

    (*a*) under the form of Acupuncture o. traditional Chinese medicine.

    (*b*) under the form of Electroacupuncture organometry of Voll.

    (*c*) under the form of Auriculotherapy of Nogier or articulomedicine.

Articular manipulation causes a general and local deconcentration.

Acupunturotherapy is a remarkable therapy which induces an entergetic stimulation.

The *neuraltherapy* induces a disconnexion of a "pertubation field".

But over and above the three important categories we should mention the indications given by S. Hahnemann in his fundamental work 'Organon'. The electrotherapy according to Hahnemann (para 280 of Organon) is as follows :

The dynamic form of the magnetic, of electricity and of galvanism does not act less homoeopathically and powerfully on our vital force than the substances called medicine.

(*a*)   The Massage therapy is indicated in para 290.

(*b*)   Balneotherapy in para 29.

So these manual and physical praxis should succeed the biotherapic medicine according to the clinic built up on the totality of the patient.

(*b*) **Biotherapic Cleansing and Drainage.** Consist in inducing the excretion of metabolities which are abnormal and accumulated on the different levels of the biological space, from the molecules to the tissues and organs.

General hygienic and biotic diatetic as well as the advice of S. Hahnemann in para 259—263 of the 'Organon' will be the first opening.

The second includes a series of biotherapic categories, as for example :

1.   *Renovated Phytotherapy.*

2.   *Gemmotherapy.*

3.   *Homoeopathic phytotherapy.*

4.   *Dynamised microtherapy.*

The practice of drainage is modern in Homoeotherapy. Exaplained by Antoine Nebel of Switzerland, it has been the object of study of Léon Vannier and A Rouy as a continuation of the Nebelian thought. It is vehemently criticised by the American Homoeotherapeutists who are "Kentists" like Gutman of New York and P. Schmidt of Geneva.

Within the limit of Homoeopathic concretology and biotherapies the practice of drainage has become revived and also the beginning of the use of Gemmotherapy, Phytotherapy and Mycotherapies.

Drainage like that of the lifting of the barrage facilitates the approach by the level of the totality of the patient. It helps the elimination of the noxious metabolities, contributes to the elimination of the products of antagonistic forces.

The drainage plays also on the organic and tissular levels and on the level of renovated phytotherapy, gemmotherapy and homoeopathic polydrainers have their sphere of action.

For a beginner in the praxis of biotheraphy, phytotherapy and clinical gemmotherapy are the two mammies of which it is easy to extract resourses.

The phytotherapy is the footstool of the beginner in biotherapy.

It is built up as ambivalent model of pharmacodynamics : induction of an organotherapic antagonistic action and of a non-antigonistic action by its symptomatic analogical potentiality.

The prescription is easy. It is the form of Galenic preparation in mother tinctures according to his pharmacopoea.

Clinical indications are simple, precise and brought to light by M. Tetau and Cl. Bergéret. The clinical gemmotherapy is situated on the organic level as corrector of enzymatic perturbations of reticulo-hystiocytary system.

As regards Homoeopathic phytotherapy, it is necessary to say here simply that it is the question of elective action on the tissue or organ which is ill, of which the perturbed function checks the elimination of noxieus substances, produced or introduced in the organism (Leon Vannier).

The essential characteristics of these biotherapies thus specified on the *second level* of biotherapic prescription, the prescriber finds the *possibility of using thus as much as autonomous entities or as elements of total biotherapic prescription.* For autonomous elements, the renovated phytotherapy has a limited field of action.

The Gemmotherapy as Phytoembryotherapy acting on the reticulo-hystiocytary system presents the characteristics of a deep action, whence there is an enlarged field of action.

(c) Setting Aright the Total Biological Space

We arrive at the *third level*, that of therapeutic induction in view of setting aright the totality of the biological space, the totality of the personality of the patient.

The *genotype* representing the hereditary patrimony of the individual and the *phenotype*, representing the totality of the actions exercised by the interior milieu on the hereditary armature of the genotype, will receive the consideratioñ of a total therapeutic and for this at first thanks to homoeotherapy.

In the molecular scale a perturbating non-antagonistic known signal used in micro dynamisation will act by effacing antagonisitc deforming effect of the biological space.

The making of biotherapic prescription will be that totalising totality of the pathological individual.

It will be considered according to *two stages* :

(*a*) The stage of the *totality* of the biological space, corti-corhinencephalo-reticulo-somatic to which will correspond the simillimum of S. Hahnemann as the elective therapeutic.

(*b*) The stage of *particular localisation of biological space.*

The correction of these *perturbations enters into the following biotherapic categories.* Homoeopathics, micro-immuno and organotherapics, micro-biomeneralotherapics and lithiotherapics, micro-metallotherapics and anthroposophotherapics.

For biotherapic prescription let us specify as follows :

The Homoeopathic remedies as structurised experimental model covers a wide therapeutic field.

It will be confronted by analogical reasoning with the symptomatic totality of a specific clinical case.

Homoeopathy alone, may induce the redress of the totality of the biological space, so far as the analogic contents are covered as perfectly as possible. It will provoke from a known symptom (*its pathogenetic characteristic*) *the same antagonistic mani-festations regarding the effects of the pathologic symptoms. It will be the work of microdose highly dynamised by inversed effect of the strong symptom in a weak symptom* (*Law of Arndt Schultze*).

It results that the most analogical fundamental homoeopathic medicine is prescribed.

Before ending this present exposition, we are going to give here a schema of biotherapic prescription.

SCHEMA OF A BIOTHERAPIC PRESCRIPTION

A. REMEDY OF THE TOTALITY OF BIO-PATHOLO-GICAL SPACE.

The simillimum of Hahnemann to be determined by analo-gical reasoning.

B. REMEDIES OF TYPOLOGICAL PERSONALITY.

(*a*) *Morpho-genetic.* Calcarea càrbonica, Calcarea phos-phorica, Calcarea fluorica.

(*b*) *Temperamental* : Sepia, Lachesis, Iodium etc.

C. REMEDIFS OF AGGRESSOLOGIC STRUCTURE.

(*a*) **External aggression**

traumatic ⎫
vaccinal ⎬ Arnica, Calendula, Hyperibum, Silicea.
antibiotic ⎪ Thuya.
chemical ⎭

(*b*) **Internal aggression**

1. *Of the genetic morbid process* (*diathesic*).

Allergic (*Psora*) : *Sulph., Lycop., Calc. carb.*

Mesenchymatosis (*Sycosis*) : *Thuya, Silicea, Nat. S...*

Tuberculinosis (*Ex-tuberculinism*), *Drosera, Pulsat, Nat. M...*

Luetosis (*Syphilis*) : *Acid Fluor., Arg. n., Aurum...*

Carcinosis (*pre-cancer*) *Hydrastic, Kreos, Condurango, Conium...*

2. *Immunologic perturbation* :
   Dynamised micro-immunotherapy
   —*Isopathy*
   —*Biotherapy.*
   (a) *Organotherapy, diluted and dynamised.*
   (b) *Hormonotherapy, diluted and dynamised Anthroposopho-therapy.*

3. *Perturbation of cellular metabolism* :
   — *Micro-bio-mineralotherapy, dynamised.* (*Schussler's salts*)
   - *lithotherapy*
   —*micro-metallotherapy*
   —*metallo-anthroposophotherapy.*

4. *Of the localised lesional perturbation* :
   —*renovated phytotherapy*
   - *clinical gemmotherapy*
   —*dynamised micotherapy*
   —*anthroposotherapy*
   —*homoeopathic drainage.*

Begin according to the necessity by one of the techniques of deblocking as described above.

The plan is conceived as a whole. It is to be considered according to the stages of evolution of illness of the patient, of the moment (time) and of the degree of intensity (space) of the pathologic contradiction.

The understanding of this tactic of the therapeutic of the moment helps to consider the strategy of the totality of analogy between the pathology and therapeutics.

The *Strategy* will consider the totality of the therapeutic plan to re-establish the health.

The *Tactic* will consider the particular therapeutic modalities according to the state of the pathological moment.

CHAPTER 2

HISTORY OF ISOPATHY

By
DR. MARC HAFFEN

The case of attempting to treat a disease by the agent which may cause of transmit the disease constitutes one of the most general and the most valid empirical acquisitions of the art of cure.

Numerous primitive peoples know that the repeated innoculations may guard against the effects of poisions and venoms. The Bohimans according to Frasschoen (The Triumph of Homoeopathy, 1908, p. 197) make an incision near the snake bite and introduce into it a pinch of the glands with venom, taken from other serpents and dried : some inhabitants of Columbia take in a similar case some serum in which the liver of the serpent is macerated.

In the far East, the Chinese people use the preventive variolisation by the compulsory wearing of the dresses of a patient in full suppuration stage or by the dried pustule, preserved one year, then introduced into the nostrils (the left for boys and the right for girls, (Huard and Wong : La médecine chinoise *ā* travers le siécles).

In the West, *Hippocrates*, who was the first to write in his Traité des Lieux de l'Homme (I, 688) : "*Vomitus vomitu curantur*" Pline (23-79, after J.C.) teaches us that : "*Est limus salivae sub lingua rabiosi canis qui, datus in potu, fieri hydrophobos non patitur*" (There is under the tongue of the rabid dog a slime formed by its saliva, which taken in drink, guards against rabies (Pline : Natural history, 1st century after J.C.). *Dioscorides of Anasarbe* (75 after J.C.) recommends to give to eat to a hydrophobic the liver of the dog which has bitten and even grilled earthworms for the treatment of worms (Dioscorides : Materia Medica, 1st century after J. C.) said that there where is the disease, there is also the remedy. He recommends to crush the scorpion where it has bitten to eat the flesh of the viper which has bitten (*Aetius—Opera medica*, tr. by Cornarius, 5th century after J.C).

Later on the doctrine of signature gave a second breath to the proto-history of Isopathy. As a particular stage in the development of the doctrine of signature, having an analogical signification mainly symbolic, primitive form of the law of similitude having rather symbolic expression, the Doctrine of signature attempts, beyond a very strict causalty, hatched in the thought some "other" relations between things disengaging what may be common to them, there "signatures". Thus a similitude between the plants and certatin "homologous" parts of the human body (as for example Nux vomica and the brain according to *Porta* (*Physiognomica*), 1558 (Naples), 1650 (Rouen). That similitude may be stretched towards the identity and *Paracelsus* (1493—1541), the "cursed doctor" according to the expression of *R. Allendy* (Allendy—Paracelsus the cursed doctor)", preconised the medicinal utility of morbid products and formulates the therapeutic by the similar : "The similars cure the the similars, the scorpion cures the scorpion, mercury cures mercury. The poison is mortal for man except, if in the organism there is another poison with which it may fight, in which case the patient regains his health (*Paracelsus : Compendium philosophae*, 1568). With this aim in view he uses very weak doses of the poison in question. In his "Archidoxes", he recommends the *fell Tauris* for the hepatic cirrhosis and the extract of the spleen for the "obstruction" of the spleen. He indicates blood serum to stop the hemorrhages

and equally preconises the therapeutic utilisation of opotherapic products. In the 16th century *Oswal Crollius* advises
the utilisation of an isopathy ; in his treatise "Signatures and
Correspondences (Crollius in La Royale chemin, tr. by M.
Boulene, Paris, 1633) he writes : "To stop the overflowing of
menstruation of women, it is necessary to take 3 or 4 drops
of the same blood, always chosing the most clear and let the
patient drink it, without her knowing and there is no doubt
it will stop the overflow.   The rat bite is cured by the powder
made of the the same rat after having burnt it.   The scorpion
carry their cure as well as all animals, and it is a fact that in
the "Provence" (province) they have the custom to crush the
scorpion between two stones and apply it on the bite and by
this means the illness goes whence it has come.   Thus, according
to *Jérome Cardan* "*Omne similia similibus confirmatur*" *in*
(*Ars curandi*, Parva, 1566).

   In the 17th century, *Robert Fludd*, nicknamed the Researcher
Jesuit of Ireland, treats the phthisis with the dilution of
the sputum of the patient.   In his *Philosophia Myosaica*
(Robert Fludd : Philosiphia Myosaica, Goudae, 1638, sheet
149, col. 2), writes "But do we not see generally the similar
of which the nature has but modified by putrifaction (Spagyric
method of preparation) has a particular noxious effect for the
similar.   Thus the worms eliminated by the organism, dried
and powdered and given internally destroy the worms.   The
sputum of a patient suffering from Phthisis cures after appropriate preparation (Spagyric method of preparation) phthisis.
The spleen of man having undergone a particular preparation
(spagyric method of preparation) is a remedy against enlarged
spleen.   The stone formed in the bladder and in the kidney
cure and dissolve the stone (Hunewald and Reirfer—Historique
de l'Isopathy, L'Hom. moderne, 1936, No. 4, p. 255).
Anthanasius Kircher in the work : *Magna sive de arte magnetica*
writes "The poisonings in general are cured by their proper
counterpoisons.   Thus the bite of the spider will be cured by

the application of a spider, the biting of a scorpion by the application of the scorpion, the poison of a rabid dog is drawn out of the body by the furs of the same dog". In the treatise of poisons (Kircher : *In mundus subterranius*, Amsterdam, 1645) he affirms : *"Ubi morbus, ibi etiam medicamentum morbo illis oppotunum"* (There where is the disease, there also is the proper remedy of the disease).

In the 17th century, Lady Montague, wife of the English ambassador at Constantinople, got her child vaccinated by the extract of variolic pus (*R. Tichner* : *Das Werden der Homoeopathic*, 1950, p. 20). Prof. Phillipus Nettr of Venise (R. Ticher—ibid) (*Ph. Netter Fundamenta medicinae theor. argentor*, 1718, v. 2, p. 646) advised the dry pus of a plague bubo for the treatment of plague. Francis Home of Edinburg, used the blood of the patient suffering from measles against that disease (in R. Tichner—ibid) (*Homoeo medical facts and Experiments*, London 1754). *Adrian La Bruyere* published in 1734 a thesis *"De curatione per similia"* on the use of galenic Simili (R. Tichner—ibid). The vaccination against pox preconised by Jenner in 1798 is taken up again under another form of the vaccin method of the Chinese.

Isopathy, we see, is a therapeutic method very ancient and universally known, but we must wait till the beginning of the 19th century and the triumph of Homoeopathy, to see its systematised use. Three great names dominate the history of Isopathy, and all the three were homoeopaths : *Constantine Hering, Wilhelm Lux* and *R.P. Collet.*

Constantine Hering (See also Document No. 1 and the end of this chapter) was born on the 1st January 1800 at Oschatz, a small town of Saxony situated between Dresden and Leipzig. His father Carl Gottlieb was an organist and composes of songs for children. While manifesting a very great taste for music, he was soon oriented toward mathematics and natural sciences which already made him famous. From 1811 to 1817 he made classical studies in the College Littan. Wishing to study surgery, he goes to Dresden then to Leipzig and becomes the assistant of the Surgeon Robbi. The latter, asked by the publisher Baumgartener to write a book exposing a complete refutation of Homoeopathy, decline to do so for want of time and charges his assistant to do well the task. Therefore Hering begins to study the works of Hahnemann and being gradually interested, finally convinced, declares himself adept of the new "medical heresy". Disapproved by Robbi and his professors, Hering however upholds his doctorate thesis (1826) taking side of Homoeopathy. The following year he goes to Surinam, in Guiana of Holland in the company of the natural scientist Weinhold. He remains six years in Surinam practising Homoeopathic medicine and works over his book containing important works on natural history. After the publication of his works in the Homoeopathic archives of Stapf, the court of Saxony ordered him to stop his researches and the practice of Homoeopathy. He therefore resigns and continues alone his work. From that time (1831) dates his celebrated study on *Lachesis* and his first ideas on the uses of homoeopathic remedies prepared from the excretions or from the pathological secretions which he named "Nosodes". In 1835 he goes to Philadelphia and founds "Academy of North America for the medical art by Homoeopathy" at Allentown, the first institution for the teaching of Homoeopathy of the world. In 1848 that school was transferred in Philadelphia (Homoeopathic Medical College of Pennsylvania). There he teaches the Materia Medica and the doctrinal principles. Finally he also taught in "Hahnemann Medical College" from 1867. Hering died in 1880 as a member of the Academy of natural science of Philadelphia, principal founder of American Institute of Homoeopathy, indefatigable experimenter. His written work is considerable ; let us cite among others his Materia Medica or "Guiding symptoms" 10 v. and his "Domestic physician '. Thanks to the impulsion of Hering, Homoeopathy received an uncomparable impetus in U.S.A.

Here are the theses of Hering, scientific father of Isopathy (A. Nebel—Contribution to the history of Isopathy, Journal Belge d'Homoeopathy, 1901, Nos. 3 and 4).

1. **Presumed effect** : The serpent poison taken interiorily must have an action (1822-1828) (in Archives fur die Homoeopathische Heilkunst of Stapf, v. 10, (1831) 2, p.) 4 and French tr. in Bibliotheque homoeopathique of Geneva, v. 2, (1833) p. 42 and 10).

—**Experiment** : The action is detailed in the essays of 28th July, 1828 and more than hundred others (Archive 10-2, p. 20 ; 13-1, p. 165, 14-1, p. i70 and Wirkungens des Schlangengifts, Allentown, 1838).

2. **Presumed effect** : The "venom" of rabies taken interiorily, must also have an action.

—**Experiment** : Experiments are solicited on the 18th June, 1930 (Archive 10-2, p. 17 ; 13-3, p. 32) but none made the experiment. The author experimented it from July 1833. The "venom" developed some pathogenetic symptoms, like all other substances.

3. **Presumed effect** : There are other products that act thus taken interiorly (Archive 10-2, p. 27 ; 13-3, p. 32).

—**Experiment** : Experiment with *Psorinum* and the pus of itch, Varionilum and vaccininum, remedies of "nosodes" prepared from excretions or pathological secretions, should be used as "Aequale's (Diluted saliva of rabid dog for a man or for an animal suffering from rabies) or as "Simele", according to the pathagenesic symptoms developed by the experiments of Nosode-remedies on healthy man (such as Psorinum, the pathogenesis of Psorinum established by Hering have not less than 439 symptoms) indicated in the psoric diathesis. Thus what is successful for a virus, may be expected from all others. Every patient would furnish from his germ his remedy and his prophylactic. The contagion would be checked in its start, and the first patient would serve to cure all the others. The plague and anthrax will no more be a terror and other scourges that are brought from the orient, will bring at the sametime the remedy.

4. **Supposed effect** : Some products of the human body and some special parts of the organism in healthy condition have a preferable action on the parts from which they are derived (Archive, 14-2, p. 98-99).

—**Experiment** : From 1834 Hering preconises the utilisation of homologous organs diluted and dynamised (iso-organo-therapy). These ideas will be taken up by Herrmann of Thalgau towards 1840.

5. **Supposed effect** : The chemical elements should have an action, such substance on such organ in which it is found as a constituent, a preferable action and influencing on the functions of these organs (Archive, 13-3, p. 65 and 14-3, p. 14).

—**Experiment** : On Calcium phosphate, fluoride, chloride, oxygen and other gases, Carbonic acid etc.... Studies on Iron, Manganum, Sulphur, Phosphorus, the Acids, the Potassium salts, Sodium salts etc... representing in this the work of Schussler on Biochemic salts.

6. **Hering** advises the utilisation as stock of nosodes a secretion or excretion (pathological or not) taken from the patient himself (as Autopsorine).

The theses of Hering, were extraordinary and in their time, would have defined the essential new method and will be the landmarks between which will oscilliate the tendency of its history.

The second great "Isopath" was the veterinary doctor Johan Joseph Wilhelm Lux (according to J. Brusch) (Uber Homoeopathie in/der veterinaermedizin—Leipzig, 1934) born on the 6th April, 1776 at Oppeln in Silesie (Germany). His father was a small businessman, cultivator and also a veterinary doctor. He studied at Brisbane and was destined to become a veterinary. In 1800 a student of Ecole vétérinaire of Berlin. In 1803, he continued his study of medicine and natural sciences at Leipzig. He received his D. Phil. in medicine in 1805, and in 1806, was appointed professor of veterinary sciences in the University. Lux became an important date in the history of veterinary medicine. In 1800 he published an article in which he concludes : "The veterinary doctor is the most important person of the state". In 1805, he brought to light without the varnish the lamentable condition of the Veterinary school of Berlin. Among his works (of which many remain unknown), we may cite :

Characteristics of the Epidemic of Bovides. (1803)

Translation of Tolnay : *Arteris Veterinaire, Compendium pathologicum.* (1808)

Study on the Teaching of Marechal Ferrand, Leipzig. (1809)

Justice of Shepherds its Relation to the State. (1815)

Popular Study on the Domestic Animals. (1819)

But Lux, from 1820 began to read the writings of Hahnemann and applied the new method in veterinary medicine, which brought him immediately some reputation. From that time he became an ardent propagator of Veterinary Homoeopathy.

He founded many homoeopathic societies and from 1830, published the first periodical on veterinary medicine, entitled *Zooiasis* (or the Homoeopathic cure destined to animals, Kollmann Leipzig) of which he dedicated the 1st volume to S. Hahnemann with the following inscription "You are the Sun which rises in the horizon of diseased animals, and as

such, I place you among the veterinaries in the temple of
Aesculapius of whom you represent the foundation stone." On
the 11th December, 1831, M. Valentin Zibrik of Szarvasend,
proprietor of the Comital Raaber in Hungary asked him in
writing a homoeopathic remedy against glanders and anthrax.
Not knowing yet any homoeopathic means against these
epidemics, his reply was negative, but he advised him to replace
the wanting Simile by the 30th dilution of a drop of the nasal
mucous of an animal attacked by glanders and to give it to
all the animals suffering from that disease. Thus he created
the stock of *Anthracinum* then *Malleinum*. In 1833 Lux
published his results in a small pamphlet entitled "Isopathik
der contagionen" or "all the diseases carry in them the means
of their cure" (Killman, Leipzig, 1833). The use of the morbid
agent itself diluted and dynamised became a general method
for therapeutic ends by virtue of the principle according to
which "Acqualia acqualibus curenur." Thus not only should
be diluted and dynamised the "known" morbid agents (as for
example Scabby of Sheeps, Tinea of animals, itch (psora) of
man, the blood of the spleen of animals suffering from Anthrax,
pus of syphilis, serum taken out of vesicles of Marochetti in
hydrophobias, lympth of Anthrax and of plague even of the
contagion of cholera) but also all sorts of products from secretions and excretions of men and of animals (dynamised fecal
matter, or humanine, vesicular calculus, sweats of feet, saliva
of epileptics or Herculine etc...). Even Lux proposed the use
of diluted and dynamised remedies that have become introgen-
ous because of over dosing (thus diluted Sulphur against the
abuse of Sulphur).

    The method, one sees well, at first applied also to contagi-
ous diseases is equally indicated for non-contagious diseases.
Thus he prepared the most varied nosodes such as Corbyzine,
Hominum, Anthraxinum, Leucorrhoea, Scabies. Equorum,
Variola hominum, Psorican.

The ideas of Hering and Lux found ardent supporter and propagator in the person one of the best disciple of Hahnemann, Stapf, founder of the Archive für die Homoeopathische Heilkunst, in 1822. He, however, made a difference between nosodes coming out of contagion of contagious diseases and the others, for which he specified the utilisation of stocks coming out of the patient himself (which later on became known as "auto-isopathy").

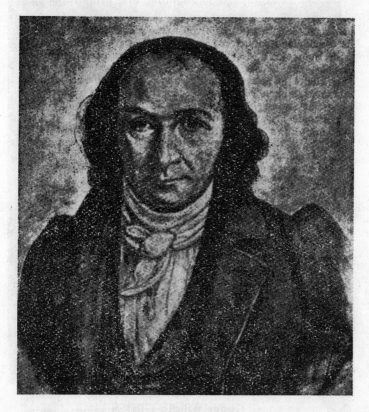

Johann Ernst STAPF

At the sametime Gross and Attomyer popularised the knowledge of Psorinum of Hering. In France Dufresne and Peochier were the mouthpieces of the new method in the

pages of their review *la Bibliothéque homoeopathique de* **Genéve.**
Weber a homoeopathic doctor and councellor in the court of
Hesse studied for many years the means of fighting isopathi-
cally against anthrax (in animals) and published in the year
1836 the most serious and scientific study on iso-treatment of
that disease (Weber : Der Milzbrand and dessen sichersten
Heilmittel, Leipzig, 1836).

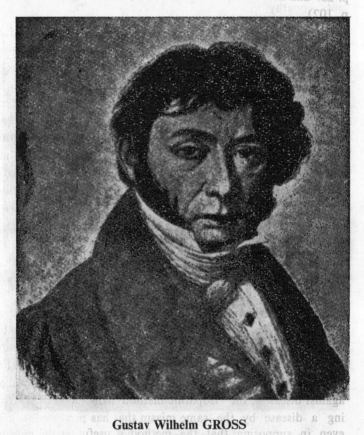

Gustav Wilhelm GROSS

He used the 30th dilution of sanious juice of gangrened
spleen (according to the specific localisation of anthrax of
animals).

A letter of C. Jolly, dentist of Constantinople written to S. Hahnemann on the 24th December, 1835, relates that Theuille homoeopathic doctor of Moscow came "to study and isopathise" the plague and obtained numerous cases of cure using 30th dilution prepared out of the serous exudation plague bubos, (in archive of homoeopathic medicine, 1837, v. 6, p. 289 and Bibliothéque homoeopathique of Genèva, 1836, VII, p. 102).

Later on J.F. Herrmann, doctor of Thalagau near Salzbourg, took up the ideas of Pliny, then of Hering, and designated as real isopathy "the medicinal power of substances of homonomus organs (in Allgemeine Hom. Zeitung, 1844, Bd. 27, p. 187). In 1848 he published "The true Isopathy or the utilisation of healthy animal organs as remedies for the analogous affections in man (Herrmann : Die wahre Isopathie, oder die Heilkraft theiericher stoffe bei Krankheiten gleichmeiniger Organe, Ausbourg, 1848) and prepared some remedies Hepatine (diluted extract of the liver of Jackal), Pulminie cerebrina—His ideas were taken up again by Brown-Squard, father of modern opotherapy.

But the new method had only a few enthusiasts and the fact that the criticism that followed were strong enough to bring a certain decline of isopathy for some years among homoeopaths.

S. Hahnemann, the founder of Homoeopathy has a slight different opinion about Isopathy. At first it was favourable, but later turned frankly hostile. In the 5th ed. of "Organon" (1833) (4th French Ed., 1856, para 55 (1), p. 144) he writes "one may admit in fact a fourth method of using medicines against diseases ; the "isopathic method", the method of treating a disease by the same miasm that has produced it. But even in supposing that the method is useful, as the miasm is applied to the patient after having modified it to a certain point by the preparation to which it is submitted, the cure in that case will be effected only by opposing *similimum similimo*". The

6th ed. which appeared in 1921 (and could not induce any fact of decline of Isopathy which goes on its course) is still more categorical (6th ed. Fr. Tr. by P. Schmidt, 1952).

"To desire to cure thus, by a pathogenic power *rigorously equal* (per idem) is contrary to common sense and even to all experiences." Similar criticisms are formulated in his book "Doctrine and Treatment of Chronic Diseases" (tr. Jourdan, 1846, p. 213). At other times Hahnemann has a clearly favourable attitude and does not hesitate to address to "Bibliothéque Homoeopathique" of Geneva the letter of Jolly relating the isopathic success of Theuille in the epidemic of plague of Constantinople. According to Jean Jarricot (Considerations histo iques sur l'Isopathic, in Actes de in Société Rhodanienne d'Homoeopathie, 1956, fasc. 2, p. 13) the reticence of Hahnemann was purely sentimental, which may be explained by the reaction of a pride of the founder of a method towards dissident disciples. According to Dénis Démarque (L'Homoeopathie Médicine de l'Expérience, 1968, p. 85) the real reason would be doctrinal, because to admit Isopathy, is to admit a "material cause" of the diseases and it is contrary to vitalism.

Genke (in Griesschlich : Manuel pour servir a l'étude critique de l'homoeopathie, 1849), veterinary doctor, is a great adversary of Lux. For him, a prolonged trituration of contagium product deteriotates its properties, except for anthraxinum, because the cantagions of anthrax is destructed with difficulty "even by cooking the skin and the staining of the skin" (Hygea, 1839, v. 2., p. 226 and 243). He even criticises severely the organic Isopathy of Herrmann.

After a period of enthusiasm, Rapou, author of the History of the Doctrine of Homoeopathy fought violently against Isopathy (Rapou—Histoire de la doctrine homoeopathique, 1847, v. 2, p. 176 and 203). We will see later on, with the argument of Rapou.

Griesselich, promotor of specificism in Germany at first favourable because he uses the Psorinum condemns openly Isopathy (Hyges, v. 3., p. 327). "What is recently called Isopathy, attributing to it some value, is only a subject of confusion, a superficial analogy less or not well understood." Further on he adds "A development of that question seems to us absolutely superfluous. Also audacious opinion raised to a law wrongly understood, should not be brought to light and it requires that one should guard himself against such an abominable madness. The positive facts that serve as foundation of Isopathy are less numerous and are easy to bring back to the principle of Homoeopathy. This judgement, considering the considerable impact of the author over his contemporaries, decided the fate of homoeopathy. The result was that most of the Homoeopaths will forget Isopathy ; however some isolated ones will continue to use some Isopathics (Des Guidi used Morbillinum ; Rapou, Anthraxinum, Arnaud, Vaccinum Cf *Isopathy and its founders*, Fouché, l'Homoeopathie moderns, 1933, No. 4, p. 260).

Concomitant with the works of Collet (from 1865) and of Krüger Nimes, Hering the founder of Isopathy, continued his researches in America and published a monograph on Lyssin (or Hydrophobinum) in the North American Journal of Homoeopathy of 1870. The same year Swan published in the New Organon two cases of tuberculosis cured by Tuberculinum (ex-Phthisine of Hering and Lux) prepared from the suppurated tubercular cavity.

Burnett of London, disciple of Swan utilised Bacillinum (dilution of the sputum of T.B. patient containing K.B.) and published his experience of five years in the treatment of tuberculosis (Burnett – Five years experience in the new cure of Consumption, Nov., 1880, London). This happened five years before Koch. Drysdale preconises Pyrogenium (product of decomposed meat) in typhus and in septic conditions. Swan recommends Erysypalinum, Diphtherinum etc... (Homoeopathic

Physician, 1892). From these numerous observation Dr. Kighel of Belgium first established a clinical pathogenesis of Tuberculinum (l'Union Homoeopathique, 1981, v. 5, No. 3, p. 85). Later on J.H. Clarke (Homoeopathic World, 1891, v. 26, p. 304) published an analytical pathogenesis culled from all the cases observed up to that time by the allopathic doctors relating to the action of Tuberculine on the tubercular patients and also on the non-tubercular patients. Mersch (Journal Bélge d'Homoeopathie, 1894, p. 236) did in 1894 a synthesis very much pruned of the two preceding pathogenesis. It is interesting to underline the chronology of these works, which were done many years before those done by Koch on the therapeutic action of Tuberculine. The phthogenesis of Tuberculinum was re-studied by Kruger (Kruger -- Therapeutique isopathique et harmonique : le virus, remédes internes, 1899) of Nimes and A Nobel of Lausanne (in Zeitschrift des Berlin : Vercins Hom. Artze, June, 1902 and tr. in Journal Bélge d'hom., 1902, No. 4, p. 149 and No. 6, p. 226).

In Germany appeared in 1861, the work of Dr. Hagero, *Medicamenta homoeopathica et Isopathica omnia*, written in Latin and which gave a description regarding the isopathics used at that time.

In France it was Denys Collet (According to Ch. Janot— Denys Collet in Homoeopathic moderne, 1936, v. 2, p. 132) who from the year 1865 began again the isopathic movement.

Father Denys Collet, a religious person of the order of dominican and Doctor of Medicine, was born on 21st Dec., 1824, at Frazi, village of Eure-et-Loire, a student of the college of Nogent le-Retrou, came to study medicine at Paris. He practised for about 12 years, during which he met father Monsabre and knocked at the door of Dominican apprenticeship of Fravingy-sur-Ozean, at the age of 40. Became a witness of homoeopathic cure and engaged himself from the year 1865 to study the new method. Himself re-discovering Isopathy he prevented an epidemic of small-pox at Flanigny in 1871 using a dilution of 4 CH of vaccin (Vaccinum). From that time being convinced of his method he took the advantage of a sojourn of many years in Mossoul, a town of Asia Minor, for the application in a large scale of Isopathy. Returned in France for his illness, he acted as a physician of a small convent and treated his community by isopathic method. Desirous to make known his method of therapeutics, he wrote and published his book, at the age of 74 (T. J. M. Collet : Isopathic, methode Pasteur par voie interne, 1898).

In 1903 his community being dissolved he exiled himself at Aubagne (Luxembourg) and died there in 1909. The book of Collet that contains a number of excellent ideas and still more unsupportable opinion, has been very well analysed by Parrot (Parrot : *Isopathie dans sa individuelle*, 1967, p. 28) of which here is the essential points : a preface disabused on the absence of the real therapeutic science precedes the "first book" by some general ideas on the life, health, disease, the death that invite the author to attempt to build up a "law" of general therapeutics which may be defined as follows : "To cure a diseased organism, it is necessary that the organism is not universally ill, that there are still some parts that are healthy and that one uses then an identical or anologous morbid agent but in relatively minimum dose, to create in the healthy parts of that organism some reactive powers, by the intermediary of nervous and circulatory system, for being reversed on the diseased part, and help them to disburden themselves of their enemy, the morbid agent" (p. 28). Further on he adds : "If the real medicine should be an agent similar to that disease, and nothing is more similar to the agent of the disease but the disease itself and because the secretions of man who is diseased are more or less charged with morbid elements which are naturally expulsed by the outlets, if one knows how to collect these elements from the secretions, one can surely have in these morbid elements some medicinal agents." Thus according to him, there are three methods of cure : Allopathy, Homoeopathy and Isopathy, each one of which is valuable to select in function of the clinical indications. In the "second book" Collet distinguishes three kinds of Isopathies : 1. "Pure isopathy" which takes the products of secretion of a patient as medicinal agent to cure the same disease. 2. The organic isopathy (at present our organotherapy) and 3. Scrotherapic isopathy" (dilution of hyper-immune serum). In fact Collet shows that the natural or artificial secretions, even the blood, may be the sources of medicines. Let us cite for example the diluted and dynamised tears in case of grave conjuctivitis, of ulcers, Keratitis, nyctalopias, of hemeralopias ; the Diphtherine, in grave anginas, the bronchial mucous in acute or chronic catarrhs, the mucosity of throat for catarrhal otitis. Similarly, urine, sweat, the secretions of human cutaneous affections, the blood and secretions of varicose ulcer, blood taken out of goitre, in case of want of secretion by causing artificially phlyctenule. He specifies the lower dilutions in acute case, the mediums and high in the chronic cases and preferably using the secretion of the patient himself. The "second book" ends by recalling the history of isopathy (let us mention that the author had the knowledges of these works well after his re-discovery) in which he criticises sentence by sentence the accusations of Rapou (Rapou : Histoire de la doctrine homoeopathique, 1847, p. 176 to 203) which is as follows : Isopathy is absurd ; 2. Isopathy is nausiating ; 3. Isopathy has inconstant results ; 4. Isopathy causes a loss of considerable time ; 5. Aequale is finally nothing but simile ; 6. Isopathy should be left out because it causes the doctors to deviate from Homoeopathy (Loc. cit, p. 179 to 193 and Parrot loc. cit, p. 58 to 65). The third book contains 42 personal cases (human and animal) as well as the rules of pharmacopraxis. Thus Collet seems to be the father of individual isopathy and his works are the starting points of a considerable renovation of the method.

The following year (1899) Kruger of Nimes published his "Isopathic and Harmonic Treatment : Virus and Venoms Internal Remedies," a work of general homoeopathic and isopathic therapeutics in which he makes a very complete study of Tuberculins. Some years later, Antoine Nebel (1870-1954) makes a real experiment of Tuberculine of Koch and he made of it a pathogenesis to which we refer even now. In 1907 Jules Gallivardin of Lyon, published his book "Allopathy—Homoeopathy-Isopathy" which is a critical examination of the "constitution de la therapeutic de jousset" (1902). He reproaches the latter for his silence on the real precursors of Pasteur, the isopaths, the students of Hahnemann. The ideas of Pasteur raises in fact a considerable interest in the circle of homoeopaths. Thus Sieffert writes "And however, effect of the serums of Pasteur absolutely conform to the law of Similitude (Sieffert : Introduction générale à thérapeutique positive, 1910). Similarly writes Pierre Jousset "After examining these facts in the light of the doctrines of therapeutics formulated by Hippocrates, we see that they are governed by the Law of Similars : That which causes stranguria in healthy man cure in it man who is suffering from it has said Hippocrates ; that which produces diphtheria, says Pastuer. And Pastuer, like Hippocrates may give us the formula of the law of indications "Similia Similibus Curentur" (Serotherapy and Homoeopathy in l'Art médicale, mars, 1906). J.P. Tessier writes "Then in whatever manner we examine the question, we see that the specific curative medicine, the serum acts in an absolutely identical manner to the disease producing a sort of medicinal disease which replaces the other and cure rapidly. Now we may affirm and say without fear that it is of course homocopathic cure (in Sieffert, loc. cit, p. 79).

In 1910 appears the fundamental book of H.C. Allen, "The Materia Medica of the Nosodes" (B.T. 1910). Allen (1836-

(1909) at first professor of Anatomy in Cleveland Medical College, then of Materia Medica in Hahnemann College of Chicago and finally the founder professor of Hering Medical College is in fact the first to have published a book uniquely meant for nosodes and one should wait till 1960, whed appears a second study of the same type, the "Materia Medica den Nosoden" by O.A. Julian (Haug Verlag, Heidelberg, 1960 and 2nd ed. 1975 and Biotherapiques and Nosodes, Ed. Maloine, Paris 1962). Allen describes by the side of classical Nosodes like *Medorrhinum, Psorinum*...a series of medicines which are sensibly different from the idea of Nosode such as its history teaches. These are studies on "Adrenalinum" which is a hormone. It is true that at the time of Allen, this one might be considered as a poison, natural and powerful but not well-known. "Ambra Grisea" is according to Hering "probably" a nosode coming from Cachalot, there is no doubt because Amber Grey is a pathological secretion of this Cetacae. "Cholesterinum" was at that time a product obtained by the dynamisation of biliary Calculus.

Finally a series of physical remedies : *Electricitus Magdetis Poly-Ambo* ; *Magnetis Poly Arcicus* ; *Magnetis-Poli-Australis* ; X-ray. These products are obtained by irridiation or saturation of lactose and cannot be included among the nosodes.

Similarly, different kinds of milk cannot be retained such as Lac-canimum, Lac felinum, Lac vaccinum, which are some normal secretions. They are rather organotherapics.

Léon Vannier found in 1912 the review "l'Homoeopathie fransaise" in which from the first number he preconises the use of Isopathy which he renamed "Isothirapie." He takes up the idea of his Master Antoine Nebel who has described some important types of heriditary or acquired intoxications in relation to such and such nosodes. Vannier was an ardent defender of individual isopaths (Cf. "Deux années de pratique isothérapique" in Bulletin de la société d'Homoeopatherapie de

France, 1929, p. 140 and l'Autothérapie Sanguine, Bulletin du Centre Homoeopathique de France, 1936, fasc. 2, p. 584) and utilises from 1927 Sanguin Isotherapy. Similarly Jules Roy makes of it a very deep study) J. Roy : Les régles de l'Isothérapie Sanguine, Bulletin de L.H.F. 1929, p. 135). Later on in 1934 J.M. Munoz publishers a very interesting study on the *modification of the blood formula by the use of isopathy and homoeopathic medicines* (in La Revue fransaise d'Homoeopathie, 1933, No. 9, p. 516).

In 1923 Doctor Lucinio Cardoso, of Rio de Janiereo, published his book "Autonosique dyniotherapy" or treatment of the diseases by their agents and their dynamised products (L. Cardoso : Dyniotherapie autonosique on traitement des-maladies par leurs agents et leurs produits dynamisés, Fr. tr. by Nebei fils, 1932). Homoeopathic doctor, professor of general mathematics and of rational mechanics in Ecole Polytechnique of Rio, Cardosa takes up the thesis of Prof. Rogers, of Chiago, and auto-isopathy. It is in fact the question of injectable auto-blood-isotherapy, very often intramuscular (Cf. Compte rendu du Dr. Rousseau, l'Hom. Moderne, II, p. 6).

In 1836 Fortier-Bernoville published an important inquiry on Isopathy and Nosodes in (l'Hom Moderne, 1936, Nos. 4 and 6). From the articles it appears that all the homoeopaths questioned, systematical uses of the nosodes and that almost half of them used individual Isotherapy. Fortier-Berneville himself preconises the use of Phlyctenular isopathy or auto-Phlyctennotherapy, provoking artificially (by using a Cantharidine paste for example) a phlyctenula which may serve as individual stock for isopathic remedy. His essay is written on the Syndrome of Parkinson, multiple sclerosis stubborn headaches, Zona, Chronic evolutive polyarthritis with more or good results.

Léon Vannier advises isopathic "**Renal** calculus" in lithiasis (l'Isopathie en renal lithiasies : Bulletin du C.H.F. 1937, II,

p. 697) while Vincent de Laurier (Isopathie, in Rovue fransaise d'Hom, 1938, p. 321) exposes his experience on "Gastric juice" in gastritis, on "Leucorrhoea" in metritis, on "Veinous blood" in migrains, on Menstrual blood (of the 1st day) in hypermenorrhoea and metrorrhoea and denounces the sometimes noxious effects of the utilisation of complex isotherapies, increasing the number of stocks. Pichet (short notes on 23 years' of the practice of Isotherapy : Propagateur de l'Homoeopathie, 1938, No. 9 p. 282) preconises like the stock vaccins of Allopathy, the vaccins of Allopathy, the utilisation of Complex Isopathics, by augumenting the number of stocks. In this way prepared "Angina complex", similarly the vaccine "Furuncle complex" (which includes a hundred of stocks of anthrax).

In 1947 appears the book of P. Brotteaux : "Homoeopathy and Isopathy" (1947, Peyronnet, Paris). The second part of the book is devoted to Isopathy, which according to him, comes out of Homoeopathy, because it is founded on the research of true simillimum. The failures of isopathy do not result out of the principle itself, but from the excretion and secretion of the patient that do not always contain the cause of the disease ; or the cause in the secretion is mixed with the latter, because according to the author, the real cause should be used as pure as possible. They also preconised the isopathy of intoxicating products consumed in great quantity such as coffee, chocolate, alcohol, tobacco and medicines like quinine, gardenal, anesthetics etc...

Einally we may note one interesting attempt of explanation of the action of homoeopathic remedies based on the theories of conditioned reflex of Pavlov.

In 1960 appeared in Germany the "Materia Medica der Nosoden" of O.A. Julian. The book was an enormous success in the Homoeopathic circle of Germany. and thanks to this book, the study of Nosodes got again a considerable impetus while it was practically non-existent there. Thus R. Voll, in the therapeutic application of Electro-Acupuncture. Organometry depended essentially on this book and gives an important place to Nosodotherapy. H.H. Reckeweg who founded his conception of Homoeotoxicosis, incorporates in his "Biotherapy" the use of nosodes. It results that thanks to these two authors, the Nosodotherapy is now widely diffused in German speaking countries. The book is "re-written" in French in 1962, taking into account the new pharmaceutic legislation, and, for this fact it contains after a general introduction, two parts : The first contains the description of new nosodes, called Biotherapics, that may be prescribed freely by every doctor in France ; the second part contains most of the Nosodes of which the prescription cannot be made for all (excepting a few). But the description of the latter are given in the hope of taking positive new steps. This book is the only modern book which gather together the informations on the present day Nosodotherapy and always serves today as a reference book.

In 1961 the National Federation of Homoeopathic Societies of France organised a vast enquiry on the practice of Isopathy (Cf. La Revue des congré, de F. Junot, in les Annales Homoeopathiques fransaises, 1969, p. 656). Thus F. Lamasson imparts his fortunate results by using his urinary Isopathy specially for the diseases of the urinary tracts, blood isotherapy in parasitosis (30 CH), Seric isotherapy in irido-cyclitis even in chronic glaucoma. P. Chavanon retraces his experience of Isotherapy in E.N.T., while M. Denis published 23 observations of isotherapic treatment of Dermatology. Doctor Iliovici takes up the interesting dispute with the intention to know *"Is Isopathy really the perfect simillimum"* ? Dano preconises the Isotherapic "Menstrual blood" in mental troubles connected with the menstrual cycle. Professor Bordet, veterinary doctor of Ecole de **Mrison**-Alfort reports his very encouraging results of urinary Isotherapy from urine (and "iso-sendiment" or "iso-calculus") in chronic or subacute cystitis without calculus and urinary lithiasis of dogs and cats. Finally here are some extracts of conclusions of Dr. Dano on that enquiry "The Isopathic medicines represent the Simillimum par excellence, the faithful image of the morbid state of the moment and may be successful there where Homoeopathy hesitates or fails even with the exact medicine. It is a powerful adjuvant of a well conducted homoeopathic treatment. The possibilities of Isotherapic method goes much beyond that what is generally thought of. An Isopathic medicine is a perfact image of the individual who has supplied its stock, *i.e.*, to say it contains the Simillimum of which any Materia Medica cannot furnish the equivalent by the application of the Law of Analogy. The reaction that it causes is therefore, perfectly adapted to the individual. It is somewhat "total" covering the apparent or unapparent troubles. Each of us can take account of it clinically, by the equilibrium that it brings on the neuroendocrinal system, on the general functions, on the mind and on the local sphere "and to concludes" it is specially in unattainable affections by other methods, that one finds one of the spheres of Isopathy".

G. Hage published a similar enquiry in 1964 (Hage-Enquete sur la pratique de l'Isothérapie "L'Hom fransaise, 1964, p. 131) which clarifies the different opinions of homoeopathic doctors who use Isotherapic method of treatment. It appears from this work that if some isotherapics seem to be effective (blood, urine, purulent exertions) the others are clearly less dependable (like the products from cutaneous exertions). According to the greater part of the doctors interrogated, Isopathy is not as much as a premordial therapeutic, but rather an *appointde depannage* before a failure of the Homoeopathic treatment.

G. Dano in his "Contribution to the therapeutic of allergic diseases and of their equivalents (Le Fransosis, Paris 1964) builds a bridge between Isotherapy and Allergology and prepares the remedy "Poummon-histamine", dilution of the lung of anaphylactised Cobaye by repeated injections of Ovalbumine. The lung of Cobaye is in fact the "Shock" organ of the antigen-antibody reaction and liberates an important quality of chemical mediators of which specially histamine is one. Dano specifies "Poummon-histamine" in allergic diseases and their equivalents such as asthma, the hay fever, the allergic migrains, allergic dermatitis, paroxystic attack of tachycardia, hyperfolliculine of allergics, as well as psychic troubles.

The book of Parrot deals finally with the present-day situation of individual Isotherapics or Auto-isotherapy. After at first devoted to the works of Collet, Parrot describes the result of an experience of more than 20 years of the method successfully studied : Blood isotherapy (injectable and by mouth), Isopathy of menstrual blood, Seric and phlyctenular isotherapy and finally urinary isotherapy, Isotherapy of pus, renal calculus and saliva (Parrot : Isotherapy dans sa forme individuelle, Ed. Doin, Paris, 1967).

Such is briefly the historic sketch of Iso-nosodotherapy or according to the name given by O.A. Julian, *Micro-immunotherapic dynamisee*. The latter has a new impetus as well in France as in foreign lands and this situation is mainly due to the works of this author.

BIBLIOGRAPHY

Here we will only mention the principal works on the method and will ask the reader to refer to the works mentioned in the body of the article.

A. RAPOU : *History of the doctrine of Homoeopathy*, 2 v., Baillere, Paris 1847.

GRIESSELICH : *Manual for the critical study of Homoeopathy*, Baillere, Paris, 1848.

D. COLLET : Isopathic—*Methode of Pasteur for internal use*, Baillere, Paris, 1898.

KRUGER : *Isopathic and Harmonic therapeutic : Viruses and Venoms as internal remedies*, Paris 1899.

J. BARBIER : *Opotherapy of the Olds*. Thesis, Paris, 1903.

H.C. ALLEN : *Materia Medica of the Nosodes* : B and T, Philla.

R. ALLENDY : *Alchemy and the medicine* : Thesis, Chacornac, Paris. 1912.

L. VANNIER : *Doctrine de l'Homoeopathie francaise*. Doin, Paris, 1931.

L'HOMOEOPATHIE MODERNE : Enquiry on Isopathy and Nosodes, 1936, Nos. 4 and 6.

R. PLANER : *Uber die Behandlung chronischer Krankheiten mit Auto-Nosoden* (Over the treatment of chronic diseases with Auto-nosodes).

BROTTEAUX : *Homoeopathy and Isopathy* : Peyronnet, Paris, 1947.

E. BUSSE : Isopathia interna et externa, 1956.

L. VANNIER : *The origins and future of Homoeopythy*, Doin, Paris, 1960.

G. DANO : *Contribution to the therapeutic of allergic diseases and their equivalents*.

O.A. JULIAN : *Materia Medica of Nosodes*, Haug Verlag, Ulm, 1972, 2nd ed.

O.A. JULIAN : *Biotherapics and Nosodes*, Maloine, Paris, 1962.

R. PARROT : *Individual isotherapy*, Doin, Paris, 1967.

L. WURMSER : What is an Isotherapic ? La documentation homoeopathique, L.H.F. de France, No. 38, 1957.

(These books are either in French or in German language. Translations are given here.

DOCUMENTS

DOCUMENTARY NO. 1

BIOGRAPHY OF CONSTANTINE HERING

(In the original book the biography of Constantine Hering was translated into French by Dr. J. Askenasi from Richard Haehl's : Samuel Hahnemann : Sein Leben und Schaffen, vol. 1, p. 465. In the present translation it has been reproduced from : Samuel Hahnemann : His life and work, published by B. Jain Publishers, New Delhi).

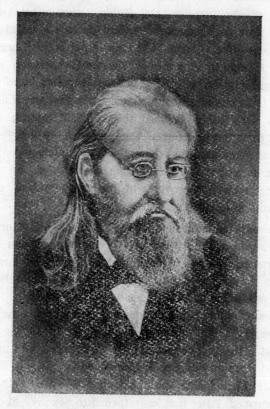

Constantine HERING

3 F

Born on the 1st of January, 1800, at Oschatz in Saxony, the son of the assistant rector there, Constantine Hering passed his school years in Zittau, whither his father had been transferred as rector. In 1817, he attended the surgical academy in Dresden and in 1820 Leipzig University to study medicine. In the early part of his sojourn in the Saxon, capital of the Muses, he made the acquaintance with Hahnemann. He attended his lectures without entering into any closer connection with the students of Hahnemann. For they were mostly older than he and as we have seen, they formed a strictly exclusive circle amongst themselves. Hering was a student and an assistant of the surgeon Dr. Robbi, who, after an initial tendency towards Homoeopathy, had become a decided antagonist to it—like Clarus. The Leipsig publisher Baumgartner had asked Robbi to write a book against Hahnemann and the homoeopathic "Heresy". Hahnemann expelled from Leipsig, was also to be completely annihilated from the scientific point of view. Dr. Robbi declined the request because he had not sufficient time, but he referred the publisher to his assistant. The latter, honoured by the publisher's offer, gave himself up to a careful study of Hahnemann's writings. In this way he became involved in provings of medicines and in practical experiments with Homoeopathy.

The results made of him, Saul, a Paul (1821). He announced his conversion without reservation to his teachers and to Baumgartener, who had made him the offer. The latter also turned to Homoeopathy later and helped to promote the movement by publishing homoeopathic works and journals. it was to be feared that Hering's convictions and his conversion to Homoeopathy might injure him in the eyes of his Leipzig professors. He therefore went to Wurzburg for a term and graduated there on the 23rd of March, 1826. In his Doctor's thesis "de Medicina futura" he confessed himself boldly to be a homoeopath. After that he returned to Saxony, in order to acquire permission to practice Medicine in his home country by a further examination. During his preparation for this, he was appointed science instructor and house physician at Blochmann Educational Institute in Dresden. This position appealed to him very much with his special interest in the natural sciences and it would not have prevented him from pursuing his own intentions.

But in the following year a distant relative from Surinam, returned home. He portrayed with such enthusiasm the natural resourses of the country that Hering and Weinhold, the scientific researcher, resolved to travel with him to Guiana. The Saxon Government and Principal Blochmann supported the project most enthusiastically so that Hering was able to depart for Surinam in 1827. Soon after their arrival the two explorers undertook a scientific journey into the interior of the country. In the course of it Hering discovered on December 15th, 1827, near Parambribo, the capital of Surinam, a man lying helplessly ill on the road-side and he took charge of him. When Hering returned from his journey, the recovered patient sought him out and took him to his master. Through his recommendation and as a result of other success-ful cures—Hering had used Homoeopathic treatment—the town governor made him his physician in Attendance. He maintained continuous connections with his home country sending thither his experiences and the results of his energetic researches in Materia Medica. From this period of his practice as a physician in Paramaribo we have letters to Hahnemann and numerous articles of Stapf's "Archiv". As a member of the research association he had been prevented from literary work on behalf of Homoeopathy and therefore he had retired from the association.

Longing for his native country induced him to return to Germany in 1833, even if only for a short visit. On his return to the New World he arrived at Philadelphia where friends prevailed on him to stay. He settled down in this mother state of the Union and it was from this time onwards that his active work for Homoeopathy—in practical healing and also in speech and writing—really began. It is astounding what Hering, in addition to his medical duties managed to achieve in organisation and literary work.

His organisation : In 1835 he founded in conjunction with Dr. Wesselhoft the "North American Academy for Homoeopathic Healing" in Allentown thirty-three miles north of Philadelphia. It was the first education institution for homoeopathy in the world. But the institution, which was financed through shares and for the founding of which support had been requested but not received from Hahnemann, could survive only for a few years. A dishonest secretary embezzled the funds, whilst antagonists of Homoeopathy assailed the institution with all the means at their disposal. In the meantime Hering had to struggle hard for his livelihood. So hard hit was he that he frequently thought of leaving the United States and approaching Hahnemann for help in this intention. The love of his home country made him return thither in 1845. He remained for a year in Saxony, apparently attaching him for ever to his native land. His new home however attracted him with greater power across the ocean and he went out once more to the United States to propagate Homoeopathy with fresh courage and renewed energy. Together with Dr. Williamson and Dr. John Jeanes he founded a new instructional institution for Homoeopathy in February, 1848—the Hahnemann Medical College in Philadelphia, which still exists and in which, until 1869 he taught as Professor of Materia Medica. This educational institution also had great difficulties to overcome before it was able by means of the generous support of homoeopathic adherents to develop into a large self-dependent institute for Homoeopathy. To-day the Hahnemann College in Philadelphia with the hospitals attached and its extensive polyclinic has become the most important homoeopathic educational institution in the world. Its buildings are valued at several million dollars. The college and hospitals are modern in their equipment and abundantly provided with materials of instruction, laboratories, apparatus, etc. The libraries comprise approximately 20,000 volumes and homoeopathic literature in every language is completely represented. For practical training the Hahnemann College offers advantages which are scarcely to be equalled in any European University. More than seventy professors and lecturers are at the disposal of approximately 300 students of medicine. The large number of cases in the hospitals and the polyclinic, with more than 50,000 patients and 6,000 accident cases treated every year, affords the professors abundant material for their clinical instruction. Besides the general hospital containing about 200 beds, the college possesses a special institution for midwifery, directly attached to it and allowing the students ample opportunity for observing obstetrical cases. In addition, numerous confinements are attended amongst the poor people in the town and these also serve for instruction.

The selection of professors and lecturers for the Hahnemann College has always been carried out with the greatest care. Only men of proved ability and eminent talents, who had made a name for themselves by their efficiency as physicians, were considered for appointment. As long as the college was in financial straits, most of them gave up their lecture fees and their salaries as hospital physicians. Now conditions are so improved that the professors, can be paid the amounts compatible with their efforts. Professors of anatomy, chemistry, pathology, etc., are paid a full salary and devote their whole time and energy to instructions and research in their special subject. The kind of spirit prevailing in the teaching staff is best shown by the fact that the Hahnemann College was the first medical institution of instruction in America to demand a three years' course of study. In the introduction of four and five years' courses it preceded all

others with its good example. By the practical training of
more than 3,500 homoeopathic physicians the Hahnemann
College has contributed more to the development and propagation of Homoeopathy than any other instructional institution in
the world.

Hering wrote an unusually large number of works. We
find a large number of volumes on medicine provings, successful cures, homoeopathic questions of dispute in the most varied
German and American medical journals. His style was
extraordinarily smooth, attractive and concise. That vacilla-
tion and contradictions occurred bringing in their train
disputations with Rummel amongst others (as for example,
concerning high potencies (Allg. hom. Ztg. v. 34, No. 4) is not
after all, astonishing. With a special interest he started a
movement in America towards the adoption of methodical
provings of medicines and advanced this cause as far as he was
able. The results were followed in Germany with the greatest
interest.

His "Homoeopathic Domestic Physician" which appeared
first in 1833 for the purposes of the missionary campaign of
the evangelical brethren in Paramaribo became such a
universal boon to the homoeopathic lay world that it has been
continually appearing ever since in increased and improved
editions. (Since 1901 the new editions have been revised by
Dr. Haehl). The twenty-seventh edition was recently published
(May 1922).

Till Hahnemann's death Hering remained in continual
touch with him. It was at the repeated urging of the Master
that Hering, together with homoeopathic physicians in Philadelphia, invested his widow with a doctor's diploma. But in
spite of his great respect and veneration for the Master he
had always managed to preserve his independent judgement.
Thus in the year 1837 he confessed :

"Generally I am considered a student and adherent of Hahnemann and I admit that I am of those who adhered to him most faithfully and venerate his greatness with enthusiasm. But at the same time, I declare also that, since my first acquaintance with Homoeopathy (1821) to the present day, I have never accepted a single theory of the "Organon" just because it is there stated."

Eighty years of age, hale and active even in his later years, Hering died of a heart attack on the 23rd of July, 1880, after returning from a visit to a patient.

As in the whole of his private life Hering was in Homoeopathy a never ceasing "worker" in the driving machinery of the new science of healing.

At his sudden departure from this life he had completed his task (of preparing a place for Homoeopathy in America) with a success which has not yet been achieved in the Old World. The first educational institutions in Allentown and Philadelphia were followed in 1850 by the homoeopathic college in Cleveland, in 1857 by that in St. Louis, in 1859 by another in Chicago, and in 1860 by one in New York, and then further instructional institutes of a purely homoeopathic tendency were continually being added. They have all been erected through private means, but all have a state grant. Now-a-days Homoeopathy is on the same footing as Allopathy in the United States. Every student who has passed the final examination of a state recognised medical school can sit for a special state examination set for the physicians in Homoeopathy.

Before the great war there were in the United States 56 purely homoeopathic general hospitals with 35 to 1,400 beds each, nine hospitals for women with 30 to 100 bedseats, eight orphanages with purely homoeopathic treatment having accommodation for 50 to 825 occupants each.

Germany was the birthplace of Hahnemann and of Homoeo-pathy. But in the propagation and practical exploitation of Hahnemann's theories as in so many other provinces, the new world with its virgin freshness and energy has far outpassed Germany and the old world. The success is to be ascribed not least of all to the inexhaustible self-sacrificing devotion of Constantine Hering.

DOCUMENTARY No. 2

BIOGRAPHY OF WILHELM LUX

French translation by Dr. J. Askenasi (Paris)

Johann Josepth Wilhelm Lux, born in 1777 at Oppeln.

His father was a small businessman, cultivator, and according to Schrader-Hering, also a veterinary. With great difficulty he did his studies in the Lycée of Brisbane and destined himself very soon for the art of veterinary medicine. In 1800 he became a student in the Civil Veterinary School of Berlin. In 1803 he came back to Leipzig to study medicine and the natural sciences.

In 1805, he obtained the diploma of doctorate of medicine and philosophic-Magister medicinae. In 1806 he was appointed professor of veterinary sciences in the University. He died in 1848 or 1849 having acquired the title : Senior Collegium Marinum.

Lux stands as one of the most interesting figures in the veterinary medicine because of his experiments contributed to the diffusion of Homoeopathy. In 1808 he published at Glogan an essay wherein he concludes : "The veterinary doctor is one of the most important class of the state." Kreutzer mentions this document. In 1805 he denounced clearly the lamentable condition of veterinary school of Berlin, thus putting the professors as well as the king in embarrassment.

While Lux was upholding his opinion on Homoeopathy he was treated as a "Spoilt head" because the time was not

---

Brusch Johannes (in der Medecin veterinaire) :

"Uber Homoeopathie in der Veterinaermedizin" ed. Dr. Willmar Schwabe, Leipzig, 1934.

yet ripe for his ideas. Only one observer of Leipzig wrote that "the writings of Lux are not without value, because they contain some truths, specially about the economic condition of the country.

With the passing of years the merits of Lux were recognised even by his adversaries.

Among the writings of Lux we must mention : *Characteristics oj the epidemic of bovide*, Leipzig, 1893 : *Translation of Tolnay* : *Artis Veterinaiae, compendium pathologicum*, 1808. *Justice of shepherds*, the relations with the state, 1815. *New method to check the epidemic of peste* : Study on the teaching of Marèchal Ferrand etc. 1809, Leipzig ; Popular study on the domestic animals, 1819.

Towards 1823 he introduced homoeopathic treatment for the animals with immediate success.

He is the founder of many homoeopathic societies. On the 14th of October, 1832 he dedicated to Hahnemann the 1st volume of his Review entitled *Zooaiasis*.

Here is his dedication :

"You are the new sun that rises in the horizon of ill animals and as such I place you among the veterinaries in the temple of *Aesculape*, of which you are the foundation stone".

Even his adversary Falke described him in 1839 as "the personality of Lux is amiable and courageous".

Many works of Lux still remain unknown.

Hering thinks that his works were very much neglected by his contemporaries, so much so that, that which is related to Homoeopathy was not reprinted because of the little importance that the officials gave to that new therapeutics.

He stopped all his activities as a practitioner towards the last years of his life, and gave himself up to the studies of pomology which he liked.

Up to the end Lux fought for the progress of Homoeopathy and he had constant and numerous adversities to win over.

DOCUMENTARY No. 3

JOHANN JOSEPH WILHELM LUX
ISOPATHY OF CONTAGIONS

or

**All the diseases carry in their substance
even the means of their cure.**

Proposed to the Congress of Homoeopathy
for their strict experiment.

Published at Leipzig, 1833, at Christian
Ernest Kollmann.

Translation : *Doctor J Askenasi* (Paris)[1]

M. Valentin Zibrik of Szarvaskend, proprietor of the Comitat R ber in Hungary asked me by writing on the 11th Decembe , 1831, for a homoeopathic medicine against *Lues boum stifera* or bovine plague (Loeserdurre) and against anthr (milzbrand).

My reply was negative, because I did not yet know the h moeopathic means for these epidemics. Nevertheless in order o honour the confidence of this proprietor, I explained to him the mystery of the nature by the highest principle of medicine which may be expressed as follows. "All the contagions carry in their substance, even the means of their cure."

---

1. This is the first French translation.

At the same time I told him, knowing that he has ideas about Homoeopathy, how a drop of blood of an anthrax and a drop of the nasal mucus of the bovine plague, *diluted thirty times*, should be used. The basis of this fundamental law was unknown at that time.

Patients suffering from frost bite find amelioration by the snow. Apples and even potatoes peeled cause to diminish their coldness by cold water. Burns are best treated by the fire. Serpent bites are treated by the venom of the same serpent. Hydrophobia in man, even very grave, is treated in Russia by the saliva of rabid dog, as is related by General Boroden in June 1829, with a rapid and certain result.

In these cases that may be multiplied easily, the natural force seems not to cure by the simillimum but by *aequale* (although in another dynamisation).

The innoculation of the cows by the lymph of the mammary pustules protects them from psora and syphilis. This vaccination remains identical.

One should potentialise with a drop of blood of the spleen of some animals suffering from anthrax or other pustules like it or syphilitic chancre, in short product of every contagious disease of cows, sheeps, cats, dogs in order to obtain a real homoeopathic cure.

It is in 1831 that Lachesis was experimented by Dr. Hering, then another experiment was carried out on healthy man by Dr. Grisselich in 1832 with Psorinum (Psoricum)—the itch. Against latent herpes, I will prescribe three grains of the latter (psorinum) with success, even for herpes squamosa.

Four members of my family were definitely cured of their toothache (dental arthritis) by the same Psorinum.

One must be very careful while treating the Ozena of horses by isotherapy, by changing the dynamisation (Potenz) between 15 to 30.

Some epidemics of the year 1832 were eradicated with Isopathy helped by some remedies in the 30th dilution like *Mercurius, Spiritus sulphuratum, China, Natrum muriaticum.*

I may be allowed to mention that the numerous prizes that I have obtained for my works in England, Holland, Germany, Austria and Turkey go to the Homoeopathic school.

Very often it is found that Homoeopathy is realised perfectly in Isopathy, *because we cure contagious disease by their own infecting substance.*

Strength and Dilution

Homoeopathy acts on the nervous system and on each organ according to its totality through the energy liberating out of the gross substance of the medicine which is a force obtained by some particular processes.

The more the substances are potentialised, the more the dormant power (energy) is liberated. Thus mineral substances that have neither smell nor taste like Silica, Gold, Lycopodium, change their qualities by diluting them to 30th, 40th or 50th potency.

Copper, Iron, Lead need to be of such high dilution.

Roots, barks and grains that have however smell and taste, act in lower dilutions, like Asafoetida, Chamomilla, Valeriana, Castoreum, Moschus etc... 12th to 15th dilutions are enough.

Contagions require higher dilutions. Contagious bites of horses require 30th dilution.

I gave to my brother-in-law O...on the 1st December, 1830 for hemorrhoids 24th dilution of *Bryonia.* Instead of one drop he took on a piece of sugar much more which developed in him thoracic pains and constipation. As *Bryonia* was indicated in his case I gave him *Bryonia 15* and everything was cured. I have seen, with other experiments that a high dilution is more powerful than a lower one ; this means that the medicinal power augments according to the gradual diminution of the matter. Since than I call it "Dilution" but "increasing the power."

THE POTENCY, CAN IT BE EXPERIMENTED WHEN ONE TAKES THE MEDICINE ?

Reply : As a rule No.

From each tube, with the medicine of which one experiments, a part of the medicinal power of the medicine, which is mixed with lactose, is lost and this the experimenter absorbs through his mouth and nose while inhaling.

He who possesses a small pharmacy or he who takes many remedies a day, finds himself in a state of constant vibration, like glasses in an almirah that resound by music, only according to their own totality and not by other sounds.

I call "essences," the extracts from vegetables and animals— Tintura fortes—these are strong extracts. The word tincture recalls futilely the high colour of wine or myritelles or aierolles and which are called essences by doctors—Essentia saturator tinctura—it is the whole power of the medicine. Everything that nature and chemistry concentrate with the end to cure, may be called "essences" concentrated of the curative power as well as the acids like Arsenicum Album, Camphora, Petroleum, Baryta acetica, Mercurisum solubilis etc…

I will also call "essences" the lower dilutions of *Silica, Aurum, Murcury* etc…

I mix the dry drugs with 1 parts of alcohol and a drachme of medicine.

I thought at the beginning of my practice of veterinary Homoeopathy to make the medicines more active, by taking 2 drops from the phial of the 29th power and mixing it with 100 drops of alcohol, and by jerking strongly and counting from 1 to 30 and I am convinced that I obtained not a simple dilution but a development of the forces of my pharmacopoea.

I mark on the corks of my tubes the potency from 1 to 30 so as that my future readers would have not to calculate in quintillions or in decillions. The power indicated is found with me in inverse proportion to the degree of the disease ; if an organism reacts strongly I give the lower dilutions only in a very small quantity, as for example in toothache in man. If the organism is sensitive or of phlegmatic or lymphatic constitution and has become weak by chronic diseases, I use higher dilutions which I renew and thus I avoid homoeopathic aggravations.

Diet, Regimen, Confidence, Belief, Fantasy

If regimen means famine cure, one may say that Homoeopathy does not know it because it allows every patient to eat according as he is hungry.

On the contrary Homoeopathy does not advise the food and drinks which are exciting like condiments, seasoned foods that resemble much more to drugs than to foods.

As a veterinarian I do not care for the regimen.

The kitchen salt has very little action on man. The high dilution of the antipsorics as well as of other medicines are not disturbed by food in man. It is not necessary to change one's habit. I do not forbid meat and sausages to dogs that they have the habit to take with their masters at table.

If the ill animals have faith in the small doses of homoeopathic medicines more than in any other medium, or if they have only an idea of their doctors and their medicines, that question should equally be put to child specialists.

It is a dangerous ignorance to attribute the homoepathic cure alone to regimen, faith, phantasy or mysticism.

The success of Homoeopathy in animals is constant and surprising which is a supplementary proof of the excellence of the system.

I practised since 1795 and up to 1822, and have treated the animals allopathically with some fortunate results. The curiosity is to a certain extent the discontendedness, as is seen in a number of doctors, and this directed me towards homoeopathic study.

In the beginning I had to meet with difficulties, some paradoxial ideas and some doubts.

For more than 10 years, I treated all the animals by Homoeopathy and I continue to follow with success this marvellous means.

Moreover, I continue experiments of new doses of different medicines which are more suitable to animals.

The positive results are so much attractive that I feel the necessity to tell them to others and it is for this reason that I have founded the review *Zooaiassis* or "Homoeopathic cure destined to the diseases of animals". The first issue is going to be published during the Easter of this year.

DOCUMENTARY NO. 4

For historical interest, we give here an extract from a book of pharmacology entitled :

Medicamenta

Homoeopathica et isopathica omnia

ad id tempus a medicis aut examinata aut usu recepta

Auctore *Dr. H. Hagero*

Lesnae : Sumptibus et typis Ernesti Güntheri

MDCCCLXI (1861)

Albinum : Albin (albino) Graecum Album. White excrements of constipated dog being ill of intestines (of dogs constipated being ill of intestines).

Alveolinum : Pus of dental alveola.

Anthracinum : Anthrakinum.

Ascaridinum : (Ascaris vermiculars L) Vermiculus totos vivas.

Balanorrhinum : Mucilageneous fluid which in Gonorrhoea is separated from glands of the glans penis.

Boviluinum : Mucous fluid that flows from nose and throat of buffaloes during pest.

Brossulinum : Syphilinum Brossulinum—pus of venerian ulcer.

Bupodopurinum : Mucous secretion of the mouth of buffaloes who are ill from epizootic claudication (scorbutic disease of the mouth).

Carcinominum : Secretion taken out of the cancer of armpit.

Cariasinum : Purulent matter of bone carries.

Ceruminum : Cerumen.

Cholelithinum : Biliary calculus.

Coenurinum Ovium : Cerebral hydatide (Coenurus cerebralis).

Condylominum : Total condyloma.

Coryzinum : Catarrhal mucosity.

Coryzinum Equorum : Mucous of the lachrymal fistula.

Dysenterinum : Anal secretion of dysentric mucous.

Emphyeminum : Pus of a pulmonary vomit.

Enteropurinum : Enterohelcosinum, ichorous pus of stools.

Enterosyringum : Fistula of "Boyau-culier".

Gonorrhinum : Spermatic liquid.

Helinum : Foot corn.

Herculinum : Foam from the mouth during epilepsy.

Herpinum : Dry and humid pustules of herpes.

Hippoestrinum : Larva of ox-fly found in great quantity in the stomach of horses in the form of bunches.

Hipposudorinum Humidum : Sweat of horse.

Hipposudorinum Siccum : Dust adhered to the sweat of horse.

Hippozaeninum : Pus or mucous secreted through the nostrils of horses suffering from humid morve.

Humaninum : Human stool.

Hydrophobinum : Saliva of rabies.

Influenzinum : Grippum.

Karkininum : The Karkininum is distinguished from those of glans penis and from those of lips, nose and uterus. Ichorous pus or humors taken out of these cancers.

Kynoluinum : Yellow mucus secreted through the nostrils and the eyes in the disease of dog which is called canine paste.

Kynotaeninum : Tenia of dogs.

Kynotorrhinum : Pus from the ear of a dog.

Lachryminum : Tears.

Laryngophtisinum : Purulent secretion of trachitis.

Leucorrhinum : Whites (White flour).

Lippitudinum : Pituitary fluid, coming out of the eyes of men in opthalmia.

Lumbricinum : Ascaris lumbricoides.

Maculahepatinum : Hepatic maculae.

Mastocarcinominum : Pus of breast cancer.

Medorrhinum : Mucous secreted from urethra in syphilitic gonorrhoea.

Meletinum : Black matters in bloody vomitings.

Metrorrhaginum

Morbillinum

Nephroposteminum : Pus of kidney abscess.

Nephrolithinum : Kidney stone.

Odontosyringinum : Purulent matter secreted from the fistula of the teeth.

Oipodopurinum : Purulent matter secreted by the hoofs of ruminants in the epizootic claudication or the sisense that destroys the hoofs.

Otorrhinum Hominum : Purulent liquid that flows out of the ears of men. Otorrhinum of deaf persons is to be distinguished from that of non-deaf persons, and Otorrhinum of ill men from Otorrhinum of scarlatina.

Ozaeninum : Humours of ozena related to carries.

Parotidipurinum : Humors of parotid secretion after an angina or an inflammation of the parotid.

Pneumolithicum : Lung stone.

Pneumophtisinum : Pus of purulent phthysis.

Podoclavinum : Corns of the sole.

Polipinum Narinum : Polypus of nose.

Prosopopurinum : Purulent matter of cutaneous pustules of the face.

Pyoninum Bobonum : Humours of bubo, that of venerian bubos and that of non-venerian bubos are to be distingui-shed.

Pyoninum Oculorum : Purulent matters secreted from opthalmic eyes ; that of cornea, and that of syphilitic cornea are to be distinguished.

Ragadinum : Raghades.

Scabiesinum : Psorinum hominum.

Scarlatinum

Scrofulinum

Sudorinum Phthisicum : Liquidfied sweats of phthisic patients.

Sycosinum : Venerian wart of men.

Sudorinum Pedum : Foot sweat.

Tinaenum : Crusts.

Ureninum : Sediment of urine of patients suffering from inter-mittent fever. One should distinguish between urininum of intermittent fever and without fever and urininum of the intermittent fever from that of urine passed during fever. The sediment collected on a filter paper is dried in a cool place.

Urolithinum

Variolinum : Purulent matter of the lymph of pustules of variola of vaccinated men (word by word : When variola is innoculated).

Varicellinum

DOCUMENTARY NO. 5

List of Nosodes that may be obtained from Nelson, London (A. Nelson & Co., 73 Duke Street, Grosvenor Square, London, WIM 6BY).

Actinomyces	30
Adenoidum	3-200
Adenoma prostrate, non-malignant	3-30
Anthracinum	6-50M
Antityphoid and Paratyphoid (T.A.B.C.)	6-50M
Arteriosclerosis	3-200
Aviaire (see Tuberculinum aviaire)	
B.C.G. vaccine	3-30
Baccillinum testiculatum (see Tub. Test)	
Bacillinum (Bacillinum Burness)	6-CM
Bacillinum and Influenzinum	12-IM
Bacillus coli	6-IM
Bacillus diphtheria (see Dipht. Bac.)	
Bacillus dispar	6-30
Bacillus Friedlander (see Friedlander)	
Bacillus pyocyanaeus (Pseudomonas acruquinosa)	3-30
Bacillus tetani (Tetanus)	6-30
Bacillus typhimurinum	30
Bacillus Welchii	30
Bilharzia	6
Botulinum	30-IM

Bowel Nosodes (see separate leaflets)

Brucella abortus   3-200

Brucella melitensis   3-200

Calculi biliary   6-1M

Calculus renalis   6-200

Calculus renalis (phosphatic)   6-200/10M/CM

Calculus renalis (uric)   200

Cancer Serum Koch (Glyoxalide)   6-200

Carcinoma (bowel)   12-30

Carcinoma (rectum)   6-30

Carcinoma Co. (bowel) (C. Intest Co.)   12-200

Carcinoma Co. (K)   12-200

Carcinoma adeno (colon)   12-30

Carcinoma adeno (stomach)   12-1M

Carcinoma adeno (bladder) (C. adeno. vesica)   12-30

Carcinoma adeno papillary (ovary)   12-30

Carcinoma adeno papillary (uterus)   12-30

Carcinoma Scirrhus (breast) C. Scir Mam.   12-200

Carcinoma Scirrhus (stomach)   12-30

Carcinoma squamous (lung)   12-30

Carcinosinum   30-CM

Cataract (immature)   6-30

Cataract (mature)   6-30

Cattle ringworm (Trychophyton)   6-30

Chicken pox (see Variola)

Cholera   6-30

Coqueleuchin (see Pertussin)

Deformans (Micrococcus deformans)   30

Cysticercosis	6-200
Denys (Tub. Denys)	12-1M
Diphtheria antitoxin (maceration)	6-200
Diphtheria antitoxin (trit.)	6-200
Diphtheria bacillus	6-200
Diphtheric membrane (maceration)	6-200
Diphtherinum (membrane trit.)	6-CM
Sclerosin (disseminated)	9-30
Distemperinum (canine)	12-CM
Dysmenorrhoea (polyvalent)	6-30
E. Coli	3-30
Empyemia	200
Enterococcinum	6-200
Epithelia syphilitica	30-CM
Epivax (see Hard pad living virus)	
Erysipelas	30
Feline hepatitis	6-30
Fox lung (see Pulmo vulpis)	
Fowl pox virus	6-30
Friedlander (Bacillus Friedlander)	6-30
German measles (see Rubeola)	
Glanders	30
Glandular fever	8x-30
Glinicum (see Medorrhinum)	
Glyoxalide (see Cancer Serum Koch)	
Gonococcin (see Medorrhinum)	
Hemolytic streptococcus (see Strept. Hem.)	
Hard pad (eyes)	6-30

Hard pad (nose)	6-30
Hepatitis, cat (see Feline hepatitis)	
Hepato luesinum	8-200
Herper zoster	6-1M
Hippomanes (Horse serum)	8-200
Nippozaeninum	6-200/10M
Hydrophobinum (Lyssin)	6-10M/CM
Influenza A England/43/472	6-30
Influenza virus A (Asia) 1957	6-200
Influenza virus A 2 (Hong Kong) 1968	6-200
Influenza virus B (Hong Kong) S-72	2x-30
Influenza virus A (Port Chalmars) 1973	2x-200
Influenzg virus A (Scotland) 1974	2x-30
Influenza haemophilis	6x-30
Influenzin-antitoxin	200
Influenza catarrhalis	200
Influenza meningoeoccus	200
Influenzin serum	200
Influenzinum	12-10M-CM
Influenzinum virus A	6-200
Influenzinum virus B	6-200
Influenzinum virus AB	6-200
Lepropsy	3-30
Louping ill vaccine	3-30
Luesinum, Lueticum (see Syphilinum)	
Lyssin (see Hydrophobinum)	
Malandrinum	30-CM
Malta fever (see Melitotoxinum)	

Marmoreck	12-1M
Measles (see Morbillinum)	
Measles vaccine	6-30
Medorrhinum (Gonococcin)	6-CM/MM
Melitotoxin (see Brucella Melitensis)	
Meningococcus	30-200
Micrococcin	30
Micrococcus catarrhalis	12-200
Micrococcus neoformans	10M-CM
Mongol nosode (Nosode M)	6-200
Morbillinum	30-CM
Mucobacter Mersch	6-200
Mumps (see Parotidinum)	
Myxomatosis	6-30
O.A.N. (hip)	6-200
O.A.N. (Osteo arthritic nosode, Osteo-arthritic synovial fluid)	6-1M
Oncolico nosode	30
Oryptococcus linguae pilosac	3-6
Osseinum	6-12
Paratyphoid A	6-200
Paratyphoid B	6-200
Parotid gland	3-200
Parotidinum (Mumps) Ourlainum	30-200
Pertussin (coqueluchin)	12-CM
Pertusis vaccin (whooping cough)	6-30
Pestinum	30-200
Pneumococcus	12-50M

Pneumonia virus pig. (see Virus Pneumonia)

Polio (mixed)   30-200

Polio vaccin (Polyomyalitis vaccin)   12-30

Polio vaccin (S.A.I)   6-30

Polio vaccin (S.A. II)   6-200

Poliomyelitis oral vaccin (Sabin)   6-30

Polypus nasalis   30-00

Psorinum   6-CM

Pyrogenium (Sepsin)   6-CM

Quadruple nosode (Bacillinum, Influenzinu,

Pneumococcus and Streptococcus)   30-200

Rachi-Luesinum   8-200

R.A.N. (Rheumatoid arthritic nosode)   6-30

Renal calculus (see Calculus renalis)

Rosen (see Tuberculinum Rosen)

Rous Sarcoma (Sarcoma)   6-30

Rubela (German measles)   6-200

Rubela virus vaccin 1970   6-30

Salmonellosis (Calf vaccin Dublin)   3-30

Scarlatininum   12-CM

Scirrhinum   6-CM

Sepsin (see Pyrogenum)

Serum anti-leptospera   6-30

Small pox pustule (see Variolinum)

Small pox vaccin (see Vaccininum)

Staphilococcinum   6-CM

Stophilococcinum abdominalis   30-10M

Staphylococcus albus   6-30

Staphylococcus aureus	6-30/10M/CM
Staphylococcus haemolyticus aureus	6-200
Streptococcus	12-10M
Streptococcus haemolyticus viridans	6-30
Streptococcus longus viridans	6-30
Streptococcus lubesis	6-30
Stredtococcus viridans (Influenza 1970)	3-30
Streptococcus rheumaticus	3-200
Streptococcus viridans cardiacus	30-1M
Swine erysipelus	6-30
Lyphilinum (Lueticum, suesinum, brossulinum)	6-CM₁MM
T.A.B. (Typhoid paratyphoid A and B)	6-200
T.A.B.C. (see Antityphoid and paratyphoid)	
Tetanus antitoxin	6-30
Vetanus bacillus (see Bacillus tetani)	
Tetanus toxin	6-CM
Tetanus toxoid	6-30
T.K. (see Tuberculinum Koch)	
T.B. (see Tuberculinum Koch Exotoxin)	
Tonsilinum (infected)	6-30
Trichomonas vaginalis	6-30
Tuberculinum aviaire	15-1M
Tuberculinum bovinum	6-CM/MM
Tuberculinum Denys (see Denys)	
Tuberculinum Kent	1M-CM
Tuberculinum Koch	6-1M
Tuberculinum Koch Exotoxin (T.R.)	6-CM
Tuberculinum Rosen	6-100

Tuberculinum Spengler	6-200
Tuberculinum testiculatus	30-1M
Typhoidinum	6-200
Vaccininum	3-10M
Varicella	6-200
Variolinum	12-CM
Vincent's Angina	6-30
Virus pneumonia pig	6-30
Whooping cough (see Pertussin and Pertusis)	
Yellow fever	6-30

Some Explanations Concerning the Use of this List

Most of the remedies can be procured "in normal Gammut." A normal gammut consists in the real Hahnemannian dilutions (done by hand) as below :

0, 1X, 3X, 4X, 6X (CH), 8X, (4CH), 6, 9, 12, 15, 30, 200, 1M (M or 1000), 50M (50,000), CM (100,000) but the latter are not prepared by hand according to the Hahnemannian method.

Explanation

1X-CM indicated that it is the question of a complete gammut *i.e.*, to say from 10 (1X) upto 100,000.

2X-30/10M, the bar/indicates on interruption in the gammut *i.e.* to say after the 30th CH, the immediate high dilution is 10,000 (10M).

The names in capital letters after the name of a remedy indicate the name or general spelling ; thus "Achilea millefolium (Millefolium) (see Millefolium).

DOCUMENTARY No. 6

A large extract of NOSODES found in the book : *Ordinatio Antihomotoxica et Materia Medica 1974*, edited by the Section medicale du Laboratoire (Biologische Heilmittel Heel G.M.B.H., 757 Baden-Baden, Postfach 729, Federal Germany) according to the works of Reckeweg who refers to the monograph of the *Materia Medica der Nosoden* of O.A. Julian.

"Ganzbesonders wird auf die Monographie von Dr. O.A. Julian (Paris) verweisen : *Materia Medica der Nosoden* (erschienen bei Karl F. Haug, Heidelberg) sowie auf die in der Homotoxinliteratur verstreuten Hinweise, die Groessenteils mitberücksichtig sind".

Anthracinum-Injeel+forte (D 15), D 20, D 30, D 200 (+Einzelpotenz D 10).

Bacillinum-Injeel+forte (D 15), D 20, D 30, D 200 (+ Einzelpotenz D 15).

Bact. coli-Injeel+forte (D 6), D 12, D 30, D 200 (+Einzelpotenz D 5).

Bact. lacis-aerog-Injeel+forte (D 6), D 12, D 30, D 200 (+inzelpotenz D 5).

Bact. protcus-Injeel+forte (D 6), D 12, D 30, D 200 (+Einzelpotenz D 5).

Bact. pyocian-Injeel+forte (D 6), D 12, D 30, D 200 (+Einzelpotenz D 5).

Bruc. Abort-Bang-Injeel+forte (D 6), D 10, D 30, D 200 (+Einzelpotenz D 5).

Carcinominum-Injeel+forte (D 15), D 20, D 200(+Einzelpotenz D 200).

Carc. hepat. metastat-Injeel + forte (D 6), D 10, D 30, D 200.

Carc. laryngis-Nosodes-Injeel + forte (D 6), D 10, D 30, D 200.

Carc. Mammae-Injeel + forte (D 6), D 10, D 30, D 200.

Carc. Urin (nur in D 200 liefebar).

Cozasackie-Virus-Injeel + forte (D 10), D 15, D 30, D 200
    (+ Einzelpotenz D 7, D 8).

Diptherinum-Injeel + forte (D 10), D 18, D 30, D 200.

Grippe-Nosode-Injeel + forte (D 6), D 10, D 30, D 200.

Hydrophobinum-Injeel + forte vide Lyssinum-Injeel.

Influenzinum-Injeel vide Grippe-Nosode-Injeel.

Klebs, pneum-Injeel + forte (D 6), D 12, D 30, D 200.

Luesinum-Injeel + forte (D 10), D 15, D 30, D 200, D 1000
    (+ Einzelpotenz D 7, D 8).

Lyssinum-Injeel + forte (D 12), D 15, D 30, D 200 (auch als
    Hydrophobinum bez.).

Medorrhinum-Injeel + forte (D 10), D 12, D 30, D 200
    (+ Einzelpotenz D 10000).

Paracoli-Injeel + forte (D 10), D 15, D 30, D 200.

Paratyphoidinum B-Injeel see Salmon, paratyphi B-Injeel.

Pertussis-Nosode-Injeel + forte (D 6), D 10, D 30, D 200.

Pneumococcinum-Injeel vide Klabs. pneum-Injeel + forte.

Polymyetitis-Nosode-Injeel + forte (D 15), D 20, D 30, D 200,
    D 400.

Psorinum-Injeel + forte (D 9), D 12, D 30, 200 (+ Einzelpotenz
    D 6), Eiter aus Kraetzpustein.

Pyrogenium-Injeel + forte (D 8), D 12. D 30, D 200 (+ Einzel-
    potenz D 5, D 6).

Salmon-Paratyfi-B-Injeel + forte (D 6), D 10. D 30, D 200.

Salmon-typhi-Injeel + forte (D 6), D 12, D 30, D 200.

Scarlatinum-Injee l ¹ forte (D 6), D 12, D 30, D 200 (+Einzel-
potenz D 5).

Staphylococcus-Injeel+forte (D 6), D 12, D 30, D 200
(+Einzelpotenz D 5).

Strept. hemolyt-Injeel+forte (D 6), D 12, D 30, D 200
(+ Einzelpotenz D 5).

Syphilinum-Injeel+jorte vide Luesinum Injeel.

Tetanus-Antitoxin-Injeel+forte (D 6), D 12, D 30, D 200
(+ Einzelpotenz D 200).

Tuberculinum-Injeel+forte (D 8), D 12, D 30, D 200 (+ Einzelpotenz D 100, D 10,000).

Vaccininum-Injeel+forte (D 8), D 20, D 30, D 200 (+Einzel-
potenzen D 200).

Variolinum-Injeel+forte (D 15), D 20, D 30, D 200 (+Einzel-
potenzen, D 15, D 200, D 1000, D 10,000).

DOCUMENTARY NO. 7

Here is an extract of the list of Nosodes that may be found with STAUFEN Goeppingen (Staufen-Pharma G.M.B.H. & Co., Goeppingen, Federal Germany). These Nosodes are under the form of injectable ampoules, dilutions and globules in decimal dilutions.

Anthracinum	D 400	Brucella melitens	D 200
Aviary	D 22	Cholera	D 400
Bac. acidophilus	D 200	Colibacillinum	D 200
Bacillinum	D 1000	Corynebakterium	
(Tuberculinum Burnett)		anarebius	D 200
Bac. Coli	D 400	Coxakie	D 1000
Bac. Dysenteriae	D 800	Diptericum	D 1000
Bac. faec. alk	D 1000	D.T.T.A.B.	D 200
Bac. Gaertner	D 600	Eberthinum	D 60
Bac. Morgan	D 600	Echinococcinum	D 400
Bac. Proteus	D 400	Encephalitis	D 400
Bac. Pyoceaneus	D 400	Enterococcinum	D 400
Bac. Subtilis	D 200	Erysipel	D 200
Bacteroids	D 200	Erysipela suum	D 200
Bang	D 1000	Fischpyrogenium	
Banti	D 400	(salt water)	D 1000
B.C.G.	D 200	Fischpyrogenum	
Bilharziosis	D 200	(sweet water)	D 400
Botulismus	D 400	Fleck fever	D 1000
Brosselinum	D 2000	Gelbfieber (yellow	
		fever)	D 400

Gonococcinum			Lupus	D 200
(Medorrhinum)	D 1000		Lyssinum	
Herpes Zoster	D 1000		(Hydrophobinum)	D 400
Hippozaeninum			Malaria	D 400
(Mallenum)	D 400		Malaria tropica	D 400
Hydrophobinum			Mallandrinum	D 400
(Lyssinum)	D 400		Malleinum	
Imferysipel	D 400		(Hippozaeninum)	D 400
Influenzinum	D 600		Medorrhinum	
Influenzinum AB	D 300		(Gonococcinum)	D 1000
Influenzinum toxicum	D 500		Meningococcinum	D 1000
Influenzinum			Manilia albicans	D 1000
vesiculosum	D 400		Morbillinum	D 400
Influenzinum			Mucor mucedo	D 1000
vesiculosum NW	D 300		Mycosis fungoides	D 200
Influenzinum			Paratyphus	
vesiculosum SW	D 400		(Paratyphoidinum)	D 1000
Klebsin (Tuberculosi-			Parulis (Straph. aur.)	D 200
dinum Klebs)	D 400		Parulis (Strept. muc.)	D 200
Klebsin (Tuberculoci-			Pasteurellose	D 200
dinum Klebs)	D 400		Pertussinum	D 400
Lamblia intestinalis	D 400		Pneumococcinum	D 400
Lepra	D 1000		Pneumococcinum M	D 400
Leptospirosis canicula	D 200		Poliomyelitis	D 500
Leptospirosis ict. hae	D 400		Poliomyelitis Stamm 3	D 500
Leptospirosis p.c.gt.W	D 200		Psoriasinum	D 800
Leucoencephalitis	D 200		Psorinum	D 1000
Listeriose	D 1000		Pyrogenium	D 1000
Luesinum			Pyrogenium avis	D 200
(syphilinum)	D 2000			

4 F

Pyrogenium ex ovo	D 400	Tuberculinum Burnett		
Pyrogenium suis	D 1000	(Bacillinum)	D 1000
Rubeoloe	D 1000	Tuberculinum Denys	D 400
Salmonella TP	D 1000	Tuberculinum Koch	D 400
Scarlatinum	D 1000	Tuberculinum	
Scirrhinum	D 1000	Marmoreck	D 1000
Sepsis lenta	D 800	Tuberculinum neu	D 400
Shiga Kruse	D 800	Tuberculinum Rest	D 400
Staphylococcinum	D 400	Tuberculinum Spengler	D 400
Staphyloccus aureus	D 400	Tuberculinum Klebs	
Staph. Koag. pos.	D 400	(Klebsin)	D 400
Stap. Strepto	D 400		
Streptococcinum	D 400	Tularoemie	D 1000
Streptococcus		Typhinum	D 1000
hemoliticus	D 400	Vaccininum	D 1000
Streptococcus		Vaccinotoxinum	D 400
viridans	D 400	Variola	D 400
Strong	D 600	Variolinum	D 1000
Syphilinum		Varizella	D 200
(Luesinum)	D 2000	Va 2-Grippe	D 200
Taenia	D 400	V-Darmcatarrh	D 200
Tetanus	D 1000	V-Grippe	D 400
Thermibacterium		V-2-Grippe	D 300
fifidus	D 400	V-3-Grippe	D 300
Toxoplasma	D 1000	V-4-Grippe	D 200
Tuberculinum	D 1000	V-5-Grippe	D 200
Tuberculinum avis	D 400	Yersin Serum	D 60
Tuberculinum			
bovinum	D 400		

DOCUMENTARY NO. 8

NOMENCLATURE OF PRODUCTS OF MICROBIAN ORIGIN IN FRANCE (1)

First Category

The real biotherapics. The list is limited to 27 products as follows :

Anthracinum

Aviary

Colibacillinum

Diphthericum

Diphtherotoxinum

D.T.T.A.B.

Eberthinum

Enterococcinum

Gonotoxinum

Influenzinum

Luesinum

Medorrhinum

Morbillinum

Paratyphoidinum B.

Pertussinum

Proteus

Psorinum

Pyrogenium

Anti-colibacillary serum

Serum of Yersin

Staphylococcinum

Staphylotoxinum

Streptococcinum

Tuberculinum

Tuberculinum residuum

V.A.B. (B.C.G.)

Vaccinotoxinum

Second Category

Serums and vaccines other than the real biotherapics but inscribed in the pharmacopoea (1937—1949—1965—1975).

1. Cahiers de Biothérapie Déc. 1976, No. 52, Page 314.

Serums :

Antibotulic serum (1972).

Anticarbuncle serum (1965)

Antigangrene serum (1972) (anti-Clostridium ocdematiens, anti C.-perfringens, anti-C. septicum and polyvalent anti-gangrene serum)

Antidysenteric serum (1949)

Antimeningococcic serum (1949)

Antirabic serum (1972)

Antirouget serum (1965)

Antistaphylococcic serum (1949)

Antistreptococcic serum (1949)

Antitetanic serum (1972)

Antivenom serum (1972) (antivipers, berus and amodytes).

Vaccines

Anatoxin botulic (1965)

Anatoxine diphtheric (1965)

Anatoxin mixed diphtheric and tetanic (1965)

Anatoxin staphyloccocic (1965)

Anatoxin tetanic (1965)

Vaccin Aatiamaril (1965)

Vaccin antimeningococcic (1949)

Vaccin antipest (1965)

Vaccin antipneumococcic (1949)

Vaccin antirabic (1965)

Vaccin antiricketsis (1965) against typhus

Vaccin antistaphylococcic (1965)

Vaccin antistreptococcic (1965)

Vaccin antityphoparatyphoidic (T.A.B.) (1965)

Vaccin anticholeric (1972)

Vaccin whooping cough (1972) (--anticoqueluchic)

Vaccin polymyslytis

Vaccin measles (1972) (...rougeolic)

Vaccin typhoid (1972).

Third Category

Serums and vaccins that do not figure by name in the pharmacopoea having a legal existence in the forms of specialities.

Example. The C.C.B. Vaccin.

These preparation may be delivered in oral unitary forms from 3 CH : tubes of granules, doses of globules, drinkable ampoules.

Fourth Category

Preparations asked for from microbian stocks or from products of microbian origin do not enter in any of the preceding catagories.

The preparation is delivered if the medical prescription is accompanied by the stock : it is considered as an auto-isotherapic preparation.

CHAPTER 3

DYNAMISED MICRO-IMMUNOTHERAPY
OR
ISOPATHY—ISOTHERAPIES

A. Definitions

It is obligatory, indispensable and necessary to begin with the definition, which is now entered in the Codex of the 8th ed. of the French Pharmocopoea.

Here is the definition :

Biotherapic

Biotherapics are medicines prepared in advance and obtained from products of microbin origin not defined chemically, from the pathological excretions or secretions, or not, from animal, or from vegetable tissues or allergens. These different substances then called *stocks* for biotherapics.

The biotherapics can be delivered only from the 3rd centesimal or 6th decimal dilutions. They can be sold only in pharmaceutic forms destined for oral use.

Experiment. The first liquid dilution and a *forteori* the following dilutions should satisfy the trials of sterility.

Isotherapics

The *Isotherapics* are also *biotherapics*, but they are prepared extemporaneously from the stocks furnished by the patient himself and of which the first liquid dilution should be sterilised.

From these "*Stocks of Biotherapics*", that have been granted a visa, the homoeopathic laboratories may produce dilutions and obtain visa ; these will then be called "Biotherapics."

The biotherapics are some remedies prepared in advance, of which there are three categories :

(*a*) Biotherapics of which the base is serum, vaccines, toxins anatoxins.

(*b*) Biotherapics having for the base pure microbian cultures.

(*c*) Complex biotherapics, defined only by the method or their preparation or by the method by which they are collected.

In this group there are some important polychrests like Psorinum, Medorrhinum, Luesinum, Pyrogenium.

Finally the biotherapics of which the stocks go from simple (from bacteria or virus) to complex (secretions or reactional excretions like pus of blenorrhagia, collection secretion of a syphilitic chancre) are prepared in advance, delivered from the 3rd. centesimal dilution or from the 6th decimal dilution.

Similarly they may be sold under pharmaceutical forms destined for oral use and never with other products.

Let us note here that in Germany, at present, the height of the dynamisation is not limited, the simple or complex injectable form may be obtained and prescribed.

Isotherapic rises up in face of Biotherapic by its *Individual character, individualised* and extemporaneously prepared from a stock of which the product comes either from the patient himself (blood, urines, pathological secretions) or furnished by the patient himself (vaccine, medicine, allergens…).

The preparation of the isotherapics is uniquely destined to the person who has supplied the stock, which will be later destroyed and will not serve again person or for any other person.

Such is at present, in France and according to the pharma-cological legislation, the actual definition of *Biotherapic* or *Isotherapic*.

The actualisation, according to the medical vocabulary of our time, suggests to us that the categories together may be designed by the name "Dynamised micro-immunotherapy."

B. Pharmacotaxi

We have shown that Isopathy has a history.

That history shows that this *Homoeopathic method* enters in the general evolutive movement of Homoeopathic medicine.

And similarly a long course with its fortunes and misfor-tunes with its grandeur and vicissitude, marks a long way which goes from Homoeopathy of S. Hahnemann to the modern homoeopathic concretology. Similarly *isotherapy* and the isotherapics have changed faces in course of years.

Again there the parallelism with Homoeopathy is striking.

The "Holy family" : Hering, Lux, Gross, Stapf found on the baptismal foundations a new therapy called by them : Isopathy.

The same mistake.

By the compound word *Isos*—Individual, and pathos — sufferings, a new theory of a pathological process is designated, while in fact it is desired to indicate a pharmacotherapic praxis concretised by the "Iso-therapy."

For having a good bearing, the whole thing was submitted to "Hofrat". Dr. Samuel Hahnemann asking his patronage.

Hering, a homoeophathic doctor, active, dynamic, enthu-siast, of German origin, emigrated in America (see Ch. 2 and Biography, documentary, No. 1) after having realised a pathogenetic experiment of the venom of Lachesis, and of which he specifies the uses against the consequences of the snake bite, realises with hydrophobinum (Saliva of a rabid dog) and Psorinum or Psoricum his first isopathics.

Lux the homoeopathic veterinarian follows, rather precedes Hering preparing the stocks of Anthracinum and Melleinum.

Thus side by side with the sagacity and meticulous experimental works of S. Hahnemann, a therapeutic method where the experimental rigour of the master is not always evident, sees light better.

A new medical theory seems to oppose to that of Homoeopathy.

To *"Similia similibus curentur"* of S. Hahnemann Lux countered with *"Aequalia aequalibus curentur."*

The principle of Analogy is opposed by that of Identity.

Here is then the reply of the Shepherd to the Shepherdress.

In the 4th ed. of "Organon" (Fr. Tr. Baillere, Paris), 1856, para 56 (1), p. 144, we read as follows :

"One could in reality admit a fourth manner of using medicine against diseases, *i.e.* to say the Isopethic method, to treat a disease by the same miasm which has caused the disease. But supposing even that the thing were possible, and it would certainly be a valuable discovery, as the miasm is administered to the diseases only after having modified it up to a certain point by the preparation to which it is submitted, the cure will take place in such a case only by opposing the *"Simillimum simillimo."*

And in the 6th edition which appeared only in 1921 in Germany thanks to Haehl, biographer emeritus of S. Hahnemann and in French in 1952 by P. Schmidt (of Geneva), he adds the following paragraph :

"To wish to cure in this manner, by a pathogenic power rigorously equal (per idem) is contrary to common sense and for this reason, to all experiences (p. 56 to p. 74, tr. by P. Schmidt).

In fact his faithful disciple Hering and Stapf have also the opinion that the *pharmacological technique of homoeopathy transforms idem into simillimum.*

The rigorism of Hahnemann undergoes some eclipses and he writes to the "Bibliotheque homoeopathique" of Geneva in view of some successes obtained by Isopathy by M. Theuiller during the plague epidemic in Constantinople.

It is besides in the same review that Dufresne, the Swiss doctor published some cases of malignant anthrax cured with Anthracinum 10 CH and 12 CH in another.

There rises in the horizon Organotherapy with the publication at Ausberg in 1848, the brochure of J.F. Hermann "The real Isopathy or the utilisation of organs of animals who are healthy as medicines for similar affections in men."

From that time Isopathy began to develop in full vigour. But following some abusive and some whimsical prescriptions, some severe criticisms appeared. These are the writings of Genke, veterinary doctor and of Grisselich that marked the steps of development.

The progress of Isopathy stopped for sometime and even had a set back.

It took up a second impulse with the book of Denys Collet "Isopathy" in 1893 in English language then with that of H.C. Allen's Materia Medica of Nosode published in 1910 in the English language. The contemporary period is that of the studies of Nobel, Léon Vannier, Fortier-Bernoville and Brottcaux.

A new impulse is given in France, rather in Germany by the work of O.A. Julian which appeared in Germany in 1969 and in the French language in 1962 and a second edition in the German language in 1975.

Then in Germany Voll (R. Voll—Medimententestung Nosodentherapie und mesenchymentschlakungstherapie, 1965) and Reckweg (Ordination Antihomotoxia et Materia Medica, 1974) gave an impulsion without precedence and even the classic Society of Homoeopathic medicine of Germany kept steps with Isopathy.

In France, Parrot published his work on Auto-Isopathy and Zissu some clinical studies.

Pharmacotaxi

In this chapter we are going to broach the three aspects necessitating a methodological research *i.e.* to say the terminology, the general classification and special classification.

1. The Terminology

The least that is said about Isopathy, Isotherapic, the Nosodes, the Nosodotherapy, the Sarcode, Isotherapic, Auto-isotherapic shows that a most bewildering confusion reigns there.

Whence comes difficult and contradictory discussion, because the terminology is not clearly defined. In the work of the same author one may find Isopathy and Isopathic used differently.

It seems to us that there is ground, after having given the actual legal definition which is current regarding Biotherapic and Isopathic, there is for the necessity of a historical study and a classification.

At the beginning most probably the term Isopathy was forged by the veterinary Dr. W. Lux towards 1831-1833 (see Isopathy of contagion published for the first time in French).

As we have said before, Isopathy is a general method of therapeutics, which utilises the morbid product itself, the "miasm" which is at the origin of the disease and should be "in an appropriate quantity, may provoke at least partly some troubles analogous to those which one opposes" (E. Iliovici) (Isopathy, the perfect simillimum).

P. Schmidt of Geneva defines the Isopathic remedies as follows : "Application of an attenuated dose of a pathogenous product for curing the disease of which it is the result. If it is used after having been experimented on healthy man, it becomes a "Nosode" (Glossary, p. 20. in S. Hahnemann's Organon of the Art of Cure, tr. of the 6th German ed. by P. Schmidt).

Isopathy is an immunotherapy according to our present day conception which we will explain later on.

For Lax, the fundamental reason that is at the basis of Isopathy is the *Law of Identity* which he expresses by the phrase :

Aequalia aequalibus curentur

For that time Isopathy and its practical corollary, rises in the rank of a therapeutic discipline having as the methodological principle the reasoning by identity. Isopathic acquires in this manner a wide and diversified dimension.

2.   General Pharmacotaxi

In order to clarify this imbroglio of substances coming from varied sources, there is every reason to make a general classification as follows :

(*a*) Biotherapics : the nosodotherapics or nosodes.

(*b*) Isotherapics.

(*c*) Allergenologics.

(*d*) Toxicotherapics.

(*e*) Organotherapics.

(*f*) Homonotherapics.

The categories taken together will be from now designed under the general Micro-immunotherapics.

(a) **Nosodotherapics or Nosodes**

This term has no legal existence in France and has been replaced by the term Biotherapic as indicated in Para A definition.

On the contrary in Germany, the term covers the totality of categories of a, b, c, d, e, f that we have enumerated previous.

What is a Nosode ?

The term is due to Hering, and has been derived from the Greek word NOSO which signifies the prefix added to the word to form an idea of disease, indicating a relation to the disease (in general).

It may also be compared with the Latin word NOXA, which means damage (Noxious).

Nosodotherapy will then be the therapeutic use of organic reactional wastes or some etiologic factors which are the sources of "damage" to the disease.

For P. Schmidt the Nosode is an isopathic remedy. "If it is applied after having been experimented on healthy man, it becomes a Nosode. In fact many of the nosodes do not possess this quality.

Allendy defines in short thus : the nosode is characterised by a pathological substance used as the medicine prepared in advance and according to the homoeopathic method of dilution.

Fortier-Bernoville characteristics a Nosode by to words : "Specificity" and "Immunity".

We explain the immunitive character later on. But with this definition, these remedies have an illegal existence in relation to the law of 14th June, 1934, which specifies as follows :

"Art. 1. The viruses, attenuated or not, and their different products of microbian origin which may serve, under whatever form, to the diagnostic, to prophylaxis or to therapeutics, cannot be delivered free or onerously as much as they will have been from the point of view of their origin, from their sources, from their appellation, from their fabrication, from the means of their identification and of their concentration as useful substances, the object of an authorisation of the government, following the advice of Academy of Medicine and of the higher Council of Public Health of France, are also submitted the same procedure as is applicable to the injectable substances, of organic origin, not chemically defined, and which may be used for some therapeutic end."

But at present, after discussions in different commissions, it is concluded that "The products for which the authorisation is asked for do not enter in any categories mentioned by the regulations above mentioned (letter of the Health Minister of the 13th January, 1939, in Les biothérapiques by L. Wurmser, Nov., 1955, L.H.F.)."

Then, with the order of "Codification of official homoeopathic preparations" published in the Journal Official of 29 December, 1948, appear for the first time two definitions which officialise and define the Nosodes and Isopathics :

Definition of Nosodes

The nosodes are some homoeopathic preparations obtained from microbe cultures, from viruses, pathological secretions and excretions.

Except on express specification of the doctor, the nosodes can never be sold to the public in kind but only from the 3rd dilution centisimal or in the 6th decimal.

The nosodes are prepared in two ways according as they come from cultures of microbes (simple nosodes) or from complex organic products.

The simple nosodes prepared from viruses or bacterias, which are not cultivable, are assimilated for their preparations to complex nosodes.

The nosodes should satisfy some trials of sterility. The first centesimal dilution and *a fortiori*, the following dilutions cultured on different bacteriological ground, should not give birth to any culture."

To regularise the preparation and sale of these products, the Journal Official specifies that "the preparation and sale of nosodes are submitted to a previous authorisation of the Government, fixed by the order under the conditions laid down by the law of the 14th June, 1934, which is to be expressed in practice by the application of authorisation to the commission of Serum and Vaccines."

Definition of Isopathics

"The nosodes of which the stocks come from the patient himself are called isopathics."

The Isopashics are prepared from :

—Blood (by puncture of the veins and in women in some particular cases, the menstrual blood).

—Urines.

—Pathological secretions which may be distinguished as :

Exudates such as liquids from ascitis, hydrocele, leucorrhoea, Cephlo-rachidian liquid.

Sputum (specially of bronchorrhoea).

Squams and transudates of eczemas.

The Isopathics are at present of real help to doctors and specially for the interested person, the patient, because with the disappearance of the French Pharmaceutical market of a number of nosodes, one may take the help of this therapeutic means.

Thus, we see that the "Nosodes" and "Isopathics" are here precisely defined.

Only, the repercussion in the daily life has from this time become less rejoicing and the tragedy began, tearing into pieces the French medical corp, creating discussions and bitterness.

In fact, contrary to the situation in 1918, inspite of having taken various steps, no reply has been given to any demand by the Commission of Serum and Vaccines.

If the order of the 21st Dec., 1948, officialises the Homoeopathic Pharmacology, it is even then apt to create inconveniences for applications for authorisation. And so the Commission refuses to receive and study the files which are submitted to it by the Homoeopathic laboratories which the Central Service of Pharmacy has been adamant to obtain control of these preparations.

(b) Isotherapics

Isotherapics is the product, that serves to get the medicines prepared according to the homoeopathic pharmacopraxis, coming from the patient himself or supplied by the patient himself.

Thus one distinguishes :

1. *Humoral products*, secretions or excretions coming from the patient himself (blood, urines, secretions and excretions which are pathogenical).

These are *auto-Isotherapics*.

2. *Microbes isolated* from the patient by culture on the appropriate ground. These are Microbian-auto-isotherapics. (see Catalogue No. 8)

3. *Allergenotherapics*. They are somewhat particular isopathics because it is the question of Allergenes, detergents, pesticides, insecticides, allergising medicines etc.

They are *Exo-Isotherapics*.

4. *Organotherapics.* As has already been mentioned dynamised and diluted organotherapics have seen light after the beginning of Isopathy of Lux, with J.F. Hermann of Ausburg.

Still the word "Sarcode" is sometimes used for the dynamised micro-organotherapics or according to Tetau and Cl. Bergeret—*diluted and dynamised organotherapy.*

According to P. Schmidt, the *Sarcode* is a remedy of natural product derived from the tissues or secretions of animals or of human beings, as for example, Cholesterinum, Adrenalinum, Lac Canimum, Pulmobovis, Urea etc. (Op. cit. p. 29).

Thereafter, it is in France, that Léon Vannier and F. Bernoville elaborated more particularly for these. indications.

Recently a clinico-immunologic study of Cl. Bergeret and M. Tetau (Organotherapic diluee et dynamisee, Ed. Maloine) has given a very good explanation of the question and through their knowledge raised it to a real *autonomous therapeutic discipline* within the general framework of the *praxis of homoeopathic concretology.*

5. *Hormonotherapy* is the particular mode of diluted and dynamised organotherapy.

It is the original work of Louis Frouché (Fontainbleau).

He has also made a study of homoeopathic clinical pathology of hormone, parathyroid, thyreotropic hormone ; of folliculostimuline and A.C.T.A.

In the present work, we will study only the biotherapics.

Specific Pharmacotaxy

A. The one which is of the Pharmaceutic order and is in conformity with the legislation in force at present, is as follows :

(*a*) **Simple Biotherapics**

These are biotherapics prepared from pure microbian cultures, which form the original stock from which will be prepared the "Stock vaccines" then the Hahnemannian dilution, namely ; Colibacillinum, Eberthinum, Enterococcinum, Paratyphoidinum, Staphylococcinum, Streptococcinum, Influenzinum, Serum anti-collibacillinum.

To the above may also be added : Leptospera I.H., and Toxoplasma-Gondii (but as isopathics).

(*b*) **Biotherapics of Codex**

Aviary, Diphtherinum, Diphtherotoxinum, D.T.T.A.B., Gonotoxinum, Yersinserum, Staphylotoxinum, Tuberculinum-T.K., V.A.B. (ex-B.C.G.) Vaccinotoxinum.

(*c*) **Complex Biotherapics**

These are complex products for which it is necessary to determine their origin (the source from where taken) ; and its nature described in a protocol giving all the guarantees of the consistancy of the preparations.

The lyophilisation helps to their preservation and assures the permenance of their stocks.

These biotherapics are : Anthracinum, Luesinum, Medorrhinum, Morbilinum, Pertussinum, Psorinum, Pyrogeninum, Tuberculinum, Residnum.

B. Those for which a clinical classification has been proposed by O.A. Julian and is accepted by Dr. Tetau.

This clinical classification, that we have described in our work Biotherapiques and Nosodes (Eq. Maloine, 1962, O.P.), has some similarity with that which has been published by Guillaume de Zissu (Annales Hom. Francaise, 1969, p. 55/143). These authors give a Classification of "Major" and "Minor" biotherapics.

According to these authors, "Major" is that which fulfils the following two conditions :

1. It conforms to a pathogenesis, that is to say, it has like every homoeopathic remedy a symptomatic experimental protocol. Its prescription obeys the law of similitude, like every homoeopathic remedy which possesses a pathogenesis.

2. It conforms to an idea of morbidity, notedly to the principles and clinical descriptions of homoeopathic intoxination : The Psora of Psorinum, the Tuberculous of Tuberculinum, T.R. and Aviary, the Luetic of Luesinum ; Sycosis of Medorrhinum. All the other biotherapics are "Minor".

Without entering into the discussion about the conception of the authors on the mode of classification, we are going to give below our classification according to the clinic of the Homoeopathic concretology.

We distinguish, and like all other arrangements also, it remains arbitrary, two categories of biotherapics (ex-Nosodes) :

(*a*) Group of "polychrest biotherapics" which exert a general action, acting on the morpho-genetic personality, temperamental, aggressologic, immunologic spheres necessitating the prescription of high dynamisation but at the same time have a loco-regional therapeutic action and require the prescription of lower and medium dilutions. They are at present :

Luesinum, Medorrhinum, Psorinum, Tuberculinum, Ruberculinum, Residnum, V.A.B. (ex-B.C.G.).

It seems to us equally, as well as the reader will be able to judge after reading the monographs and according to our own clinical experience that Collibacillinum and Anti-collibacilary serum, find their place in this group, as well as Toxoplasma gondii and Leptospira I.H.

(*b*) Group of biotherapics applied to lesional perturbations which are localised at some loco-regional immunological sites.

To this group applies the question of purification, cleansing and elimination of antigens created by the organism.

In this class enter all the other Biotherapics already mentioned in the pharmacological classification (besides those mentioned under the denomination "polychrest").

A remark is required here

What we have written above concerns the Biotherapics having at present legal pharmaceutic existence in France.

But we may add as follows :

—In the present work some nosodes are to be found that cannot be prescribed in France, but a large number of them have a legal existence in Germany, in England, and in some Latin American countries and in India.

—It may then be hoped that a modification of pharmaceutical legislation brings more understanding.

And then everything will go well.

If the whole does not break down under the weight of assaults of some "scientists", which are far from being scientific, they can never understand Heraclitas for whom there is no absolute truth but a *truth in the being*.

Let us hope.

CHAPTER 4

HOMOEOPATHIC AND BIOTHERAPIC PHARMACOTAXY

We have thought it necessary to inform the doctor equally about that in which the pharmacist is more interested.

It is useful in the state of our scientific and intellectual exigency to have a sure and clear information in order to avoid some obscurities.

Here is then the :

Preparation of Homoeopathic and Isotherapic Medicines

The Homoeopathic preparations are some medicines obtained by the method of succusive dilutions called Hahnemannian. These preparations are designated by Latin names of drugs, substances or compounds used, followed by the indication of the dilution. The following abbreviations are used :

For Mother Tincture ... ... M.T. (θ)

For Decimals ... ... D, Dec. or X

For Centesimals ... ... C or CH

preceded or followed by figure of the dilution.

The granules, globules, powder doses and tablets impregnated bear the denomination of the dilution used.

A. THE RAW MATERIALS

In order to continue to prepare the dilution according to the Hahnemannian principle one starts from the basic substances which are as follows : Mother Tinctures, Macerations,

Biotherapics, Isotherapics, Chemical products, minerals and their compounds, organic products, opotherapic preparations.

I—Mother Tincture

The Mother Tinctures are liquid preparations resulting out of a dissolving action of an alcoholic liquid on the drugs of vegetable or animal origin.

The Mother Tinctures of vegetable drugs are obtained by maceration in alcohol of different degree of concentration, of fresh plants, stabilised fresh plants and very rarely dry plants. It corresponds to 1/10 of their weights in dehydrated drugs, excepting the tincture of Calendula which corresponds to 1-20.

The Mother Tincture of drugs of animal origin are also obtained by maceration in alcohol of different degrees. In some cases, they have for vehicle a mixture of water and 95° alcohol and of glycerine. They correspond to 1/20 of the weight of the drug put to the preparation.

1. *Choice of drugs.* For the Mother Tinctures of vegetable substance it is preferably collected from their natural habitat :

—The entire plant at the time of flowering.

—The leaves after complete development before flowering.

—The flowers immediately after complete blooming.

—The stalks after development before flowering.

—The barks of plants including the young and the resinous type at the height of their pith.

—The woods of young plants at their pith.

—The roots of seasonal and biannual plants at the end of their vegetative period, and those of a longer life during their 2nd and 3rd year before lignification.

—The fruits and seeds at their maturity.

For the Mother Tincture of animal products, the raw material is constituted of healthy living animals (except Coccus cacti and Cantharis) which are collected during a particular period of their evolution ; or some part(s) of their organism, or certain secretions of them.

2. *Preparations.* On a medium sample of the drug, determine the humidity by dessication at 50 degree for 24 hours.

Place the raw material in a recipient piling it lightly in alcohol having the necessary strength. Close the recipient.

Let it be macerated for three weeks and shake frequently, then decant by pressing, mix the liquid thus obtained and adjust the Mother Tincture to the concentration desired by addition to alcohol having the necessary degree of strength. Mix, let it stand at rest for 48 hours in a cool place, then filter.

3. *Experiment.* The experiment of Mother Tinctures are identical to those prescribed for the tincture or alcoholatures mentioned in the pharmacopoea.

4. *Conservation.* Conserve in some recipient well corked and in a cool place.

II—Different Macerations

These preparations are the result of the dissolving action of certain vehicles : glycerine, different oils etc. on some vegetable and animal substances. They are obtained by maceration or digestion and correspond to 1/10 or 1/20 of the weight of the dehydrated drug.

III—Biotherapics

The biotherapics are medicines prepared in advance and obtained from the products of microbian origin not chemically defined, excretions and secretions pathological or not, animal or vegetable tissues and allergenes. These different substances bear then the name of the "stocks" for biotherapics.

The biotherapics cannot be delivered except from the 3rd centesimal or 6 decimal. They cannot be sold except in pharmaceutic forms for oral use.

Experiment. The first liquid dilution or a *fortiori*, and the following dilutions should satisfy the experiment for sterility.

IV—Isopathics

The isopathics are also biotherapics, but they are prepared extemporaneously from the "stocks" furnished by the patient himself and of which the first liquid dilution should be sterilised.

V—Chemical Products of Mineral or Organic Origin

—Simple or compound substances.

—Chemical compounds of natural origin.

—The products or mixtures defined only by their method of preparation.

We should like to add the following precisions :

The preparation of Biotherapics (Nosodes) vary according to the substance. As much as it is possible it will be described in course of each monograph (v. 2.)

However, we will describe below the preparation of Lysate forming the "stock" of actual biotherapics. When in any one of our monographs, there will be the question of Lysate, it will be understood that it is the question of this type of preparation Lysate.

The microbian biotherapics are obtained from lysated microbian suspensions, originally estimated 10 milliards per milimetre of considered germs.

The preparation of these lysates are done according to a technique common to all these nosodes.

One proceeds by congelation at a temperature of 30 to 40 degree, maintained for 24 hours, of the bacterial suspension prepared from the preserved stock by lyophilisation.

Then the congelation is left for being decongealed and rest at pius 20 degree for 20 hours and the whole operation congealation—Decongealation is repeated three times. It is then centrifuged for a sufficient time to obtain a complete sedimentation of the lysated bacterial debris. The floating suspension is then collected, put to filteration on Seitz and kept in refrigerator.

Thus a suspension of endotoxins of germs is obtained which is necessary to be detoxified by heating at 75 degree for one hour and at an interval of 24 hours. This stock solution is then divided asceptically into sterile ampoules. It does not contain any preserving agent or any stabilising agent.

Every biotherapic requires a sterility test which should be done on the first liquid dilution obtained the concentration of which depends on the nature of the "stock".

B. DILUTION AND TRITURATIONS

The dilution and triturations are obtained according to the Hahnemannian method by the division of the basic substance in a condition fixed as below, in liquid or in solid base respectively.

They are called Decimal or Centesimal according to the successive operations of divisions are done at the ratio of 1/10 or 1/100. The number of operations thus done define the height of the dilution and triturations obtained and is expressed in the following table :

Dilution	Concentration			Decimal scale		Centesimal scale	
1/10	10	p. 100	10·1	1st	Dec		
1/100	1	p. 100	10·2	2nd	Dec	1st	CH
1/1000	0·1	p. 100	10·3	3rd	Dec		
1/10000	0·01	p. 100	10·4	4th	Dec	2nd	CH
1/100000	0·001	p. 100	10·5	5th	Dec		
1/1000000	0·0001	p. 100	10·6	6th	Dec	3rd	CH
1/1 (18 Zeros)			10·18	18th	Dec	9th	CH

Preparation

(a) Centesimal dilution

Have a series of phials and new corks well washed in water and dried, in a number of corressponding to the number of centesimal dilutions to be obtained.

Put in the first phial a part in weight of the basic substance add one hundred parts in volume the appropriate vehicle, shake at least one hundred times. The dilution thus obtained is 1 CH.

Take one part in volume from 1 CH, put in the second phial containing 99 parts of vehicle. Jerk equally 100 times. The dilution thus obtained is the 2 CH. Operate in this way upto the desired dilution.

(b) Decimal dilution

Operate in the same manner but according to the decimal series.

(c) Tituration. Decimal or Centesimal.

Triturate for a long time and carefully in a morter the solid active substance, reduced previously into fine powder with a small quantity of lactose used as vehicle. Continue the trituration in the same conditions adding gradually the remaining lactose. The respective quantity of active substances and tactose are calculated in a manner to obtain the first decimal tituration or centesimal trituration. Take one part of that trituration and triturate as above with nine or ninety-nine part of lactose to obtain respectively the 2nd decimal or 2nd centesimal, operate in this way for obtaining the 3rd decimal or centesimal. After which pass into liquid base and continue as before for the dilutions.

C. PHARMACEUTICAL FORMS

All the pharmaceutical forms may be utilised for the homoeopathic preparations. However some forms are particularly used : Granules, Globules and Doses.

Granules and Globules

For preparing the medicinal globules and granules one uses inert globules and granules in the form of small rounds of saccharose or a mixture of saccharose and lactose of a weight of 0·05 gr (about) for the granules and 0·003 gr. to 0·005 gr. for the globules. These inert globules and granules are impregnated by shaking them with alcoholic medical dilution, then dried in a temperature lower than 50 degree.

The globules and granules take the denomination of the dilution with which it is impregnated.

Doses

These are the units of doses presented in habitual forms (ampoules, capsules) or in a particular form of dose-globules, or dose-powder.

As regards more particularly the biotherapics (and Isotherapics) their presentations are in granule tubes or dose-globules having the standard dynamisations as follows : 4 CH, 5 CH, 7 CH, 9 CH.

Let us mention that Anticollibaciliary serums are presented in the form of drinkable ampoules in 3 DH, 5 CH, 7 CH, 9 CH.

Finally in authoritative prescription without being able to modify the presentation one may obtain the dynamisations 15 CH or 30 CH.

CHAPTER 5

PHARMACODYNAMICS OF DYNAMISED MICRO-IMMUNOLOGY
OR
Isopathics and Biotherapics (ex-nosodes)

One of our teachers, Paul Langevin teaches us that it is necessary in all scientific researches, to start from the empiric, from observation of phenomena in order to try later on to interprete them and to return to practice with the aim of an experimental verification.

In the present state of our medical knowledge it is *immunology* which may help us to understand the *mechanism of action* of Isopathy.

Immunology is defined as the study of humoral and tissulo-cellular reaction of the organism in response to its environment.

Immunotherapy is its practical consequence and is transformed among others into vaccinotherapy.

The *immunologic mechanism* is described as an antagonism an antagonistic conflict between Antigen-Antibody, these two *units forming a contradictional unit.* Antigen or immunogene is generally, a substance foreign to the organism and it is the "possession of a lymphoid system, related to the sangum and lymphatic circulation which helps the organisms of vertebrates to respond, to react in a "specific manner to the aggression" (G.L. Daguet : Elément d'immunology medical—Flammarion, 2nd ed. 1972).

The *Antibody* "are protein synthesised in the living organism under the influence of an antigenous stimulation" (G.L. Daguet loc. cit.).

Thus specified, the conflict Antigen-Antibody may provoke two kinds of responses of the organism :

(*a*) A protective effect which is at the basis of the sero-and Vaccino-therapy and our dynamised micro-immunotherapy with our Biotherapics (ex-nosodes) and Isotherapics.

(*b*) A *pathogenous* effect which may be direct or indirect :

—*direct*—by a cellular lysis-hemolysis type.

—*indirect*—by a series of immunopathological mechanisms, anaphylaxy and allergy type.

It follows that there exists a complex process of interaction between the virulence of the foreign substance (micro-organisms or others) and the mechanisms of resistence of the host.

This host, is the *morpho-genetic* condition of the organism, and is called the *ground*.

Thus we have described the essential constituents of immunology.

It is in this context that we should try to elucidate the mechanism of action of Isopathy and of the Biotherapics and Isotherapics.

We are indebted to H.H. Reckeweg who has undertaken a biochemical study of the disease and immunologic reactions of the organisms to the aggression (Dr. med. H.H. Reckeweg : Homotoxicologie : Ganzheitschau einersyn these der Medizin Aurelia verlag, 1975).

According to this author, from the biochemical point of view, the phenomenon of disease should be studied as the reactional expression of the organism towards "Homotoxins" or "Anthropotoxins" (exogenous or endogenous).

Homotoxins (homo-man, human) or Anthropotoxins are the pathogenous agents capable of provoking in the human organism some patho-physiological actions and pass through a series of *six* phases, viz :

1, Excretion phase.

2. Reaction phase.

3. Phase of precipitation or of "deposition", follows a phase of cesura or *biological break* and ends in the phases of :

4. Impregnation.

5. Degeneration.

6. Neoplastic syndrome.

The first three phases are humoral having the excretion function, with reserved even unfavourable prognosis, and require a gross biotic therapeutic "substituant". Such is the picture of patho-physiological process, drawn in bold outline, in consideration of its biochemic action according to Reckeweg.

We are now going to take up the problem of Biotherapics and Isopathics.

Reckeweg describes the reactions of the organism under the form of "the system of the Mass defence" rather according to us *contradictional reactional process* of the five mechanisms that are its expression :

1. The Reticuloendothelial system of Aschoff is responsible for the production of antibodies and the function of accumulation and of disposition of toxins.

2. Hypothalamo-hypophysio-cortico-suprarenalian axis.

It induces in a greater part the reactional phase of the mesenchyma.

The stimulation of this axis by the toxins provokes secretion of corticoides in the direction of inflammatory zone and the *contradictional process*, the secretion of cortisone which opposes the inflammation.

This corresponds to the syndrome of *adaptation of selye*.

3. With the neuro-humoral reflex system of Speransky Reilly we have the third form of rection.

It is the sympathic-parasympathic antagonism.

It corresponds to *irritation syndrome* of Reilly and excitability of the neural receptors by a toxin may be shown experimentally by a dilution going up to 10^0.

The therapeutic action of biotherapics as well as of homoeotherapics is placed in this process.

4. *The 4th process* intervenes with the *detoxicating function of the liver*.

The liver is the origin of the formation of antitoxins in the form of enzymes and here intervenes similarly the neutralisation of acids and of toxines and endogenes.

5. Finally comes the action of connective tissue with the formation of leucocytes and the *Antigen-Antibody reaction*.

The cellular formations such as fibrocytes, reticulocytes, histiocytes participate in the analysable chemical substances which are responsible for reflexological reactions and reconstruction of tissues.

The connective tissue has as known at present, three essential characteristics :

It intimately participates in the pathology of the organs in the constitution of which *it is deeply integrated* ; it is the seat.

For the deposit of toxins in the form of Homotoxin (formed by two toxins neutralising each other), and of inflammation as reactional process towards the reconstruction of the normophysiologic ; and it has *etiologically specific* pathology, besides its own clinical and evolutional forms which is called "connectivities".

But it is on the level of inflammatory processes that Recke-weg tries to detect the action of the Biotherapics.

According to homotoxicology, the inflammation is a process of *drainage* of homotoxins. The inflammation then, according to the author, will have a useful biological action that may be induced by the biotherapics in an *anti-homotoxic direction*.

Thus the therapeutic action of biotherapics is understood to be the intermediary of the mechanism of inflammation.

Inflammation is expressed by the well-known rubor-tumor-calor-dolor (redness-tumefication-heat-pain) and which has, for its biochemical respondant, the action of the different factors, notably histamin, acetylcolin, noradrenalin, also por-phyrin and other intermediary homotoxins.

At this stage the components of albumin (peptids and poly-peptids) following the enzymatic action, hyaluronidasis, play an important pothogenous part.

If the development of the acid phase is blocked by an intempestuous therapeutic intervention, there will result a contrary reaction, which is alkaline, and checks or stops the formation of fermentation activity of hyaluronidases and instead of the hydrolysis reaction, there follows the formation of "unta-med peptides" which are the extremely toxic synthetic product, particularly antigenic.

The patho-physiological development of inflammation impli-cates an acid reaction and hyaluronidasic enzymes contribute to the hydrolysis as well of the intercellular substance as of homo-toxins in order to end in their elimination.

The elimination of homotoxins is done through the vessels of *lymphatic system.*

If the quantity of homotoxin in the connective tissue is very much important the action of hydrolysis of the hyaluronidasis is at fault.

The completion of this hydrolytic action, is useful and necessary to deblock the mechanism of elimination of homotoxins, is the work of the bacterias.

Thus the strepto-staphylo-meningo-pneumo-and gono-cocci and many others intervene by their power of production of hyaluronidasic enzyme. At this stage, the *non-antagonistic part*, biologically useful for bacterias, decisively contributes to the hydrolysis of the connective tissue but, being *antagonistic process* they prepare in this manner for themselves, the ground offering them the best condition of life.

Here one will understand fully the significance of the famous phrase of Claude Bernard "the germs is nothing and the ground is everything" because this homotoxic ground is, in fact, an excellent bouillon of culture for the microbes.

The rejection of homotoxins by the connective tissue which is the state of hyaluronidasic hydrolysis, and the bacterial phagocytosis are the normal process of the evolution of the inflammation manifested in the form of elimination of pus, mucosities, and other rejections.

A blockage has for its consequence a re-intoxication.

By the sudden change of the biochemic milieu, a pathophysiological *phase of excretion* is suddenly transformed into a *phase* of impregnation, otherwise injurious.

This sudden change is the result of antibiotic treatment or *chemiotheraphy* and shows that if it is necessary, there also arises a necessity of a biotic intervention by the help of Biotherapics, Isopathics, and Homoeotherapics and others.

The re-toxic impregnation, resulting out of a suppression of a pathophysiological process, means that the toxic element, such as the "untamed peptides, the endotoxins of the bacterias and the chemio-antibiotics cause a sudden hyaluronisation (phenomenon of a "sudden start") of connective tissue.

5 F

This reaction results from the biochemic point of view of the *sudden change* of the acid into basic reaction and the sudden cessation of hyaluronidasic activity.

It will therefore be the work of biotherapics to induce the therapeutic effect in view of the elimination of the untamed peptides or to reabsorb the blockages caused by the same injurious peptides.

This reaction is concretised *by the appearance of the antigen* (untamed peptides)—*antibodies* contradictional unity.

Such polypeptides are found in different pre-clinical stages.

Thus after a severe stage of influenza, treated by toxic medicines, the "untamed polypeptides" supervene, either by precipitation or hyalinic sedimentation in the tissue formerly inflamed, the pulmonary infiltrate which is thus reabsorbed or condensed during a pneumonia treated by antibiotics.

Face to face with them the organism forms some antibodies which are auto-antibodies.

These auto-antibodies have a contrary action towards the peptides which are untamed and have analogous protein structure, but their injurious action goes equally to manifest itself against the cells of the organism.

Let us cite : The lesion of hepatic parenchyma entrails troubles in the hepatic cells ; the lesion of renal parenchyma with massive proteinuria or glomerulo-nephritis ; lesions of muscles of the heart may cause a degeneration of myocardia, of the arteries with thrombo angitis ; of the thyroid, of the brain etc.

Thus an auto-immune pathological chapter sees light.

On this sphere the role of Biotherapics intervenes.

The organism cannot itself eliminate, by its own means the "untamed proteid" even by the formation of antibodies often induced more and more by the molecules of sulfanamides, antibiotics, febrifuges, etc.

In order to help the formation of specific antibodies against the peptids, one introduces, in the form of specific stimulant, one or more biotherapics (ex-nosodes) or rather a chemiotherapic or diluted and dynamised allergens.

This is what Fortier-Bernoville has lapidarily expressed as specificity and immunity.

These will intervene equally the action of Biotherapics, Organotherapics or Hormonotherapics opposing the secondary action of auto-antibodies situated on the liver, kidney, heart etc.

Experience shows that the dynamised Biotherapics have an action, *protective* or reparative, against the deep lesions consecutive to the action of these antibodies.

There are cases where the organism has lost control on its auto-antibodies. These auto-antibodies wear, we may say, the "same uniform" as that of the protein proper, and it results that they are not recognised by the organism's own "system of mass defence".

The tendency of the organism is to react against the destruction caused by these auto-antibodies and the process can be made easy ; thanks to the action of *Biotherapics* (ex-nosodes).

The Biotherapics direct, at that time, their action against the diseases of antibodies, because they contain the *simillimum*.

They have an exciting action on the system of mass defence by inducing an analogous reaction against certain toxins that are similar to those against which the organism already defends itself but insufficiently under the form of diseases of the antibodies.

Thus, it is now being more and more understood that many diseases like erythrodermatosis, nephrosis, myocardosis, agranulocytosis etc., are consequential to the sudden suppression of the acute inflammation and to the formation of antibodies.

The Biotherapics possess in their structure a part *analogous* to these substance which are in the origin of these diseases.

The latter is characterised by the absence of an analogous substance for forming antibodies before neutralising the auto-antibodies.

Then, it becomes understandable that the mechanism of action of Biotherapics and Homoeotherapics, by a *specific mini excitation*, activates the "system of mass defence".

But from the fact that many homotoxins may participate in the course of the process of the use of many biotherapics or homoeotherapics and find from thence their biological justification.

The mechanism of action of Biotherapics and homoeotherapics seem to have found, by enzymology, a new scientific dimension.

As for example when a carcinotoxin, such as Methylcholantrene, is injected in the peritonium of a rat, a neoplasma is formed.

If now the same substance is injected in the form of a dynamised dilution in 3 or 4 DH the curative effects are seen, as has been proved by the experiment of Connay and Burns (Mediziniche Klinik, 59, 1964, No. 48, p. 1811).

The injection of 3 or 4 DH of Methylcolantrene in 0·1 to 1 mg for 1 mg H_2O in the peritonium of the rat helps to observe the formation of an enzyme on the liver, which is capable of detoxicating other carcinotoxins as for example 3-Methyl-4-Methylamino-Azobenzol (the yellow colouring of butter).

There we find *an analogy therapeutic proof*, Biotherapic, Homoeotherapic or Hormonotherapic or a Carcinogenous substance with which we may determine, in dynamised microbes, some anticarcinogenous action, specific or analogous against other carcinogens.

According to Reckeweg as we have explained above, the disease is the expression on biochemic level of the reaction of the "defence" of the organism against the homotoxins.

Because we do not know always the exact homotoxin which is in the origin of the defence of the organism, a similar or analogous toxin is used in the form of Biotherapics to direct the therapeutic affect against the analogous homotoxins that possess the same biochemic receptors as that of these homotoxins.

Because all the biological reactions are conditioned by analysable chemical substances, which are even the foundation of homotoxicology, it becomes necessary to search for these homotoxin substances for discovering the relations of the disease and the remedies that cure it.

It follows, then, that the therapeutics by analogy contributes to the regenerescence of blocked enzymes which may be verified by the change of the homotoxic phase.

If we are face to face with a degenerative phase following the enzyomatic deterioration (as for example in the case of an antibiotic treatment) after the administration of an Analogous, biotherapic or homoeotherapic, the enzyme may be normalised.

The enzyme begins anew their function, which has for its consequence to make effective again the whole "system of mass defence" and there comes the process of detoxication. This may be observed in the processes of *regressive vicarisation* in the *inflammation* where organism liberates itself again from its homotoxins.

There is, therefore, every ground to induce the functioning of "system of mass defence" of the organism by the analogical medicines in order to provoke the enzymatic process to work again and thus assure the detoxication.

In order to realise it, one should take the help of Biotherapics.

The concept of Homotoxicology and of Homotoxins helps thus to establish the scientific foundation of Biotherapics on Biochemical basis.

CHAPTER 6

THEORETICAL STUDY OF
MICRO-IMMUNOTHERAPY
OR
ISOPATHY

Conformism, as says our master Rene Leriche has a hard life and the advantage of convenience.

It is always painful to modify our intellectual habit and that effort is troublesome.

Then it is refused by convenience. It was necessary for us "long and painful efforts" to take up the research of the concretology of dynamised immunotherapy or isopathy.

These theoretical researches have not the exigency of "an absolute truth before which one should kneel down" (Karl Marx).

Well, on the contrary they are submitted to criticisms. Constructive criticisms are required in order to contribute to the perishing of the old and the arrival of the new.

We have shown that Homoeopathy of S. Hahnemann, that of 1810 with the "Organon" and that of 1828 with the "Chronic Diseases" shows that evolution, even a radical change, is revealed. It is manifested by the damming up of the absolutism of simillimum and the appearance of the three etiopathological processes, of the three "miasms", Psora, Sycosis and Syphilis.

Because to these morbid processes, *two new ideas are added the Etiology and the Homoeotherapaic specifics of these miasms.*

From then opens a new era.

It was in 1830, that the therapeutic discipline, the elder daughter of Homoeopathy, was born without any confusion, misunderstandings or any bitter controversies.

The desire to substitute the formula of S. Hahnemann,

"Similia Similibus Curentur"

with the formula of Lux

"Aequalia Aequalibus Curentur"

however, created all the confusion and diverse controversies were raised on the ideas of "Similia" and "Aequalia". This will be dealt with later on the significance of "Analogous" and "identical".

For W. Lux, his "Aequalia" has an etiological meaning and even for this reason it will be the perfect simillimum.

This affirmation of our time finds the support of Leon Vannier who says :

"The true simillimum is not what corresponds identically by its pathogenetic symptoms to the morbid symptoms of the patient, but it is the remedy of the same nature as that of the cause that has produced the troubles observed.

"I am very sorry that I cannot be exactly of the opinion of the masters who came before us."

"No doubt the therapeutic perfection for a homoeopath is to find out the homoeopathic remedy, the most analogous to what comes nearest to the observed clinical picture, it is there the "simillimum" of Kent and Nash."

"According to me the true simillimum cannot be prepared by the causal element which has determined immediately or in long time the troubles that we should treat. The toxinotherapy should take its place by the side of pure Homoeopathy. Isotherapy should complete Homoeopathy (Individual homoeopathy or organotherapy) (Courses of C.H.F., 9th March, 1948, v. 5.).

To which E. Iliovici replies "It does not in any way appear to me that Isopathy is the perfect simillimum" (Annales Ho. Fr. No. 3, Dec. 1961, p. 64/65).

But it is not the advice of R.P. Collet for whom "If the real medicine should be an agent similar to that of the disease nothing is more similar to the agent of the disease but the agent itself" (Isopathy. Ed. Vigot, Freres, 1920).

And let us turn to our master for a reply in his Organon.

"The fact that Isopathy is submitted to the technique of preparation according to the homoeopathic pharmacopraxis, the cure would in this case take place by opposing "Simillimum simillimo.""

1. "The cure by *Idem* is contrary to commosense and even to all experiences" (Organon 6th ed., para 56a, P. Schmidt).

The doctrinal intransigence of S. Hahnemann with some hesitations and fluctuations was repressed, as is understood through the fight of his time between pure Homoeopathy and Allopathy, sometimes well wishing, but perfidious (Hufeland) or brutal, arrogant, caustic and biting.

S. Hahnemann who knew Plato, is Kentian by his doctrinal exposition. But it seems that he was not familiar with the logic of Hegel, specially with his dialectics.

As a result the notion of Analogy remains in the restricted field of Kent's "Categorical" and ignores the contradictional movement that implicates dialectic thought.

The idea of Analogy in 1810 is of a monist integral purism, absolute and imperative.

Stumbling against the clinical reality and against the contradictional concord from 1816-1817, he makes a *dialectic jump*, without knowing in 1828.

It is a qualitative jump of a singular importance.

In his work "The Chronic Diseases" hit two new statements are to be noted :

"The categorisation of the three great miasmatic states."

2. The Causal, Etiological specificity resulting as a consequence of the *therapeutic specificity* of each of the miasm.

To the categorical monism of the Analogous, it is a dualist contradictional unity—Simillia and the similimo—(Aequalia) which is introduced in Homoeopathic doctrine.

It is from that date of historic moment, Hahnemann causes a dialectic mutation in his medical philosophy.

I reconstruct the foundations :

(*a*) By *qualitative* modification of a monist spiritualistic concept—"only the vital force untuned"—into a dualist spiritualistic concept—vital force plus specific cause.

We know, in philosophy, some doctrines that are related to it like that of Descartes and Spinoza.

The gravity of the situation in Hahnemann, having a certain philosophic culture, ought to have understood the reflexive bearing. Admirable and honest clinician, who has described with much vigour the clinical aspect of "miasmatic" entities, on the contrary, has missed the importance of casualty, and this has created many difficulties in the growth of homoeopathic movement.

Whatever it may be, it is from 1928, the memorable date in the history of Homoeopathy that the doctrine and practice of Homoeopathy have a new development.

To say *casuality*, is to say *Etiology*, therefore "Isopathic", under the reserve that "Morbid cause is directly represented there in a pathogenically active manner" (E. Iliovici, Loc. cit.) which is not and which will not always be the cause.

From this fact there are the fortunes and misfortunes of Isopathy, its success and its failures, its sometimes spectacular clinical results and its famous failures. But as it is noted by G.L. Rau in his beok "New Organon of Specific Medicine" or

"Exposition of Homoeopathic Medicine" (J.B. Baillere, 1839) a number of reputed Homoeopathic doctors during the life time of Hahnemann and whose names are inscribed in the field of Homoeopathy made a therapeutic application and note of its favourable results.

He cites thus that "Batzendorf and Aegidi assure that the attenuated vaccin renders the vaccin not only more benign but also shortens even the duration of the disease. Weber has cured with Anthracinum a number of animals suffering from Anthrax...Attomyer reports a case of tenea cured properly by this method, *and one is lost in conjectures on the question of knowing of such a substance is an ison or a simillimum* (Loc cit., p. 221).

For Swan according to P. Schmidt "The dynamisation of an Isopathic product makes it homoeopathic to the disease which has produeed it" as if an if an *Ison* (idem) moves towards an analogous by a simple physical manipulation.

It is the total confusion between the significance of the concept of Identity and of Analogy of Hahnemann up to our time.

Hahnemann at first called his new medical practice *Specific Medicine*.

It is towards 1800 he uses the term *Homoeopathy*.

In 1830, after the ideologic fracture regarding absolute monism of simillimum and the daulistic conception of "Miasm" and of the causality, the term "Specific" or "Homoeopathic specific" appears in the surface again.

In the thought of Hahnemann Homoeopathy, rather Homoeopathicity remains but is distinguished by the unique analogical specific.

For W. Lux it is *Isopathic specific* :

For *Hahnemann* :

Psora—Sulphur

Sycosis—Thuya

Syphilis—Mercury

For modern Isopathy :

Psora—Psorinum

Sycosis—Medorrhinum

Syphilis—Lyphilinum (Luesinum).

And the homoeopathic doctor will combine the homoeo-pathic specifics with Isopathic specifics.

The *etiological idea* is not concordant according to the ideas of Hahnemann and Lux.

For Hahnemann, and Denis Demarque seem to have well detected the origin of the difference (l'Homoeopathie : medi-cine de l'experience) (1968, p. 15). "It is the philosophy of *Vitalism* which is at the root of the misunderstanding."

And Denis Demarque has noted "We will see him criticising bitingly the doctors who admitted material morbific cause of the disease and try to evacuate the injurious substance (Loc. cit.)

But for Lux "All contagious diseases carry in their own products of contagion, the means to their cure" and even for D. Collet, with religious and spirtualistic formation, therefore, suspecious of a "vulgar materialism", "Isopathy is a medicine that cures by the help of medicinal agents that are identical to the morbid agent."

Therefore, it is clear that Hahnemann himself is the origin of the ideological conflict without knowing, as has previously been explained.

We are not going to take up here our long discussion on "vitalism" and "neo-vitalism." However a very short approach has been made in our Introduction to the chapter on the

"Theory of a knowledge of a contradictional monist concretology."

Let us here specify only what one may think at present and in a very concise manner has been expressed by Fr. Jacob in his works "The Logic of the Living"—"To *accept the unity of the Physico Chemical Process on molecular level is to say that vitalism has lost all its function.*"

For more information we refer the reader to the works of the writer "Recherches theoriques at partiques en Homoeopathi", t. 1 and 2 (Librairie, Le Francois, Paris).

Let us say only that for Hahnemann alone *an immaterial power*, the "vital force" is at the origin of the disturbance of the health.

Afterwards, even if the isotheurapic practice indicates some favourable therapeutic results, S. Hahnemann thwarts this new therapeutic because it is "contrary to the commonsense" (see. Organon, 6th ed.)

Finally if Isopathy is there, it is only an other simillimum.

It is even in this spirit that the modern authors (Iliovici, Zissue, Demarque and others) give to Isopathy its right of existence in the field of Homoeopathy.

"The term Isopathy has a wide acception."

"The analogy that it implies is related either to the external pathogenous cause or to the patient or to both".

"In any way Isopathy should satisfy the principle of simillitude" (...) and further on "and even if not proved by a pathogenesis, Isopathy is submitted to the laws of the latter (E. Iliovici : Isopathic, the perfect simillimum, in Annales Hom. Franc. No. 3, Dec., 1961).

For Denis Demarque Isopathy has the benefit of an ambiguity. "Although its therapeuticas interent is considerable and helps to unite the Hahnemannian conception of morbid ground to the classical works on the material exogenous pathogenous causes" (Loc. cit, p. 95).

The case is the same with Zissu ; because the "major nosodes should obey a pathogenesis, its prescription should obey the law of similars and finally obey a conception of morbidity on the principles and clinical descriptions of homoeopathic intoxination, *i.e.* Psora for Psorinum ; the tuberculinism for tuberculines, T.R. and Aviary ; Syphilis for Luesinum : and Sycosis for Medorrhinum'' ("The minor biotherapics and nosodes in current practice" by Drs. Guillaume N Sissu, Annales, Hom. Franc 1969, p. 55/143).

The theory of "vitamin" of Hahnemann and the neo-vitalism" of his successors stumble against the real, and harmonious against the etiology of material expression of Isopathy of W. Lux, and against its biological and immunobiological contents.

Moreover, the want of comprehension of the ideas of "Analogous" and "Idem" is manifest. It is better one restricts the idea of "Analogous" to Hamoeopathic analogous and finally the "content" is confounded with the "form".

Content : It is the Homoeopathic pharmacotherapic model of a particular experiment.

Form : It is the container, it is analogous.

On the contrary Isopathy expresses *Idem* while in fact there is only an etiological sense.

What is really this *identical*, this *identity* ?

For Heraclitus, the Greek philosopher, "One cannot take bath in the same water."

"It is not possible to touch twice a perishable substance in the same state, because it docomposes and reconstruct anew through the rapidity of the change, rather it is neither anew, nor afterwards but well at the sometime it appears and disappears" (Haraclitus by Jean Brun, p. 136).

Fr. Engels says that "infact there is not a strict identity between A and A, but contains in it the distinction of a difference".

"For the natural science in the stage of generalisation, the abstract identity is totally insufficient, even in whatever particular field it may be, and although roughly it is eliminated from the practice, in theory it continues to dominate the brains ; most of the learned men still imagine that identity and difference are unconceivable contraries, and not of incomplete poles that have truth only in their reciprocal action by the inclusion of the difference in the identity". (Fr. Engels : Dialectique dela Nature, Ed. Sociale, Paris, p. 218)

Really speaking there is no identity in two moments of the same event but a dynamic and productive difference.

To take into account of the difference in the identity is to see everything is at the sametime itself and another, that it contains at the sametime itself and its contrary and that everything leads to its contrary.

Since the fundamental cause of movement and development of things and phenomena is not external but internal ; it is found in the internal contradictions of the phenomena themselves. The external causes are not thus the conditions of changes, but the internal causes are the basis of the changes and the external causes act by the intermediary of the internal causes.

Thus the Static sense of Identity loses its appearance of being formal to acquire the appearance of "contradictional" of the dialectic logic.

The *identical* has no more a formal significance, no more a formal unity. It has the contradictional significance of contraries, because it has a tendency to be transformed into its contrary under some determined conditions, *which is in fact called the identity.*

To speak otherwise, the two contradictory aspects co-exist in the unity conditioning the existence of the other and the one is converted into the other. It is this *reciprocal transformation* which is called the "identity", and has nothing in common with the formal and primitive idea of the identity of the identical in Isopathy.

It is the analogical reasoning which will put the *concrete model* of the Isother. py (Bio- or Iso-therapic), *analogous to pathological model* by judging the dissemblance and resemblance of the two models.

An analogous remedy has a double action in the pathological process *viz* :

—to induce the decay of the antagonic processes.

—to induce the re-establishment of non-antagonic process towards the normo-physiological by the intermediary of analogical isopathic model in existence.

It is on this level that there is every reason to understand the content of the container, the content of the Analogous, and that it cannot be only that which is determined by the homoeopathic pharmacotherapic model.

The whole error lies there and it is to be underlined here that there exists as well an analogical pharmacotherapic isopathic model.

This model has, therefore, its specificity of immunological content.

Thus it will be the object of analogical reasoning.

To be more clear :

The homoeopathic medicine is ruled by analogical reasoning.

In order to proceed to this reasoning two analogical models are put forward :

(*i*) The pharmacotherapeutic model.

(*ii*) The pathological model.

The analogical reasoning is applied to determine the relation of semblance and dissemblance.

The content of the pharmacological model may be determined by many processes and of substance to become changed pharmacotherapeutic.

Thus S. Hahnemann has established a *particular* experimental protocol by the pharmacological experiment of a substance, administered in attenuated dose to a normo-physiological subject in order to obtain a specific symptomatological response.

In a second time he proceeds by analogical reasoning for the establishment of concordances and discordances between the medicinal model and the pathological model.

There, it is the question of reasoning which enters in the research of a similitude.

Later on, after having found the relation of resemblances and dissemblances, one *induces* that the *therapeutical effect* will be manifested if the symptomatic simillitude of the two models coincide.

But, it is the Praxis which will verify the good foundation of the analogical reasoning.

The complex of this attempt is called Homoeopathy.

What is then isopathy and isopathic ?

It will also be the unfolding of analogical process.

One will have to have submitted a pharmacological and pathological model to the reasoning of analogy.

The pharmacological isopathic model (Biotherapic—Isotherapic) will have its specific content. It is an immunobiotic substance having for its characteristic the significance of the antagonistic complex represented by *proteins* and *hapthenes* of different stocks : bacterial, viral, vegetable, animal, reactional. allergenes, chemiotherapics, vaccinotherapics and autobiotherapics.

This pharmacological model will have two characteristics : it expresses an *etiology* and has a pathological *symptomatology*.

This constitutes its *specific content*.

This pharmacologic model will be put in the *analogical relation* with the pathological model.

And the same process of analogical reasoning is going to be unfolded.

The biotherapic will have to induce the therapeutic effect ; there will have been induced an analogous reaction against toxins that are similar to those against which the diseased organism, the pathological model, already reacts.

The concordance and the discordance are to be studied and according as the symptoms of the two models concord the therapeutic effect will be induced.

It is again the praxis that will verify the one well founded. Let us note equally what follows : The property of a good number of biotherapics, is that they contain in their structure, as is shown by H.H. Reckeweg, a part analogous to the substances that are found in the pathological model and which are at the origin of the processes (see Chapter 5).

Finally, from then one finds himself in the *real*, in the *concrete*, without having to lose oneself anew in the "transcendental similitude" of Zissu (p. 33, Appendix, t. 3, M.M. Hom. constitutionnelle).

Let us repeat.

The contents of Homoeotherapic and Biotherapic models have each one their *specificity*.

Similarly, *Homoeotherapic content* is the resultant of an experimental research.

The *Biotherapic content* is the result of an immunobiotic process.

Only the containers (and *ipso facto* the contents) are both submitted to analogical reasoning.

Thus they enter from then in a vast symposium of *analogical therapies*.

And because of this fact Homoeopathy rather homoeopathic concretology acquires a new height.

Since then it will be not only a simple praxis of specific therapeutic but a scientific medical theory having the characteristic to consider the diseased man in his behavior.

Homoeopathy or homoeopathic concretology is a revolutionary ideology, because it is the science of the suffering individual in his concrete particularities and his own nature.

It corresponds to the exigency of Claude Bernard for whom "The theories are relative in the state of our knowledge and they vary...according to the progress of our knowledge. (C. Bernard : Principles of Medical Experiment, p. 263)

If one desires a perenneity of Homoeopathy or of homoeopathic concretology one will paraphrase Heraclite saying :

—*Homoeopathy is in the constant becoming.*

CHAPTER 7

EXPERIMENTAL RESEARCHES

Bibliography

Plazy M. : Modern experimental research in Homoeopathy. Ed. Coquemard—Angoulème, 1967.

Julian O.A. and Launay H. : Psycho-pharmacological experiment on animal according to the law of Analogy and Identity of Homoeopathy by Reserpin and the Cicuta virosa.

Cahier de Biothérapique—2nd year—No. 8, Dec. 1965—and —Annales de thérapeutique psychiatrique—t. 3, p. 310, 318, 1967, Presses Universitaires de France, Paris.

Tétau M. and S. de Luna :

Experimental data on the action of "Tuberculinum" in homoeopathic dilution.

Rev. Monographic Dolisos, 1956.

Pharmacological and psycho-pharmacological study of Nepenthes in *O.A. Julian* : Recherches théorique et Pratiques en Homoeopathie, 1965, Librarie Le Francois, 91, Bd. St.-Germain, 75006 Paris.

Tétau J. and Tétau M. :

Pharmacology and psycho-pharmacology of Thuya.

Les Annales Homoeopathiques francaises, 2 année, No. 8, May, 1960.

Vincent S. :

Some experimental proofs of the activity of homoeopathic remedies.

Revue Bélge d'Homoeopathie No. 2 and No. 3, V. IX, 1975.

Wurmser L. :

Evolution of research in Homoeopathy. La Documentation Homoeopathique No. 47, L.H.F.

INTRODUCTION

Experimental research began about 100 years ago.

The short bibliography given above is due to the fact that we are going to give in this chapter very briefly a description of some experiments only in order to objectivate the value of Isopathy on the clinical sphere.

Proving the Law of Identity

There it is the question of going beyond the objectivation of a simple action of the homoeopathic dilution for proving an orientation, a selectivity and specificity of that action. Different authors try to show that a given substance is susceptible under certain conditions to behave once it is diluted and dynamised as an antogonist of the same substance given in gross dose.

These researches have been done on animals and plants.

A– Experiment on Animal

1. *Study of biological activity of the Homoeopathic dilutions of Folliculine.*

Devraigne, Bagros and Boiron have studied in 1952 the biological activity of the homoeopathic dilutions of Folliculine on rat. The authors have shown that when it is injected in rats castrated by Benzoate of Oestradial in weak doses of the gamma order, the maximum of the frequency of Oestrus was retarded 24 hours by folliculine 7 CH.

When a strong dose of oestradiol is injected which normally inhibits the oestrus in an witness animal, it is seen that in rates treated by Folliculine 5 CH, there is a shortening of that inhibition phase and a regulation of the phase of the cycle.

Some experiments have been done with up to 30 CH. When every two days 1 gamma Oestradiol is given to adult rats, it is registered at first a stimulation, then an inhibition, then anew increasing stimulation with the time of the Oestruses. Administration of Folliculine 30 CH to animals thus treated counteracts the inhibition, consequently the increase of Oestrus continues. These experiments were multiplied by varying the quantities of Oestradiol and the modalities of the application of Folliculine 30 CH.

More than 2000 animals were used in the maternity of the hospital Lariboisiére, in the service of Dr. Pierre Devraigne and from this experiment 3 important facts were possible to show as results :

(1)   The homoeopathic dilution of Folluculine causes in the animals some conditions, some pharmacodynamic effects which can be controlled.

(2)   The biological resposes registered according to some experimetal protocols, have helped to determine the antagonist action of strong and weak doses of the same substance.

(3)   It was possible to show experimentally on the animal the biological action of 30 CH (much beyond the Avogadro number).

2 . *Study of the elimination caused by a toxic substance under the influence of dynamised infinitesimal doses of the same toxic substance.*

The merit of this very beautiful research originally goes to Mlle. Wurmser who in 1955 with Prof. Lapp of Strassbourg studied in the animal the cinetic of the elimination of Arsenic under the influence of the same toxic diluted and dynamised. Some researches of the same order have been afterwards taken up on Bismuth and Lead.

The experimental protocol chosen was very simple. For Arsenic and Bismuth the animal selected is cobaye.

The normal elimination curves were set up on witnesses who were injected with a known dose, not lethal, of the toxic in soluble form, and one observes the quantity eliminated in different micturitions until any detectable trace of the metal disappears.

Then the animal is let at rest and from time to time is verified whether the urine contains any trace of the mental.

Two kinds of experiments were attempted :

(*a*) The animal is injected with infinitesimal doses in course of the same spontaneous elimination *i.e.* to say from the very beginning of the intoxication. The quantities found in the different urinations help to compare the rhythm and intensity of the eliminations thus provoked in relation to the samples (witnesses).

(*b*) Some experimental witnesses are realised with some distilled water or with some other substances, in order to verify the specificity of the action of the infinitesimal doses utilised.

The state of Arsenic in the organism is well known. After the application of a strong but non toxic dose of Arsenic, elimination through urine is observed. About 35% of Arsenic is eliminated during 90 hours following the injection. No elimination through the intestines is produced.

At the end of that period no trace of Arsenic is detectable in the urines, at least it is less than gamma 1. The Arsenic is fixed in some organs (liver), on the nails, hairs etc.... and as it is shown by Prof. Poncet on the spongy tissues of bones.

For these experiments, the cobayes are prepared by an injection of 1000 gamma of Arsenic.

The Arsenic is measured in each urination.

The animals are treated by infinitesimal doses of Arsenic either just after the administration of 1000 gammas of Arsenic or after a period of rest of 3 weeks, 7 weeks or 3 months after the first injection. To do so the dilution 4 CH, 5 CH and 7 CH are used in an interval corresponding to that of the therapeutics of human beings.

The results obtained are interesting.

Under the actions of the dilutions (4, 5, 6, 7 CH *i e.* 10^{-8} 10^{-10} 10^{-14}) injected after 3 weeks or 7 weeks of rest, the metal appeared again in the urine and the quantity thus eliminated may rise up to 10% of the metal fixed in the organism.

If the substance in dilution is given from the very beginning of the intoxication and during the whole duration of the spontaneous elimination, the quantity eliminated increases and may reach up to 40% of the metal injected, against 35% without treatment.

These works were taken up again by Cier, Boiron and Mouriquand in pigeons of which have been studied the urinary elimination of the toxic and the variation of the vestibular chronaxic index.

The metals studied were Arsenic and Ammonia. As in the cobaye the elimination of Arsenic represents 31 to 34% of the dose administered and the latter was graduated during 5 days. At the same time the vestibular chronaxia rises suddenly from 2 to 3 sigma from the 5th day which followed the injection. It is maintained for 60 days and comes to normal at the end of 90 days. However if an infinitesimal dilution (7 CH) is injected 6 weeks after the starting of the intoxication, it is observed that in a few days the chronaxia returns to the normal, and parallelly the Arsenic is seen to reappear in the excreta, in the proportion of 12 to 17% of the Arsenic which remained fixed in the organism.

With Antimony the result was identical.

Same experiments on the radioactive antimony have helped to measure the radio-activity of the excreta. There again it is ascertained that under the infinitesimal doses of radioactive antimony there is clear increase of the elimination of the activated element. On rats, some 15 CH dilutions prepared from the blood of an intoxicated rat, have been shown to be active.

The sensibility of animal can equally be shown by the injection of different substances (Hemophilic pertusis, Dextran, certain endotoxins etc...)

It is by utilising the sensibilisation with *hemophilus pertusis*, a Cier and Coll. researched the preventive effect of the dilution of *histamin* or of *lung histamin*. In *vivo*, one observes a real protection since one obtains a toleration to serosol of Histamin similar to that of a non-sensibilised witness. *In vitro* (R. de Schulz Dale) the dilution of Lung-histamin shows to be active while those of Histamin do not appear to act.

M. Tétau and S. de Luna have also done some researches of Psychopharmacology with Thuya.

Operating on some conditioned animals, the author verifies that some important doses of Thuya perturbs the psychic equillibrium of rats who loose their "conditioning". These intoxicated animals see their troubles disappear under the action of a dose of Thuya 9 CH with the restoration of the conditioning.

A second experimentation concerning Nepenthes has been taken up by Julian, M. Tétau and ne Luna.

Experimentally they found no stupifying result, but noted a trouble of readaptation to the test done on rates previously prepared. However the experiments are less conclusive than with Thuya, because Nepenthes has never produced deconditioning effect similar to that caused by Thuya.

Parallelly a *pathogenesic experiment on* man was conducted by Dr. Julian.

Baranger and Coll. have done researches on the influence of different factors on the therapeutic effectiveness of Homoeopathic dilutions on lucemia of birds. Some male chicks leucemised by the virus E.S.H. were treated by Cantharidine.

This remedy has proved active in up to 45 CH.

B—Experiment on Plants

Professor Netien of Lyon and his assistant Mme Graviou proved in the year 1965 the activity of infinitesimal doses of Copper Sulphate on plants intoxicated with the same substance.

The principle of this experiment is as follows :

The dwarf beans were made to germinate on some buckets full of earth ; 3 times a week a solution of Copper Sulphate 20 mg/l is sprinkled on them for two months. The plants develop, flower and bear fruits. Then some grains treated are collected which were the materials for experiment. Then one observes the germination of these treated seeds in relation to some seeds not treated after having imbibed a portion of them by simple distilled water for 24 hours, another portion treated with Homoeopathic dilution of Copper Sulphate 5 CH, another portion with 7 CH, another portion with 9 CH and still another portion with 15 CH.

After 3 days of observation no difference has been noted regarding the growth of the lots. The young plants are then placed on bi-distilled water put in culture-phials, each plant corresponding to a differenciated lot. At the end of 3 days the bi-distilled water of 4 of these phials is replaced by a dilution of Copper Sulphate of the same concentration as that has been utilised, for the impregnation before the germination, *i.e.*, to say either a 5 CH, or 7 CH, a 9 CH or a 15 CH.

On the 11th day photographs are taken and it is verified that in relation to the witness plants a very marked increase of the development of the plantules treated by the homoeopathic dilution of Copper Sulphate.

This increase is marked specially on the shooting of the roots and the stimulation is as much more important as on the rise from 5 CH to 15 CH. Some analogous observations have been done on the 15th day and on the 18th day of the experiment.

Therefore homoeopathic dilution of Copper Sulphate has a positive action on the growth of bean-seeds that are the issues of plants intoxicated by the same Copper Sulphate.

If the same experiment is done on the seeds issues of non-treated beans the results are much less convincing. It therefore seems that the diseased plant of which the metabolism has been perturbed in relation to the exogenous element, occurrence of Copper Sulphate, is the best revealer of the homoeopathic dilutions.

It helps to show a demonstration of the Law of Identity and one enters into the sphere of pathopharmacology illustrating the works of Claude Bernard : "One knows since longtime that the medicine do not act on the patient in the same manner as in a man having good health".

These researches are examined thoroughly by Nitien, Graviou and Boiron who have more strictly studied the positive action of 14 CH of Copper Sulphate.

C—Proving the Law of Identity with Possible Extension of the Law of Simillars

Here it is necessary to cite the works of Prof. Cier of Lyon. This author has shown at first, in order to be within the framework of the researches of the type of Lapp and Moriquant, that a 7 CH of Antimony is capable to mobilise the Arsenic already fixed in the tissues of a prepared animal. There we are no more face to face with the Law of Identity although Antimony and Arsenic are two elements chemically very near to each other, having many analogies on the biological sphere. We come nearer to the Law of Analogy.

Afterwards he was set upon the treatment of experimental diabetes by some infinitesimal dilutions of Alloxane, a substance which in toxic doses may produce diabetes by the degeneration of beta cells of the islands of Langerhans that are responsible for the production of insuline.

Cier has at first shown that Alloxane 7 CH acts on the Glycemic regulation by checking more rapidly the occurrence of hyperglycemia caused by the injection of a solution of glucose.

On the rats, the administration of Alloxane 9 CH has for its effect to inhibit partly diabetigenous effect of a dose of 40 mg/kg of Alloxane. Besides always in the rat Alloxane 9 CH has been found curative after an injection of diabetigenous Alloxane. And it seems well that activity of the Hahnemannian dilutions of Alloxane while the treatment is at the sametime preventive and curative, acts in experimental diabetes when it is caused not only by Alloxane but also by other diabetegenous substance specially some inflammatory agents such as (EDTA) Ethylene-diamine-tetracetic.

It should be noted that these researches were completed by histologic analysis of the tissues taken from the surface of the pancreas of rats treated and the examinations done have helped to objectivate the protective action of Alloxane (CH or 7 CH on the cellular surface). The beta cells of the islands of Langerhans of treated rats are normal while those of rats not treated are lacunary and degranulised.

In the psycho-pathological laboratory of "Ecole pratique des Hautes Edudes" directed by Prof. Baruk, member of the Academy of Medicine with the contribution of J. Launay head of the laboratory O.A. Julian has undertaken a series of experiments during 1963-1965 in order to contribute to the verification of the law of Identity and the law of Analogy.

We are going to give here the experimental part concerning the Law of Identity (Complete exposition is to be found in Nouvelle recherches théoriques et pratiquas en Homoeopathy, t. 3, Le Francois 91, bd. St-Germain 75006, Paris). The experiment has been conducted on some rats and cobayes in *two phases* :

(*a*) Determination of psycho-motor troubles and of the catalepsy with Reserpine in increasing doses.

(*b*) Verification of the Law of Identity (Isotherapy) by chronic -sub-intoxication with Reserpine in hahnemannian dilutions for 3 weeks, 3 injections a week. After one week an acute intoxication is produced by Reserpine in catatogenous doses.

1—**Experiment on Mouse** : (*A*) *Determination of catalepsy by reserpin.*

The optimum catatogenous dose seems to be 4·5 mg/kg causing the following phenomena :

lh. 10 after injection : Slowness of the psycho-motor, with numbness and reduction of the spontaneous activity.

lh. 45 after injection : Catalepsy of a duration of about 24 hours.

36th after the injection : Return to normal state.

(*B*) *Experiment of the Identity*

We have used Reserpine 7 CH, 9 CH, 15 CH, 30 CH, diluted and dynamised in bi-distilled water in order to avoid the interference of Alcohol and a lot of withnesses receiving bi-distilled water.

(*a*) *Action of the chronic sub-intoxication.*

By using the dilutions of 7 CH and 9 CH one observes from the 1st to the 3rd injection : Slowness of the psychomotor, and a catalepsy for 24 hours with weakening of **the** general condition, lustreless and humid hairs.

Return to the normal at the end of 24 hours.

By the dose of 15 CH : Excitation phase with hyperactivity and aggressiveness during 4 days, after the 2nd and the 3rd injections. Then return to the normal.

In the 30th, nothing was noted.

(*b*) *Acute intoxication by Reserpine at 4·5 mig/kg.*

By 7 CH : Slight delay of 15 minutes of the appearance of the slowness and of the catalepsy in comparison to the witness.

By the dose of 9 CH : *Important delay of 2 hours.*

By the dose of 15 CH : Slight delay of 30 minutes.

By the dose of 30 CH : Same phenomena as that of the witnesses that received bi-distilled water.

Concerning the lethal toxicity it is noted : Strong lethality except in 9 CH where it is of 10"

2—Experiment on Cobaye

A. *Determination of the Catalepsy by Reserpine*

We have retained the dose 6 mg/kg.

B. *Experiment of the Indentity*

We have used Reserpine in 7 CH, 9 CH, 15 CH, 30 CH and a group of witnesses receiving bi-distilled water.

(*a*) *Action of the chronic sub-intoxication*

In doses of 7 CH, and 9 CH, it is noted from the 3rd injection : psycho-motor slowness, lustreless hairs, less frequent cries which are less acute.

In the dose of 30 CH : nothing to note.

(*b*) *Acute intoxication by Reserpine 6 mg/kg.*

In all the dilutions (7 CH, 9 CH, 15 CH, 30 CH) it is noted : labile catalepsy, less marked, many more cataleptic sleeps at the end of $2\frac{1}{2}$ hours for 9 hours.

This experiment indicates that an experimental verification of Isotherapy is conceivable and verifiable in laboratory. It indicates also that even beyond the Avogadro number, a biological corticosomatic action may be noted.

Finally, let us mention that an experimental pathogenesis in rats and cobayes can be noted.

Here we close the experimental chapter, because the intention was only to elucidate the notion by some well conducted scientific experiment.

CHAPTER 8

CLINICAL PRAXIS OF THE DYNAMISED MICRO-IMMUNOTHERAPY OR ISOPATHY

In the field of dynamised micro-immunotherapic concretology, the biotherapics are to be considered according to some modalities in different steps.

(a) The aggressologic step.

(b) The step of immunological perturbation.

Let us study these two steps closely.

(a) The aggressologic step

It is distinguished as :

—*External aggression* : Vaccinotherapy, antibiotherapy, Chemiotherapy.

—*Internal aggression* : It includes the three miasms of S. Hahnemann, the three important morbid processes : Psora or Allergoso ; Sycosis or Chronic mesenchymatosis; Chancre disease (syphilis) of Hahnemann or Luetosis (see Ch. 6).

(b) On the step of immunological perturbation

It is the original clinical indication of dynamised micro-immunotherapy with Biotherapics and Isotherapics.

Thus the field of the application of the therapeutics of dynamised micro-immunotherapy is delimited.

But before starting the practico-clinical study of these two particular fields, it is necessary to precise the complex bivalent *clinical significance* of Biotherapic (Ex-Nosode).

It is necessary to know that ceratain *Biotherapics* may specially have a *double quality.*

1. *Homoeotherapic quality.*

2. *Biotherapic quality.*

To be more clear, every Biotherapic having been submitted to pharmacological experiment according to the methodology of Hahnemann will be *Homoeopathic*.

These homoeotherapic qualities imply the application of the law of homoeopathic simillimum taking into account homoeopathic semiology. It means that in a patient it is necessary to consider the "symptoms" that he feels personally, that his entourage remarks, and what the doctor observes himself.

They include :

1. Subjective symptoms.

2. Objective symptoms.

3. Accidental, causal and peculiar symptoms (Para 6, Organon, Schmidt).

In a word the totality of symptoms is the principal and the only thing with which the doctor should occupy himself, in a morbid individual case, the one that should be fought with the force of his art, in order to be able to cure the patient and to transform him into health (Para 7, Organon, 4th ed., tr. J.L. Jourdan.)

In fact, the homoeopathic practice, which takes into account the *totalising totality* of the patient in his pathological becoming, does hardly differ when a Homoeotherapic or an Isotherapic is prescribed.

The second modality in the clinical application of Biotherapic is the idea, *the etiological quality.* It is that which is *specific* for an Isopathic of W. Lux, *i.e.* to say for a Biotherapic or Isotherapic.

It is at the known or supposed etiology that one aims.

In summary : The same pharmacological substance, a biotherapic, has a double therapeutic quality : Homoeotherapic

6 F

and Immunotherapic. The first quality belongs to those of Biotherapics having been the object of a hahnemannian pathological experiment.

Now we are in a position to enter into the study of the two steps mentioned above.

A. Aggressological Step

1. As regards external aggressology the couple Biotherapic-Isotherapic will act as specific stimulant which will induce an active mini-excitation of the "mass defence system" (of H.H. Reckeweg) in view of the elimination of "primitive peptides" or the resorption of the blockages caused by the same "primitive peptides."

It is there one would have to play a part of a therapeutist of importance, alone or associated with Homoeotherapics or Biotherapics.

It will act thus in vaccinal complications (see O.A. Julian : Prevention and treatment : bio-homoeo-therapic of vaccinal complications 1973, Libraire le Francois, 91. Bd. St. germain, Paris.) and also as sensibilising specific or anaphylactic.

2. As regards internal aggressology, the biotherapic will act in morbid processes, the "miasms" of Hahnemann as much as signal of specific perturbation in view of effacing the deforming effect on the molecules in the Spatio-tissular site of a given biological space.

Since then Psorinum will be the specific, the *molecular therapeutic signal* of the old Psora of Hahnemann at present to us *Allergoso.*

The case will be the same, with Medorrhinum in Sycosis of Hahnemann or chronic mesenchymatosis of H. Benard, in the Luetosis with Luesinum (=Syphilinum).

3. *Immunological perturbation* : It is a therapeutic field of wide diversity.

Here the tiological idea dominates the therapeutic indication.

There also the Biotherapic is of value for its possible double action : Immunotherapic and Homoeotherapic, if it has been the object of pathological experiment.

It is here one distinguishes Polychrest biotherapic having local therapeutic action as well as a possible specific general action in the depth of the pathological processes.

This therapeutic action on etiological level is directed to two different pathological conditions *viz* :

(*a*) A state of acute or subacute immunological perturbation in evolution.

(*b*) A chronic stage which is manifested either by a symptomatology corresponding to a slow evolution or to a stage of mending as much as a sequale of an *old Anamnestic infection*.

In the field of therapeutic activity, thus specified, one sees that the exigencies of some authors rise up.

P. Schimdt, the famous Kentist, formulates in the following manner the indications in the clinical application :

If a reactive or reactional remedy like *Sulphur*, *Nux*, *Cuprum* or *Opium*, to city only a few, may be given when a case does not react to the chosen remedy according to the art and doctrine, the formal indication of a nosode according to long experience of Hahnemannian homoeopaths is legitimate in the following five circumstances :

1. *When a well selected remedy have given some effects, but these do not continue or do not persist, or the beneficial action stops.*

2. *When the disease relapses continually, although ameliorated with every dose of the medicine* : repeated coryza, hayfever, periodic return of some affections. If it is the question

of pulmonary affections which relapse constantly, one will more willing give Tuberculinum for example ; if it is the question of mucous secretion, one should think of Medorrhinum ; in the presence of a tumefication, tissular proliferation one should think of Syphilinum etc...

3. *When there has been suppression in consequence of an abortive treatment* : Suppression of an eruption, of a discharge, of sweat, of menses and when the indicated remedy does not act.

4. *When a patient presents the characteristic symptoms of their pathogenesis, i.e. to say their experimentation on healthy man, as Homoeopathy requires it* for the application of every remedy. It is the homoeopathic indications of Nosode.

5. *Finally according to the anamnesis of the patient, if he presents only in part of the pathogenesis of Nosode, or when a patient has suffered of a microbian infection, as for example old Scarlatina, diphtheria, measles, syphils, tuberculosis etc... which one may find in the personal antecedents of a patient who does not progress any more.*

(*Cahiers du groupment hahnemannian de Lyon*, 3rd, serie, cahier No. 5, p. 168.)

Henry Duprat who seems to be somewhat disdainful towards Isopathy expresses himself as follows : "The help of Isopathy should be taken recourse to when the remedy seems to be insufficient, inactive, in cases where a correspondence in our Materia Medica cannot be found and above all in cases of high gravity, where it becomes our duty to attempt everything to save the patient."

Denis Demarque, while accepting that Isopathy has been proved to be effective, speaks in reserve while writing that one should not make of it a method of routine, applied without discrimination and should know to specify the indications for it (l'Homoeopathie médicine de l'Expérience, p. 95).

Those indications were formulated by *Guillaume and Zissu* in the following manner :

(*a*) When the intoxication in cause is found in the antecedants, the nosode assures a kind of immunisation against the intoxication.

(*b*) When the simillimum which has been well chosen does not "hold" or when there is an identical relapse.

(*c*) When an eliminatory suppression results because of an intempestive treatment or for an exogenous cause and that the well indicated simillimum however does not act.

These indications are of those of "Major nosodes" according to these authors.

For the "Minor nosodes" they will be used basing on two ideas :

(1) On etiological idea. A patient has a morbid condition since a Diphtheria, a mumps etc...and whatever may be his treatment of which the simillimum, the same clinical morbid condition comes at long intervals...*Morbillinum* or *Diphtherotoxicum* find there an indication for selection.

(2) On a clinical idea. If in a patient is found a totality of morbid symptoms similar to the symptomatology produced by the aggressive agent, the latter diluted as particularly indicated.

(Guillaum and Zissu : Les Nosodes et Biothérapiques mineurs en pratique courante—*Annales Hom. Fr.* 1969, p. 55-143 and ff.)

One may see that some homoeopathic authors, and we have mentioned only a few, make of Isopathy a *therapeutic complimentary* to Homoeopathy in which rules as absolute master, the pathogenesic remedy of Hahnemann.

However some discordant opinions are seen and we have mentioned that of Léon Vannier above.

There is an other enthusiast of Isopathy, P. Brotteaux, who in his book "Homoeopathy and Isopathy" (Peyronnet, Paris, 1947) writes :

"Facts superabundantly prove, that the real law is that of identity, the law of similarity is simply approached." There is of it a consequence. As says Roy, Isopathy is "Homoeopathy maxima" where the law of simple analogy has become rigorous similitude (Hom. fr., 1928, p. 259).

And Brotteau goes further to formulate this sentence, "Homoeopathy is an approximation of Isopathy."

It seems to us to have shown, that with our analysis of the Homoeopathic concretology and Isopathic concretology, that with the clarification of our ideas about Analogous and Identical, a new theoretical understanding, help us to make of these two antagonists some analogical entities, each having its own characteristics.

- There is no more conflict, there is only a question of going ahead.

The two therapeutic modalities enter in the vast field of Analogotherapy.

The indications for clinical application, that of P. Schmidt of Zissu and others are perfectly valid under the condition of recognising the value of the field of therapeutic activity of Homoeopathy and dynamised micro-immunotherapy. These are *Biotics* analogotherapic therapy. Their aim is to re-establish the "health" which has been the most dear wish of S. Hahnemann according to the para 1 of the Organon.

In conclusion, we repeat our formulation.

The clinical indications of micro-immunotherapy is situated on two levels.

1. That of aggressological structure. 2. That of immunological perturbation. Homoeopathy and micro-immunotherapy have their respective applications by their own pecularities.

These two therapeutics come out of the same course of thinking.

CHAPTER 9

IMMUNOTHERAPIC OR ISOTHERAPIC PRESCRIPTION

A. PHARMACOTHERAPY

The prescription according to an acute and sub-acute condition or in chronic cases are to be distinguished for Pharmacotherapy.

The Acute Stage

Prescription of a biotherapic will be done according to the *etiology* of the pathological case in question.

This will be according to the expression of P. Schmidt, the treatment by the "idem," the identical, *i.e.* to say by the substance pathogenous agent, virus toxin etc...which is the probable cause of the disease (which is surely not always exact) (Glossary, Organon, p. 23).

Thus one will prescribe :

Morbillinum in measles.

Pertussinum in whooping cough.

Anthracinum in Anthrax.

Staphylotoxinium in furuncles, or Pyrogenium etc...

Well, within the framework of our concretological clinical conception there will be ground to prescribe according to the specific symptomatology of an individualised case, either a second biotherapic, or one or two Homoeotherapics.

In fact a furuncle will require the prescription of Staphylococcinum alone or with Anthracinum or Pyrogenium. But the etiological prescription requires according to the pathological condition and to the evolution of the disease; a homoeotherapic prescription of Belladonna, or Hepar Sulphur. at the beginning, Apis or Tarentula if there is a tendency to phlegmons with burning, Merc sol. if the resorption is late, Echinacea or Lachesis if the infection aggravates Calcarea sulph. to help the evolution and Silicea to stop the suppuration.

Here one perceives the static stage of Isotherapy which surrounds only the etiological motivation and the dynamic state of homoeotherapy which covers the individual "in progress" of his pathological evolution.

There is a constant and a variable :

Take the case of an Erysipelas : It requires the constant : Anthracinum or Pyrogenium and the variable Bellad-Apis-Rhus tox-Naja-Hepar sulph.

Herpes requires the constant : Vaccinotoxinum or Staphylococcinum and the variable Ranunculus bulbosus-Arsenicum-Rhus tox-Croton tig.

The few examples make clear the prescription of dynamised micro-immunotherapy in the acute conditions and its place in the vast system of Analogotherapy.

The Chronic Stage

In the chronic stage the therapeutic application is to be considered according to the necessity of a biotherapic prescription of the total man.

The immunotherapic remedy is to be added to the constitutional and temperamental remedy. The Sulphur patient of H. Bernard requires Psorinum, the Phosphoric, Tuberculinum, the Fluoric, Luesinum.

The old anamnestic etiology will also be considered while prescribing.

Here are some examples :

Dr. Poisson (Observation de malades gueris par le Nosode Paratyphoid-B, Annales Hom. Francoise, 2nd year, No. 1, Oct. 1959) has reported the case of a patient presenting a grave syndrome of deneutrition and post-traumatic depression where all Homoeopathic and Allopathic treatment failed and it is a dose of Para-typhoidinum-B 9 CH which miraculously transformed and cured the patient.

My regretted friend Dr. Pfister of Saverna, with whom I did my first course in Homoeopathy in 1935, was reposted in Journées homoeopathiques Alsaciennes in May, 1938, cured a case of an epilepsy with unilateral sciatica of standing of many years with Eberthinum, selected because of typhoid antecedants.

Dr. H. Bernard (observation d'un cas de Psorinum, Hom. Mod., 5th year, No. 20, 16 Dec., 1936) reports a case of chronic bronchitis with sensitiveness to cold, with unhealthy skin, and lesions because of scratching, with one dose of Psorinum 200 K.

In the daily practice of chronic cases, the microimmunotherapic prescription should be integrated in a biotherapic prescription :

Here are some examples :

1. Eczema of a baby (Summary)

Baby, 10 months, impetiginous eczema with some furuncles on arms and abdomen.

Treatment : 5 drops Mezereum 3 DH in the morning, 5 drops of Graphitis 4 CH at night while going to bed ; 1 dose of Anthracinum 7 CH, twice at an interval of 8 days. Cure in 15 days.

2. Enurisis (Summary)

Boy of 6 years and a half, lean, micro-polyadenopathics, nervous, anorexic, urinates between 1 to 2 a.m.

Treatment : Every 19 days in the following order :

1 dose of Silicea 7 CH ; Drosera 7 CH, Calcarea fluor 7 CH, Mermoreck 200 (K) (cannot be prescribed now, is to be replaced by V.A.B. 7 CH).

The other days : Before meals, Morning and Noon 8 drops of Dulcamara 1 XH ; Aveda Sat. at 17 hrs., 5 drops of Equisetum 3 DH ; while going to bed Causticum.

Two months after good amel.

2. *Treatment* : Every 10 days Calcarea fluor 7 CH ; Tuberculinum 7 CH ; Silicea 7 CH, the remaining treatment not changed.

3. Facial Nuralgia (Summary)

Man of 43 years, facial neuralgia since 3 years, longlimbed type, mean, nervous.

Different allopathic treatments without result.

1st treatment : Every 5 days 1 dose in the following order : Arsenic 9 CH, Causticum 7 CH, Spigelia 9 CH ; Tuberculinum 9CH.   Every day : Morning 10 drops of Causticum 4CH, Spigelia 4 CH.   While going to bed 10 drops of Arsenic 4 CH ; Kalmia 3 DH. After one month excellent amelioration.

2nd treatment : Every 10 days 1 dose in the following order : Arsenic 7 CH, Hypericum 7 CH ; Aconite 7 CH ; T.R. 9 CH. Every day : Morning while waking up 10 drops of Kalmia latiforia 3 DH ; while going to sleep 10 drops of Arsenic 10 DH, Ledum 3 DH.

Complete cure without relapse.

4. Raynaud's syndrome (Summary)

Man 68 years, fingers of the feet white as if "dead", Agg. by humid cold.

Heavy eyelids, swollen. Towards the age of 20 had 3 gonorrhoeal infections.

Treatment : Medorrhinum 7 CH and 5 CH alternated with Secale 7 CH and 6 CH. Complete cure after one month.

5. Cyclothymia—Depressive Melancholy (Summary)

Man 32 years, fat, strong, anxious, depressive crisis, weeps, digestive troubles. Tried suicide twice. In full depressive condition.

Treatment : Tuberculinum 9 CH, one dose every 5 days. The other days Mag phos 1 DH (trit), in the morning ; Aurum 5 CH and Chelidonium 4 CH in the evening. After one month, goes very well.

Finally we may say that the Pharmacotheraphy of a Biotherapic is situated, as we have said many times, according to the etiological modality of dynamised Micro-immunotherapy or according to Homoeopathic modality, also the two are associated in the same remedy.

B. PHARMACOLEXY

Pharmacolexy means the selection of the remedy.

In the framework of clinical homoeopathic concretology as theory and general praxis we preconise a polyvalent medical concretism.

In a particular case, choice of the remedy, according to a "unicist" or "pluralist" conception, is done in the presence of the concrete therapeutic application concerning the individual who is ill in his totality.

It is for this reason that one understands easily the need of prescribing an Anthracinum with a Pyrogenium, an Oscillococcinum with Streptococcinum or Staphylococcinum, and so on.

The quarrel Unicist-Pluralist is a false quarrel, because it is situated in the *abstract*. A living being, healthy or ill is a whole in himself and his environment. He is one and multiple.

As regards dynamised micro-immunotherapy, it is enough to read the Chapter 5, where we have indicated that in a morbid process many homotoxins may participate. Hence the necessity, real, concrete, and practical to prescribe many biotherapics, as well as many homoeotherapics.

C. PHARMACONOMY

It is the question of the prescription of Dynamisations and their modalities of indications.

Dynamisation

According to the French Legislation of Pharmaceutics one can prescribe currently as far as biotherapic remedies prepared in advance are concerned, the dynamisations 4 CH, 5 CH, 7 CH, 9 CH.

On the contrary, as regards authoritative prescription, 15 CH and 30 CH are used.

Each biotherapic is a simple unit and is presented in the form of globules, granules and doses in drinkable ampouls.

Only the Anticollibacillary Serum can be delivered in 3DH, in drinkable ampouls.

Modalities of Indications

The high potency 15 CH or 30 CH is used when it is a question of inducing typo-aggressological process in the sphere of important morbid processes or anamnesic modality.

In the last case the 7 CH or 9 CH may also be prescribed.

We have specified several grades of dynamisations. Thus one may prescribe simultaneously or in rapid succession 7 CH, 9 CH, 15 CH, 30 CH.

The lower and the medium potencies are to be prescribed when it is the question of its use as *specific signal.*

Its action will be directed towards the level of lesion of tissues of organs.

Pertussinum 5 CH will act in the acute process of whooping cough and may be prescribed in 15 CH or 30 CH if one wishes to act on the cortic-visceral perturbation.

Medorrhinum 5 CH will be prescribed for gonorrhoeal articular rheumatism, the 30 CH for inducing the setting aright of the cortico-visceral perturbation.

The *Pharmacopollaxy* which means the repetition of the remedy is modulated according to the acute and the chronic stage of the patient.

4 CH, 5 CH, or 7 CH or 5 CH plus 7 CH combined are to be repeated every hour, and according to the evolution of the case, the doses are espaced.

The 9 CH, the 15 CH or the 30 CH, are to be prescribed in chronic cases, one globule every 7, 15 or 30 days.

But there may be some clinical situations where the prescription of high dynamisation in granules may be used daily.

INDEX

A

Aconite—156
Acute cases—42
Adrenalinum—44, 99
Aggravation—62
Allergology—48
Alloxane—142
Ambra—44
Ammonia—138
Angina complex—46
Anthracinum—34, 36, 39, 46, 62, 125, 153, 155, 157
Antimony—138
Apis—153
Apples—62
Argent Nit—24
Arnica—24
Arsenicum—136, 137, 156
Aurum—24, 157
Auto-isopathy—35, 49
Auto-psorine—32
Avena Sat—156

B

Bacillinum—39
Belladonna—153
Bismuth—137
Blood—29, 42, 46, 47, 48, 62

Blood serum—27, 47
Brain—27
Bryonia—63
Bubo—29, 32
Burns—62
Butter yellow colouring—118

C

Calcarea Carb—24
Calcarea Chloride—32
Calcarea Fluor—24, 32, 155
Calcarea Phos—24, 32
Calcarea Renal—45
Calcarea Sul—154
Calendula—24
Cantharidine—45, 140
Carbolic acid—32
Causticum—156
Chelidonium—157
China—63
Cholesterinum—44, 99
Chronic cases—42
Condurango—25
Conium—25
Corbyzine—34
Croton Tig—154
Cuprum—149
Cup. Sulph—140
Cyclothemia—156

(161)

PART II

MATERIA
MEDICA OF
BIOTHERAPICS
(EX-NOSODES)

ANTHRACINUM

BIBLIOGRAPHY

Hering :

Stapfs-Archiv für die Homoöpatische Heilkinst, 1830, Bd. 13.

The Guiding Symptoms of our Materia Medica. v. 1., p. 334-347.

Homoeopathy, 1933, p. 299.

Dufresne P. :

Bibliothéque Homéop. de Genéve. Janvier et fevrier 1837, Hygea. v. 6, p. 351.

Allen H.C. :

The Materia Medica of Nosodes. Boericke and Tafel, Phil., 1910, p. 351.

Boericke W. :

Pocket Manual of Homoeopathic Materia Medica.
Item-1st ed. German, 1972, by M. Harms.

Allen H.C. :

Key-notes and Characteristics of the Materia Medica with Nosodes. Jain Publishing Co., New Delhi, 110055.

Clarke J.H. :

A Dictionary of Practical Materia Medica. London, 1955, v. 1, p. 118.

Denis M. :

Observation de Furonculose. Annales Homoeop. fr., 1968, No. 3, p. 249.

Julian O.A. :

Materia Medica der Nosoden. Haug-Verlag, 2nd ed. 1975, Heidelberg.

Biothérapiques et Nosodes. Maloine, Paris, 1962.

Renard L. :

Anthracinum. L'Hom. Moderne, p. 592, No. 8, 1933.

Schmidt P. :

Les Nosodes (avec bibliographic). Cahiers groupement Hahnemannien de Lyon, ser. 3, Cahiers No. 5., p. 155-178.

Weber G.A. :

Rapport sur Anthracinum. Reclam 1836, Leipzig.

Margaret Burges-Webster. :

"Le Recorder" from 1932.

HISTORY

We owe to J.W. Lux the first preparation and the therapeutic use of Anthracinum. He made mention of it in 1833 in his *Isopathick der Contagionen*. Towards 1831 it was Charles Hering who communicated, perhaps first before Lux, the use of Anthracinum. This Nosode was prepared by Dr. G.A. Weber (not to be confounded with Pharmacien Weber of Paris, as it seems to have been done by Dr. P. Schmidt of Geneva) who made an alcoholic tincture with the spleen of a sheep, suffering from carbuncle, a process mentioned also by Clarke.

The preparation of Lux was dynamised up to the 30th.

But the process of preparing has changed in course of time.

Lux reports in the third book, page 83 of *Zooiasis* an observation of Hahnemann 1834, regarding a worker of a farm, affected by a malignant anthrax of both the hands whom he gave two drops of the 30 C, to an other worker of the same farm who had only two pustules, Hahnemann gave only one drop. Both men were cured.

STOCK

At present the preparation of the Biotherapic anthracinum is done from a lysate obtained without addition of antiseptic, from the liver of a rabbit suffering from Anthrax. The stock is supplied by the Merieux Institute.

The lysate corresponds per centimetre cube to 0.001 cm^3 of a suspension of the liver of the rabbit suffering from Anthrax. It is presented in the form of ampouls of 1 cm^3 from which is prepared the dilutions—homoeopathic dynamisations.

METHOD OF PREPARATION

1. Collection of Livers infected with Anthrax

Some rabbits having the weight of 2.5 to 3 kg. received subcutaneously $1/10$ cm^3 of a culture of 24 hours on ordinary bouillon of the virulent stock of *Bacillus Anthracis* C$_2$.

The animals are watched over. They are killed in the last stage of agony (generally on the third day). The liver is taken out. The proof of Anthrax infection is done by putting in evidence the bacteria in the blood of the animal.

2. The Technique of Preparation

(*a*) *Preparation of the suspension at 1/100* :

The liver is made free from fibrous and fatty matter, then the weight is taken. They are cut into pieces. Then the pieces are crushed in a mixer after having added to it some quantity of distilled water. The suspension obtained is diluted in distilled water at the rate of 10 grams of the liver to 1000 cm^3 of water.

(*b*) *The obtaining of the lysate* :

The initial dilution 1/100 is congealed at 20° then decongealed in ordinary temperature, the latter is carried out four times continually so as to cause the breaking of the cells.

(*c*) *Sterilisation and distribution of the initial dilution* :

The previously obtained lysate is filtered on Seitz C$_5$ filtre, then sterilised by passing through Seitz E.K.S. The filtered liquid is then divided in fractions of 10 cm^3 in sterile phials.

(*d*) *Stocking of the initial dilution* :

The fractions of 10 cm³ of initial dilution is lyophylised in such a way that it may be preserved without decomposition. Each phial contains a quantity of the lyophilised product corresponding to 0·10 cm³ of lysate. The dilution is characterised by its technique of preparation and by its controlled tests.

(*e*) *Dilution* :

The contents of each phial is taken again in 100 cm³ of distilled water so as to cause the concentration of the final products to 0·001 by cm³ of lysate.

Control of the Product

(*a*) *Sterility*. 2 ml of the iysate is inoculated in 20 ml of thioglycollate medium. The culture may not be perceived even after one day's incubation at 37°.

(*b*) *Inoccuousness*. 2 ml of lysate is injected subcutaneously to 5 white rats weighing 20 g., 5 other rats receive 0·75 ml intraperitonially. The mortality should be nil. If one of the animals dies the experiment is repeated and if something happens, the lysate should be rejected.

CLINICAL CORTICO-VISCERAL PROTOCOL
OR CLINICAL PATHOGENESIS

No experiment of this product is done according to the Hahnemannian methodology. The description below results out of the clinical experiences of Lux, Hering, G.A. Weber, Dufresne and Peschier of Geneva.

It was Dr. Käsemann who used first in human medicine, in a case of gangrene, in the year 1853, then Rau in 1858 for a case of anthrax.

1. Generalities

Here it is the question of a patient who becomes suddenly septicemic with asthenia, emaciation, intense thirst, developing towards a state of prostration.

High fever with an anxious state, delirium of nearing death.

2. Nervous System

Adynamic condition, excessive sensitiveness. Delirium.

3. Skin

It is the most characteristic seat of Anthracinum. Ulceration with intense burning which is intolerable.

At first there is a local indurated inflammation of subcutaneous tissues. Afterwards a *bluish*, violet coloured vesicle, which becomes black, and from which there is an ichorous, foetid and irritant secretion.

The ulceration may end in gangrene, having intense putrid smell. This condition is accompanied by corresponding adenopathy with big and painful lymphatic ganglions.

Complications : There may be hemorrhages of thick black blood rapidly decomposing.

Evolution : The affection may become rapidly grave and toximic.

4. Digestive System

Hard lignous swelling of parotides and submaxillary glands. Predominantly right side.

Intense thirst.

Diarrhoea with liquid stools having foetid smell.

POSITIVE DIAGNOSIS

Anthracinum is characterised by the following tripod :

1. Indurated vesicular inflammation.
2. Intensive burning pain.
3. Irritating and foetid secretion.

DIFFERNTIAL DIAGNOSIS

Anthracinum may by compared with :

Argentum metallicum : (Dr. O.A. Julian—Etudes homoeopathiques, cliniques et thérapeutiques. Le François, Paris 75006).

Sensation to painful excoriation, pruriginous, burning ending in a bloody secretion. It is to be used in 10 DH or 7 CH by sub-cutaneous injections.

Arsenicum album : Patient, restless, anxious, worse, after midnight to 3 a.m., burning pain, better by heat.

Tarentula : Pain forcing the patient to walk ; better by smoking.

Carbolic acidum : General foetiodness, sensation violent burning pain, but short lasting.

Pyrogenium : Horrible putrid smell of the secretions, dissociation of pulse and temperature, delirium, restlessness, cardiac collapse.

Lachesis : Great sensitiveness to touch, dark blue infiltration sometimes livid, with tendency to ulcer and gangrene. Black blood non-coagulating or coagulating very soon.

It is necessary to mention also *Carbo vegetabilis, Crotal., Echinacea, Euphorbium, Secale.*

CLINICAL DIAGNOSIS

Carbuncle : Secretion of foetid pus (Ars. alb.)

Septicemia : Prostration, adynamia, thready pulse, hyperthermia, collapse, delirium (Pyrogenium).

Gangrenous phlegmon (Ars., Lachesis).

Panaris (whitlow) (Pyrogenium, Tarent).

Furuncles, Anthrax Erysepelas.

Acne.

Inflammation of the parotids and submaxillary glands. Acute Gastro-enteritis.

POSOLOGY

Dynamisation : 4 CH, 5 CH, 7 CH, 9 CH.

Lower dilutions are to be repeated many times a day. The high dilutions 7 CH and 9 CH, every 3 to 5 days.

COMMENTARY

Our experience allows us to advise Anthracinum as an important remedy.

This remedy alone is not sufficient to cure some of the affections mentioned above.

Its action is better when used very early and in high dilution, either 7 CH or 9 CH, one dose every evening, for three days. If accompanied by *Belladonna* and *Hepar sulphur* at the beginning of the affection its action becomes much better ; afterwards with *Tarentula* and *Arsenic album.* All these medicines are to be used in medium dilutions : 4 CH or 5 CH.

Finally I associate it with *Argentum metallicum*, 5 CH.

To end, here is a case by M. Denis (Annales Hom. fr., No. 3, p. 249, 1968).

A Case of Furuncle

In 1962, a patient of about 50 years old came to consult us for a generalised furuncle, suffering from the age of 25. Everything was tried : Vaccin, Sulfamides, Antibiotics.

Lastly O.T.A. has caused an amelioration of the furunculosis but having found that he is becoming deaf an ENT was consulted who advised to stop O.T.A.

Blood analysis shows glycemia to 2 gr. traces of albumin and glucose in the urine.

The patient was in full explosion of furuncles ; a dose of *Anthracinum 30 K* and *Uranium nitricum 4 CH* and because of the pains *Tarentula cubensis 4 CH*.

Spectacularly, the furuncles diminished. A dose of *Lachesis 30* was used basing on the modalities, then a dose of *Lycopodium 30 K*. These two remedies brought a great amelioration. The patient told us that he was suspected of syphilis and was treated and that since then the furuncles appeared.

Serology done several times was negative. Nevertheless *Luesinum* 200 was prescribed without any effect. The patient is continuing *Uranium nitricum 4 CH* and is at present in perfect condition.

We are following up the patient and perhaps later on we will be able to give you more information.

AVIARY

BIBLIOGRAPHY

Cartier Fr :

Thêrapeutique des voies respiratoires. Baillére et Fils, 1920. Paris.

Bernard H. :

Nouveau Traité d'Homoeopathie. v. II, 1947, Coquemard Angoulême.

Voisin H. :

Matiére Medicale du Praticien Homoeopathie.

Clarke J.H. :

A Clinical Repertory of the Dictionary of Materia Medica, London, 1904.

A Dictionary of Practical Materia Medica, London, 1955, v. I, p. 235.

Kollitsch. P :

Homeopathie. Matiére Médical Therapeutique. Maloine. Paris. 1955.

Julian O.A. :

Materia Medica der Nosoden. Haug-Verlag. Heidelberg, 2nd. ed, 1975.

Biothérapiques et Nosodes. Maloine, 1962.

STOCK

It is the question of Aviary tuberculine used mainly by the veterinary doctors for a diagnostic aim. It enters into the category of biotherapics. The preparation of the Aviary tuberculine is mentioned in the codex which specifies in the article on Tuberculine that for the diagnosis of tuberculous affections due to bacillary Aviary and therefore more particularly in veterinary medicine, one may prepare an uncultured Tuberculine, without addition of antiseptics, with the *Mycobacterium tuberculosis*, var. "Aviary."

Its preparation then does not differ in any way from that of Tuberculinum if it is not of the nature of bacilli utilised (see Tuberculinum).

It is perhaps better to indicate that the action of Aviary does not develop at 100,000 IU in gramme required for uncultured Tuberculine. The Biotherapic Aviary is identical to the old Aviary nosode, the stock which is used being the same.

HISTORY

The Aviary tuberculine or Bird tuberculine was used, according to Cartier, by Pierre Jousset towards 1900, in human tuberculosis.

According to P. Jousset the therapeutic results in that affection does hardly seem fortunate. On the contrary Cartier specifies the prescription of Aviary in *Non-tubercular* diseases of the respiratory system.

He published an article, "Aviary and Bacillinum" in the Revue Hom. Fr., and presented in 1896, a communication in the International Homoeopathic Congress under the title, "Des virus tuberculeux en thérapeutique Homoeopathiques" (Some tuberculous viruses in Homoeopathic therapeutics).

He insists on the indication of Aviary in the acute pulmonary affections and established also a difference between Bacillinum and Aviary. While he indicates Bacillinum in case of muco purulent expectoration of adults or of old, he assigns clearly to Aviary "a place in the broncho-pulmonary diseases of children and in acute affections of adults, such as influenza, simulating some actue bacillary symptoms".

He prescribes the 100th dilution in repeated doses in a portion containing 5 to 10 drops a day.

Cartier thinks that Aviary is a marvellous medicine in infantile therapeutic as in broncho-pneumonia and measles.

Then in l'Art Médicale appeared an article by *Source* of Havre and *E. Vannier* of Rouen concerning a grave case of infantile broncho-pneumonia cured by Aviary.

Clarke gives a short clinical pathogenesis in his Dictionary of Materia Medica. In contemporary French homoeopathic literature some short indications are to be found in the Matiére Médicale du Practicien Homoeopathie of *Dr. Voisin*, in Traité d'Homoeopathie de H. Bernard and that of Kollitsch.

O.A. Julian has included a monograph in his book Biotherapiques et Nosodes as well as in the Materia Medica der Nosoden of which a second edition is published in 1975.

CLINICAL CORTICO-VISCERAL PROTOCOL
OR CLINICAL PATHOGENESIS

1. Generalities

Asthenia, Anorexia, Emaciation.

Cervical micro-adenopathy.

Broken down condition of Bernand-Jacquelin type (Tubercular condition of old homoeopaths).

2. Nervous System

Frontal Headache with hot forehead ; the root of the nose is painful.

Troubles of perception with obnubilation.

Meningeal convulsive attacks.

3. Cardio-hemo-vascular System

Tachycardia with rapid and bounding pulse.

Circulatory troubles of the extremities, cyanosis,

Thermoregulation : General uneasiness accompanied by chill, diffused muscular pains, fever, oscilliating between 39ᶜ to 40°.

4. Respiratory System

(a) *Throat* :

Irritation of larynx and of the trachea.

Hoarseness.

Congestion of the larynx with dyspnoea.

(b) *Lungs, pleura* :

Pain in the upper part of the lungs.

Thoracic wall painful.

Dry and painful cough.

Polypnoea with beatings of the nasal wings ; cyanosis ; obstruction.

5. Sense Organs

(a) *Nose* :

Pain in the root of the nose.

Anosmia.

Continual sneezing followed by watery hypersecretion.

Muco-purulent catarrh.

(b) *Eyes* :

Congested conjunctiva with lachrymation.

(c) *Ears* :

Acute catarrhal or purulent otitis.

Acute mastoiditis.

6 Skin

Redness or paleness of the face.

Palms hot and sweating.

POSOLOGY

Dynamisations : 4 CH, 5 CH, 7 CH, 9 CH.

In acute cases 4 CH or 5 CH, repeated every 2 hours.

In the chronic cases prescribe 7 CH preferably.

DIFFERENTIAL DIAGNOSIS

Among the classical homoeotherapics let us mention *Ferrum phos.*, *Pulsatilla*, *Sulphur iod.*, *Arsenicum iod.*

Among modern homoeotherapics let us cite :

Mimosa pudica : Irritation of the mucous of the nose and conjunctiva. Thoracic pains, dry cough, pain and tickling in the throat.

Luffa operculata : Fronto-occipital headache. Inflammation of nasal mucous, dryness of larynx and tongue.

Galphimia glauca : Hypersecretion of oculo-nasal mucous, sneezing, hypersensitiveness to the changes of weather

Finally *Aviary* may be associated with *Oscillococcinum* and *Serum of Yersin.*

(For all these medicines refer to O.A. Julian and Collab. Matière médicale d'Homoeopathie, Paris, 1971, Le François, 91 Bd. St., Germain, 75006 Paris).

CLINICAL DIAGNOSIS

1. Generalities

Influenza.

Measles and its pulmonary and meningeal complications.

Jacquelin Bernand syndrome.

Ganglionary primo-infection.

2. Neuro-endocrino-psychic System

Meningitis in influenza (Adjuvant treatment).

3. Respiratory Apparatus

Capillary bronchitis.

Broncho-pneumonia.

Pulmonary congestion.

Infantile asthma with fever.

4. Sense Organs

Acute rhinitis ; acute sinusitis.

Acute blepharitis ; conjunctivitis of influenza.

Acute otitis.

Mastoiditis.

COMMENTARIES

The want of an experimental pathogenesis is to be regretted because *Aviary* is a very valuable remedy, specially in acute affections of respiratory tract. Its action is sure and faithful. (O.A. Julian)

It should be prescribed with adequate homoeotherapics in rhino-pharyngitis, influenza with tracheo-bronchitis, pulmonary congestions of children and of aged persons.

It is also to be used in cervical adenopathies of children and in asthma of young children.

Voisin indicates it in acute otitis, and in broncho-pneumonia; H. Bernard recommends it in tuberculosis of bones and of ganglions and in infantile asthma ; Kollitsch in dragging pulmonary congestion.

BACILLINUM OF BURNETT

BIBLIOGRAPHY

Boericke W. :

Pocket Manual of Homoeopathic Materia Medica, p. 101, 1927, NY.

Materia Medica and Repertorium. Verlag Margarete Harms-Leer, 1972., p. 88.

Certier F. :

Thérapeutiques des Voies Respiratoires. Baillére et Fils, 1920, p. 107.

Clarke J.H. :

Dictionary of Practical Materia Medica, London, 1965, p. 237 and 239.

Julian O. A. :

Biothérapiques et Nosodes, Ed. Moloine, 1962.

Materia Medica der Nosoden, 2nd. ed., 1975, Haug-Verlag, Heidelberg.

Tyler M.L. :

Homoeopathic Drug Pictures. London, 1952, p. 830.

HISTORY

It is Burnett who baptises and experiments with this nosode of which the preparation was made at his request by Heath, starting from the sputums of tuberculous patients after having been assured of the presence of B.K. by a microscopic examination. Burnett also experimented, according to Clarke, an other Nosode *Bacillinum testium*, prepared from the testicle of tuberculous patients.

(180)

In U.S.A. Bacillinum was utilised, in high dilution frequently repeated as a preventive of tuberculosis.

There is no real pathogenesis of *Bacillinum*. The experiment of Burnett is essentially clinical.

The symptoms are very similar to those of *Tuberculinum bovinum* of Kent. Fincke and Swan gave an outline study on a nosode prepared with the pus of the tuberculous abcess. This product was sometimes called *Bacillinum* of Fincke and seemed to have been confused with the *Tuberculinum* of Hering.

Bacillinum is not at present sold in French pharmaceutical market.

At Nelson of London may be found *Bacillinum* (Bac. Burnett) 6-CM and *Tuberculinum testiculatum* 30 to M.

STOCK

Lysate of sputum of tubercular patient, in which the presence of B.K. is microscopically verified.

CLINICAL CORTICO-VISCERAL PROTOCOL OR CLINICAL PATHOGENESIS

1. Generalities

Lability of symptoms, child or adult having the "craze for travelling".

The patient has a deep-seated headache ; an eczema of the eyelids ; coughs and spits.

2. Nervous System

Adult : Bacillinum is a depressed patient, sad, irritable, is better nowhere, constantly changes places, country, doctors. He has a craze for movement. He feels uneasy in his own room, like a stranger.

Has *frequent chill*, does not known how or where it comes. *Violent, deep,* depressing headache, better by complete rest, and is aggravated by the slightest movement of the head.

Localisation : Suborbitary, right side, irradiating towards armpit.

Sensation as if there is a tight iron band around the head. (Cactus)

Trembling of hands.

Sensation of coldness, humidity, as if the dress is wet above the dorsal vertebra.

Child : Bacillinum is *always* in *movement*, distracted, emaciated.

Timid, is easily afraid, specially of *black dogs.*

Often wakes up, has a weak body, irritable.

Complains of headache, specially after school tasks.

Headache of students, aggravated by the least exercise, mental exercise, has defective eyesight. (Myopia)

Sleep : *Adult.* Absence of sleep during headache.

The patient sleeps during the day, is *restless at night.*

Child : Restless sleep, with dreams and nocturnal hallucinations.

3. Eyes, Ears

Eczema of the eyelids ; eczema of the ear passage. Impetigo behind ears.

4. Respiratory System

(*a*) *Nose* : Small painful furuncles, situated specially on the nasal orifices. Discharge of foetid pus, greenish. Ozena.

(*b*) *Lungs* : Bronchitis with jerking and fatiguing cough, spasmodic. Pricking pains in the larynx causing cough. Abundant mucus or muco-purulent expectoration. Cough worse at night but very often the patient does not wake up. Cough while sleeping.

5. Digestive System

(*a*) *Mouth* : Toothache.   Teeth sensitive to cold air.   Roots of the teeth are painful.   Abundant dental tartar.   Teeth shoot up badly in children.

(*b*) *Stomach* :   Gastric flatulence with pinching pain under the right ribs.   Appetite diminished or augmented, in the latter case gradual emaciation.

(*c*) *Abdomen* :   Bloated,   meteorism,   indurated   inguinal adenopathy.   Blackish, acquous stools, alternating with stubborn constipation.   Sometimes intestinal hemorrhage. Morning diarrhoea, urging, accompanied by sweats and nausea.

6. Uro-genital Apparatus

Urine, pale, abundant with whitish sediment.   Nycturia.

Dysmenorrhoea, very painful with abundant long continued menstruation.

7. Loco-motor System

General weakness of the back.

Left knee painful, aggravation in the beginning of movement, then amelioration by continued movement, a walk for example.

8. Skin

Impetigo of the head ; pityriasis versicolor, squamous eczema, generalised pruriginous eruptions.

Weeping eczema of the head, behind ears in the folds of the skin.

On the face, specially on the left cheek, some small button like eruptions ; juvenile acne, which persists for long time (Anthrac.) *Alopecia* of the head.

9. Fever

Fever with flushes of heat and perspiration.

10. Modalities

Aggravation : By movement, cold air, at night and in the morning.

Amelioration : By change of weather, continued movement.

POSITIVE DIAGNOSIS

Bacillinum is characterised by :

Patient having the craze for movement.

Headache, deep headache, aggravated by movement.

Eczema of eyelids. Impetigo.

Chronic cough with abundant muco-purulant expectoration.

DIFFERENTIAL DIAGNOSIS

Lac caninum : It is a remedy of changing places, crosswise.

Belladonna : Beginning and ending suddenly. Hypersensitiveness to light and headache, better by tight bandage.

Graphitis : Is indolent, apathetic, obese, constipated and eruption with honey-like secretion.

Chamomilla : Has night cough which does not awake the patient while sleeping, but Chamomilla is a restless patient, too much sensitive to pains, has intolerable pains.

Pulsatilla : A mild type, weeping, having labile character, changing, with a hyposthenia, dyspepsia and troubles of venous stasis. Catarrhal irritation of the muscous membranes with thick greenish yellow excretion, non-irritating.

Natrum muriaticum : Is depressed, with chronic headache, anemic, emaciated, medial fissure of the lower lip and great desire for salt.

As well as *V.A.B.* and *Tuberculinum* (See articles).

POSOLOGY

Dynamisation : May be found with Nelson, London, *Bacillinum Burnetts* 6-CM and Bacillinum testiculatum 30-1M.

CLINILAL DIAGNOSIS

The indications of Bacillinum are very polymorphous because of its spectrum of action extends by the intermediary of nervous system to many regions.

(*a*) **General Diseases**

Denutritional state. Emaciation.

Troubles of growth in children having hereditary tuberculosis.

Tubercular condition (Bernand-Jacquelin syndromes).

Rachitis, Scrofula.

Addison's disease.

(*b*) **Nervous System**

Idiot. Hydrocephale.

Mental unstability.

Student's headache.

Insomnia of children.

(*c*) **Eyes, Ears**

Eczema of eyelids and of the auditive conduite.

(*d*) **Digestive Apparatus**

Dental caries, specially of children.

Intestinal tuberculosis.

(*e*) **Respiratory System**

Tubercular laryngitis.
Chronic bronchitis.
Humid asthma.
Bronchiectasis.
Pulmonary abscess.

(*f*) **Genito-urinary Apparatus**

Uneasiness. Salpnigitis having tuberculous etiology.
Inguinal adenitis.

(*g*) **Loco-motor System**

Arthrosis of knees.

Rheumatism of Poncet-Leriche.

(*h*) **Skin**

Alopecia, impetigo, pytiriasis versicolor.

COMMENTARY

Here we should also mention *Bacillinum testiculatum* or *Tuberculinum testiculatum* (Stock : Testicular tuberculosis), which according to the indications of Burnett, is to be prescribed in male genital tuberculosis, inguinal adenitis and tuberculosis of the mesenteric glands. *Bacillinum* is favoured by Kent and Clarke.

Cartier uses it freely in abundant bronchial secretion. According to the indications given by Margaret Tyler to Dr. Renard, the latter prescribes one dose of *Drosera 7 CH* followed after 15 days by a dose of *Bacillinum 9 CH* in tuberculous conditions.

Voisin considers it as a medicine acting rapidly but not faithfully.

Our own experience is favourable for Bacillinum in children who do not grow well, tuberculinic weakness, and bronchiectasis of children. In the latter case the action of Bacillinum is clearly favourable. The V.A.B. (Ex. B.C.G.) may be substituted by *Bacillinum*, which is at present discontinued in France.

BOTULINUM

BIBLIOGRAPHY

Consult the General Biliography at the end.

STOCK

On principle it is the question of Clostridium Botulinum toxin elaborated in putrified meat of porc. There is no experimental pathogenesis because the substance is extremely toxic. One may doubt whether the Botulic toxin really existed in the products used.

This badly defined product seems to be a kind of Pyrogenium, is not now sold in France.

CLINICAL CORTICO-VISCERAL PROTOCOL OR CLINICAL PATHOGENESIS

Use of this medicine is done basing on the pathological symptoms collected from persons intoxicated.

1. Expressionless face, as if a "mask" after a paretic state.
2. Liquid secretions from the nose.
3. Great thirst, dysphagia.
4. Double vision (diplopia), ptosis.
5. Gastric pain ; abdominal meteorism.
6. Retention of urine and stools.
7. Respiratory paresis, of speech and walk.

DIFFERENTIAL DIAGNOSIS

Benzinum nitricum : Diminution of blood coagulation. Asphyxia of exremities ; eye troubles, mydriasis, nystagmus, rolling of eyeballs.

(187)

Gelsemium : Paresis or spasmodic paralysis of the lower limbs. Mental and physical weakness with tremblings, paresis and paralysis. Absence of thirst. Urgent desire for stools.

Lathyrus : Paresis and spasmodic paralysis of the lower limbs.

Causticum : Chronic state with emaciation, paresis, and paralysis of the upper eyelids, of optic nerves, of vocal chords, of the bladder and intestines, of hands.

CLINICAL DIAGNOSIS

1. Heine-Medin disease.
2. Facial paralysis with ptosis "a frigor"
3. Dyphtheric paralysis.
4. Chronic uremia.

POSOLOGY

Prepared by Nelson, London, in 30—1 M.

BRUCELLA MELITENSIS

BIBLIOGRAPHY

Nussbaum Fournier :

Brucella Melitensis. : l'Homoeop. fr., 1935, p. 799.

Julian O.A. :

Biothérapiques et Nosodes. Maloine, Paris, 1962.
Materia Medica der Nosoden. Haug-Verlag, Heidelberg.
1975, 2nd. ed.

Schmidt Roger :

Brucella. Un Nosode rarement employé. Annales Homoeop.
Fr. 1959, No. 2., p. 113.

HISTORY

Nussbaum Fournier of Perpignan, communicates a study of undulating fever in course of which he prescribed *Tuberculinum* with great success and the *Melitine* the use of which is very delicate. He also uses blood, urinary, and suderal Isopathy.

It is in 1959, when asked by H. Dupart that Roger Schmidt, President of the American Institute of Homoeopathy carried out a study of Brucella.

STOCK

The Melitine is a filtrate of a 21 days old culture of the microbe of undulating fever utilised for the diagnosis of the affection.

POSITIVE DIAGNOSIS

1. Febrile state with *profuse sweat* by the least effort and at night.

2. *Muscular and articular pains,* specially of the lower limbs.

3. Anorexia, emaciation.
4. Headache, irritability, nervousness.
5. Emotive unstability, insomnia.
6. Lymphothymic states, vertigo.
7. Constipation, dry and hard stools.
8. Vesicular eruptions.

Amelioration : By heat and in the sun.

Aggravation : By prolonged exercise, in hot room, by sea breeze, by humidity, during storm.

DIFFERENTIAL DIAGNOSIS

Natrum muriaticum : Emaciation with anemia, cachexia. depression, headaches, constipation, sensitiveness to cold, desire for salt, mapped tongue.

Gelsemium : General weakness with tremblings ; headache with heaviness ; weakness of limbs, slow pulse.

Ferrum phosphoricum : Febrile states with full, rapid and soft pulse, thirst and sweats that does not ameliorate.

CLINICAL DIAGNOSIS

1. Chronic Malta fever.
2. Myalgia.
3, Subacute polyarthritis,
4. Orchitis and orchy epididymitis.
5. Neurasthanis.

CLINICAL CASES

Two cases of Roger Schmidt, p. 115-116 in Annales hom. Fr., No. 2. 1959.

Case 1 : Acute case

M.W.F.R.......a butcher of 43 years old, called me on the 18th October, 1948, for high fever 103.°4 F in the evening which lasts since three days. Profuse sweat on the upper part of the body, preceded by shivering which jerks him from head to foot. During the fever he is very restless, is hungry, and has the desire to drink cold water. The diagnosis was very easy because the patient said, while telling me his history, having been treated for an acute brucellosis a few years ago, in 1935 and that 50% of the workers of the same firm were affected. At that time M.W.R. should stop his work for a year. The fever, he said to me, caused to fall all his hairs, that fortunately grew again on. In 1940 and 1941, he had two new attacks that were treated by serum. In 1949, a new relapse complicated with anemia, which was treated by *Penicillin* and *Vaccins*. He tells me that since that time he always feels weak. I sent him to the Hahnemann Hospital where my diagnosis was confirmed by the agglutination test although the culture of urine and blood was negative. *Gelsemium* 6, ameliorated the fever in 24 hours *i.e.* to say the temperature did not rise above 99° 5 F. One week later, the patient had a diarrhoea with profuse sweats which was rapidly ameliorated by *China 6*. During the following month he took weight by 8 pounds and was feeling better than he never was. My intention was to complete the cure by the Nosode but I had not the chance for it, because in order to be able to begin again his work M.W.F.R. was forced to see the doctors of the company who treated him before.

Case 2

Mme. H.B....of San Diago, married, age 69 came to see me in September 1950, and complained of some gastric troubles from which she was suffering since several months ; she was also suffering from wind, vomiting, regurgitations, as well as from a stubborn constipations.

Constantly depressed and weak, she became nervous, restless and had shiverings. She felt sudden weakness, had vertigo by the least movement. She was under the care of another doctor for many months. Unfortunately there was no amelioration. While she was young she suffered from a perforated appendix. Physical examination negative, except a distended abdomen, an arterial tension 160/75. hyperkinetic pulse, and a marked secondary anemia. Weight 141 pounds, height 5′ 1″.

After her return to San Diago she asked me to prescribe by correspondence. *Arsenicum, Sulphur, Nux vomica, Carbo. veg., Kali phos., Carbo. sulph.* did her some good but these variety of remedies shows that the case was jumbled when it is difficult to get a simillium. Finally in July, 1951, I had the idea that this may be a case of Brucellosis ; the sudden attack of fever and sweats, loss of weights (7 pounds), the persistence of some symptoms indicated the diagnosis. I gave her *Brucella melitensis 10 M.*

Without any delay the patient informed me that this was the first remedy that gave her almost instantaneous result. This is the typical response of a homoeopathic remedy. She soon took up weight, but after six weeks she complained anew of serious vertigo and the stubborn constipation that were cured by *Brucella melitensis 30*, and for 3 months her condition was satisfactory.

On the 6th December, 1951, she had fever anew with profuse sweat and complained of abdominal pains. I gave her *Brucella 10 M* which caused a moderate aggravation but clearly ameliorating during two weeks, with a maximum temperature of 100°F during the day, which ended in a long period of amelioration which lasted for 3 years.

CANCER NOSODES

Consult : General Bibliography.

At present, because of the historical interest, it is felt necessary to mention here the different Cancer Nosodes. However, these are not in much practical use now and according to some homoeopaths their use is not to be encouraged.

Some nosodes are homoeopathically prepared from cancer tissues :

1. *Epitheliomine* : Extract of epithelioma.

2. *Scirrhinum* : Extract of squirrhe.

3. *Carcinosin* : Extract of any kind of cancer.

It is Cahis of Barcelona who utilised the cancer toxin and *Pan cancro* in different dilutions and mixtures.

Then it is Dr. Nebel who prepared Micrococcin in 30, 200, MK from micrococcus of Doyen. The author obtained some favourable results on condition that the patients should have been well drained and correctly followed.

Then Dr. Nebel prepared *"Onkolysines"* from a stock of *Onkomyxa Neojormans* and with those Onkolysines the author had favourable results but he always took good care to do a homoeopathic drainage of the heart, kidney and intestines.

Jean Roy of Paris has, in his turn specified Oscill ococcinum but it was revealed that its uses are more favourable in otitis after influenza.

Finally Dr. Rubens Duval specified a whole series of extract of cancer tumors, of histologic varieties and in weak doses 10—21 in the form of gloubles.

(193)

Such are the historical informations in short concerning cancer nosodes.

A renewal takes shape at present in quite a different sense with researches of Foubister, pediatrist of Royal London Homoeopathic hospital, regarding Carcinosin or Carcinosinum about waich ample information is to be found in articles on Carcinosin.

Let us note that Reckeweg of Germany prepares at present the stocks of the following nosodes :

Carcinosinum—Injeel + forte (D 15), D 20, D 200 and unitary dynamisation D 200.

Carc-hepat. metastat -- Injeel + forte (D 6), D 10, D 30, D 200.

Car. laryngis—Nosode--Injeel + forte (D 6), D 10, D 30, D 200.

Carc. mamae—Injeel + Forte (D 6), D 10, D 30, D 200.

The first stock is indicated in all the forms of neoplasma, The others are specifics.

They form a part of biotherapic treatment by biotherapics specified by H. Reckeweg.

CARCINOSINUM OR CARCINOSIN

BIBLIOGRAPHY

Foubister M. :

Carcinosin. British homeop. Journal, 1954.

Templeton W. :

Carcinosin. B.H.J., April 1954.

Julian O.A. :

Biotherapiques et Nosodes, Maloine, Paris, 1962

Hui-Bon-Hoa J. :

Carcinosinum. Etude pathogenesic et clinique. Annales Homeop. fr. October, 1962, p. 5.

Solvey M. :

A modern look at Corcinosins. Journal of the American Institute of Homoeopathy, v. 68, 3 Sept., 1975, p. 159.

HISTORY

Templeton made an experiment "provers" in 1952-53 with 9 subjects and 8 witnesses. The 30th and 40th dilution used.

Some clinical researches were done by Foubister who gave a clinical pathogenesis, later on taken up again by Templeton.

STOCK

At present in foreign markets (England) are found some stocks received from operation theatre of Royal **London** Homoeopathic Hospital of which here is the list :

1. *Carcinosin-adeno-stom.* (Adeno carcinoma of the stomach), dilution 6 CH to 30 CH.

2. *Carcinosin-adeno-vesica* (Papillary adeno-carcinoma of the bladder). Dilution 6 CH to 30 CH.

(195)

3. *Carcinosin intestinal comp.* (Intestinal cancer of different stocks). Dilution 6 C.I to 30 CH.

4. *Carcinosin scir. mam.* (Scirrhus of Mamae). Dilution. 6 CH to 200 CH.

5. *Carcinosin squam. pulm.* (Pulmonary cancer). Dilution 6 CH to 30 CH.

6. Carcinosin (1st stock used by the author). Dilution 30 CH to 1000 CH to 10 M, 50 M, CM.

The multiplicity of preparations is the reason for warning the doctors to prescribe to a patient a nosode in relation to an organ which should not be suspected of a neoplasma. Thus one may prescribe pulmonary Carsinosin to a patient having a pulmonary affection but one is sure that there is actually no cancer formation.

The preparations of Nelson come from America of which the stocks are undetermined.

CLINICAL CORTICO-VISCERAL PROTOCOL OR CLINICAL PATHOGENESIS

1. Generalities

The prescription of this nosode should be absolutely forbidden to a patient actually having cancer or suspected of having a cancer.

According to Foubister, this nosode finds its indications specially as a remedy of ground and of which the therapeutic effect is on the constitution of children or of adults having pernicious anemia, or of cancer.

Predisposition to diseases like pneumonia, and whooping cough of babies.

Carcinosinum is indicated specially in Carbonic constitutions of Leon Vannier and Sulphur constitution of H. Bernard.

Individual having pale colour of the skin, sclerotic blue, and carriers of naevi.

General symptomatology :

Children having numerous acute infantile affections.

Slight hyperthermia, which is temporary after the absorption of Carcinosin in children.

Action of carcinosin .

Action, deep and of long duration.

Children having the colour of milk-coffee, with sclerotic blues, numerous naevi and suffering from insomnia.

Children having tendency to acute pulmonary affections (pneumonia, whooping cough). Knee-elbow position during sleep in children (Medorrhinum, Calcarea phosphorica, Lycopodium, Sepia, Tuberculinum, Phosphorus).

2. Nervous System

(*a*) **Psychic** :

Intellectual torpor.

Thinks with difficulty ; indifference ; *apathy.*

Worse by conversation.

Tendency to suicide. Dislike consolation.

Children have great *fear*, sensitive to reprimands, but is sympathetic to others.

Particularly sensitive to music and to dance.

Fear in the pit of the stomach with the desire to vomit.

Obstinate : Desire for travel.

Child, mentally deficient with loss of interest, understands with difficulty.

Meticulous character (Arsenicum, Anacardium, Nux-vomica, Graphitis) ; whimsical (Tuberculinum), likes to look at storms (Sepia).

(*b*) **Nervous** : Insomnia. Takes long time to fall asleep. Restless sleep.

Headache before storm. Beating headache with cerebral constrictions.

Sleeps in knee-pectoral position up to nine months.

Sleeps on the back with hands on head in case of young children.

Bizarre tics ; blinking of eyes ; tears skin around the nails.

Grimaces.

3. Digestive System

Sensitive gums, toothache.

Aversion to salt, milk, eggs, fat meat, fruits or desire for the same materials.

Digestive troubles in children. Diarrhoea or constipation and autonomia.

Pain of the palate, worse by hot drinks.

Tendency to constipation.

4. Cardic-hemo-vascular System

Violent cardiac palpitation.

Sensation of constriction of the heart.

Thoracic oppression with desire for deep respiration.

5. Respiratory System

Asthma ameliorated on sea-side.

6. Uro-genital System

Albuminuric hematuria.

7. Locomotor System

Trembling of the muscles of thighs, of arms and back.

Pain, weakness, fatigue, numbness of thighs, better by a short sleep.

Pain in legs, ameliorated by heat and by moderate movement, aggravated by rapid movement.

8. Skin

Numerous naevi.

Acne of the face.

9. Modality

Amelioration by stormy weather, in the evening, on sea-side, by a short sleep.

Aggravation on sea (very often it is the amelioration which is to be noted), while undressing, speaking, laughing.

POSITIVE DIAGNOSIS

Family antecedant : Cancer, diabetes, tuberculosis, pernicious anemia.

Personal antecedants : Whooping cough, pneumopathies in lower age.

Amelioration or aggravation on sea-side.

Desire or aversion for salt, milk, eggs, fats, fruits.

Genou-pectoral position during sleep.

When a homoeopathic remedy is prescribed, it does not act or does not act well.

DIFFRENTIAL DIAGNOSIS

Tuberculinum, Medorrhinum, Natrum muriaticum, Sepia, Alumina, Phosphorus, Calcarea phos., Luesinum, Lycopodium, Sulphur, Psorinum, Arsenicum, Nux vomica, Anacardium, Graphitis.

CLINICAL DIAGNOSIS

Allergic (psoric) condition ; tubercular condition.

Pre-cancer state.

Learning late ; retarded student.

Characterial troubles.

Trisomic 21 (mongolism).

Insomnia of children and old men.

Diathesic conditions. Diabetes, chronic tuberculosis, anemia. Depressive state with tendency to suicide.

Chronic hepatosis ; migraine ; sexual weakness ; masturbation of young people. Tics.

Parasitosis ; Constipation ; Dorsalgias ; Sacralgias ; Sciatica.

POSOLOGY

Dynamisations :

The English authors recommend as follows :

Carcinosinum   : 6 CH, 12 CH, 30 CH, 200 CH, M.

C. Adeno vesica : 6 CH, 12 CH, 30 CH.

C. Adeno stom. : 6 CH, 12 CH, 30 CH.

C. Intestin co.   : 6 CH, 12 CH, 30 CH.

C. Scir. mam.   : 6 CH, 12 CH, 30 CH.

COLIBACILLINUM

BIBLIOGRAPHY

Vannier L. :

Colibacilline, l'Hom fr., 1933, fev., No. 2, p. 132-134.

Jullian O.A. :

Biothérapiques et Nosodes. Maloine, Paris, 1962.

Lefort :

Aspects de l'Homoeopathie—chapitre : Particularité psychiques de Colibacillinum. La mémoire. Edition Franése, 1963, p. 246-265.

Hui Bon. Hoa J. :

Revue des livers. Annales hom. fr., nov., 1963. Indications de Colibacillinum. d'aprés le Dr. Gosh.

Baruk Henri :

Traitè de psychiatrie. t. II, p. 891-895 ; p. 1093-1096. Masson et Cie, Paris, 1959.

Vannier L. :

L'isothérapie dans les maladies des voies urinaires. Revue bélge d'hom., 1949.

Lefort :

Particularités psychiques de Colibacillinum. Bulletin, Soc., Homeop. d'Aquitaine, No. 7, avril 1954.

Wurmser L. :

Biothérapiques anti-colibacillaires. Bulletin C.H.F., 1961, p. 27-33.

Vannier L. :

et Poirier/J. Precis de Matiére médicale homoeopathique Doin, Paris, 1958.

Jeannes, Tetau M, et Fouche L. :

Expèrimentation pharmacologique de la Folliculo-stimuline hypophysaire diluée. Annales hom. fr. No. 4, 1972.

Fouche L. :

Micro-hormonothérapie dynamisée : la Folliculo-stimuline.

Course de 2e année a l'Institut d'Enseignement et de Recherche de la Société Médicale de Biothérapie.

STOCK

The biothérapique *Colibacillinum* is prepared from the lysate obtained with the addition of artiseptic from the culture made out of a mixture of several Colibacilli stocks.

Escherichia coli belong to entero-bacterias of which there are two groups : Escheria and Shigella.

Escherichia coli was isolated in 1881 by Escherich from fecal matters of new borns.

PREPARATION

1. Stock Used

Three stocks of Escherichia coli, Marcy 423, 430, 431.

These stocks have the classical character of the type.

They are controlled from the point of view of the morphological type, biochemic and antigenic character.

Mobile sticks, Gram negative, round soft, opaque.

Lactose, glucose, arabinose, xylose, maltose, mannite, rhamnose plus G. citrate— ; I+, M+, VP—, H2S − ; Gelatine 0, coagulated milk.

They are preserved in lyophilised condition.

2. Medium of Culture

(a)	Maceration of chopped meat	500 g
	Water	1,000 ml

Put in contact for 24 hours, then filtre after having heated in autoclave for 30 mts. at 100° and 30 mts. at 110°.

(*b*) Add :

Peptone	12 g
Sodium chloride	5 g
Powder gelose	30 g

(*c*) Adjust the pH at 7, 2 by the addition of Sodium.

(*d*) Put on autoclave at 110° for 20 mts.

(*e*) Distribute in tubes in Roux boxes.

(*f*) Sterilise at 110° for 20 mts.

3. Inoculation and Culture

The three lyophilised stocks are put back again in solution then inoculated on inclined tubes in a medium described previously. After 20 hours of culture on stove at 37° the colonies are examined to ascertain the characteristic types of these cultures and the purity of the stocks.

The culture of each tube is washed in a volume of 5 mg solution of 9% Sodium chloride, then taken in droppers for inoculating on Roux boxes containing 1,200 ml of the same medium.

The Roux boxes are in their turn put on stove at 37°. After 48 hours of stay on the stove the boxes are examined individually in order to be assured of the purity of the colonies.

Then to each is added 25 to 30 ml of sterile water. After suspension of the microbian culture by manual balancing the bacterial suspension is adjusted to 20 millards of germs per mililitre by the addition of sterile water.

The suspension thus obtained is heated at 56° for 45 mts. then placed immediatly in refrigerator at +4°, +5°.

4. Lysate and the Getting of the Endotoxins

The bacterian suspension is transferred in a recipient of resistant pyrex glass. It is then congealed at a temperature of 30° to 40° for 24 hours. Then the suspension is left to be decongealed and left at + 20° during 20 hours. The total operation congealing-decongealing is again resumed 3 times *i.e.* 4 operations in all.

It is then taken centrifuged in some sterile tubes at a speed of 6,000 t/m for a time sufficient to obtain a complete sedimentation of the lysated bacterian debris.

The floating suspension of endotoxins is then collected for filtration on Seitz EKS and preserved in refrigerator at +3°, +5°.

5. Detoxification

The suspension of endotoxins is added to an equal volume of distilled water and heated at 75° for one hour and at an interval of 24 hours.

6. Distribution

Then it is distributed in sterile ampouls.

Trial of the non-toxicity : To 5 white mice weighing 20 gr, 2 mlg of the lysate is injected subcutaneously ; 5 other receive 0·5 mlg intraperitonially. The mortality should be nil. If one animal dies, the experiment is recommenced and if the same thing happens the lysate should be rejected.

Sterility : 2 mlg of lysate is inoculated in 2 mlg of medium of thioglycolate. The culture may not be proved even after 7 days of incubation at 37°.

HISTORY

The clinical pathogenesis of Colibacillinum was given by Léon Vannier under the heading Isotherapy, p. 132-134 of l'Homoeopathie francaise No. 2, February, 1933.

Léon Vannier saw in the works of Prof. H. Baruk which was first communicated on the 30 October, 1932, and appeared in the Bulletin medicale, the possibility of "Isotherapic use of Colibacillinum.

Afterwards Allendy used Colibacillinum in psychic affections of Coli origin.

Fortier Bernoville issued a special issue of l'Homoeopathic Moderne on Colibacilline, No. 16 of 15th November, 1934, with the collaboration of A Pretet, Kollisch, Allendy, F. Bernoville and M. Martiny.

La société médicale homoeopathique de Normandie of which Dr. O.A. Julian was the founder and general secretary has also devoted a special issue of Archives Homoeopathiques de Normandie No. 15, 1958 on this subject.

CLINICAL CORTICO VISCERAL PROTOCOL
OR CLINICAL PATHOGENESIS

We are going to sketch a clinical pathogenesis basing ourselves on the clinical works and clinical experiences of H. Baruk, of Vincent and of Homoeopaths like L. Vannier, Allendy, F. Bernoville and their contemporaries.

1. Generalities

General fatigue and depression which goes on aggravating with digestive and urinary troubles.

Psycho-motor weakness.

Permanent worn out condition.

Quasi Permanent asthenia with somatic and mental weakness.

2. Endocrine psychic System

(a) **Psychic** : *Empty feeling in the head, great timidity, indecision.*

Always hestitating, cannot decide on anything.

Amnesia of recent happenings with great difficulty to find out the right word.

Constant mental *confusion* because of the loss of memory.

Forgets proper names.

The patient complains of loss of memory. Sometimes it is due to an old urinary or intestinal trouble. Everything has started from that time.

Uses very often one word for another.

Depressive melancholia.

Obsessional neurosis.

Confused deliriums.

Schizophrenic states, loss of contact with his environment and with his own reality.

(*b*) **Nervous** :

Frontal and suborbitary headache, worse by humid coldness, after contrariety and strong emotion.

Unilateral swelling of the upper eyelids, sometimes left, sometimes right. To L. Vanniér it is a key-symptom which is contested by F.-Bernoville.

Catotonic condition with somnolence and oneiric dreams.

Heavy somnolence ; hypersomnia.

(*c*) **Endocrines** :

Hyposurrenalism, progressive asthenia, lumbar pains.

Hyperthyroidia : Chilly, specially post prandial or nocturnal chill.

3. **Digestive Apparatus**

(*a*) **Mouth, tongue, pharynx** :

Flax tongue, coated, rosy with a median band (L. Vannier) extending from the root to the point.

United glossy spots without papillies on the median strip. White tongue.

(*b*) **Stomach, intestines, abdomen** :

Capricious appetite or anorexia.

Very slow digestion with the sensation of the stomach remaining heavy for a long time.

Post prandial bloating.

Sensation of intense coldness with chill immediately after meals.

Worse after injection of milk.

Big sensitive liver. Gall bladder, painful.

Slow intestinal transit.

Flatulence, intestinal spasms.

Heaviness and drawing in the intestines.

Rumbling in right caeco-colic region.

Expulsion of putrid gas.

Constipation.

In babies and young children, profuse weakening diarrhoea with hypothermia, bradycardia, dehydration.

4. Cardio-hemo-vascular System

Hypotension, tendency to weakness, even collapse.

Paleness, anxiety, vertigo, sweats, sound of the heart become muffled, and lowering of the arterial tension.

Thermoregulation : Fever with great weakness.

5. Uro-genital Apparatus

(a) Urinary :

Troubled urine with bad smell, does not become eclear after rest.

Frequent micturition of little quantity everytime, painful with the sensation of burning at the end of the flow.

The sensation as if he must go again to pass urine immediately after micturition.

Painful sensation in the region of kidney.

Pain along the urethra, costo-lumbar pain, painful to palpation.

Aggravation of urinary troubles in cold humid weather.

Heat and burning after urination.

Sometimes hematuria.

(b) **Genital** :

Man : Erection and ejaculation sometimes painful, with the sensation of burning in the urethra after coition.

Woman : Heaviness of the lower abdomen with bi-lateral ovarian pains.

Algomenorrhoea.

Yellow leucorrhoea, slightly irriating.

Sexual relation becomes difficult, with vulvo-vaginal burning sensation.

6. **Locomotor System**

Polyarticular pains ; swelling of small joints of legs and hands.

7. **Modalities**

(a) *Aggravation* :
By cold, humid cold ; on sea-side, after rest, by milk.

(b) *Amelioration* :
By heat.

(c) *Laterality* :
Right, not characteristic.

POSOLOGY

Dynamisation : 4 CH to 30 CH.

Prescription of several dilutions at a time will help to get a rapid and better result.

POSITIVE DIAGNOSIS

Asthenia, timidity, amnesia (uses one word for another).

Slow digestion, intestinal spasms and gurgling in the right. Caeco-colic region.

In babies : diarrhoea with dehydration.

Frequent micturition, burning, with pain in the costo-lumbar region of the right side.

Irritation of genital organs (vulvo-vaginitis ; urethritis with burning pains).

Key symptoms :

Swelling of upper eyelids.

Tongue with a median glossy zone without papilliae.

DIFFERENTIAL DIAGNOSIS

Regarding classical Homoeopathy we must think of :

Psorinum (see article). *Medorrhinum* (see article), *Anacardium, Lycopodium, Sepia, Thuya,* etc.

Regarding modern Homoeopathy :

Thymol : Syncopal tendency, state of aberration, temporal headache : frequent micturition, with imperious urging ; leucorrhoea.

Folliculinum : Anxiety. Abdominal meteorism, repeated cystitis, alternate diarrhoea and constipation.

Folliculostimuline : It has been specified by Fouchet in 9 CH in all acute or chronic manifestations of colibacillosis. But the prescription should be 2 to 3 subcutaneous or intramuscular injections a week.

Cynodon dactylon : Cortico-somatic weakness, heavy sleep, abdominal flatulence, urethral pain after micturition with the impression that the micturition is not complete ; irritating, acid noisy stools.

CLINICAL DIAGNOSIS

1. Generalities

Allergoso-tuberculinic condition with dragging chronic enterorenal infection.

Syndrome of worn out condition of Jacquelin Bernand.

Chronic colibacillosis ; tuberculinosis ; typhoid fever (Gosh).

2. Neuro-endocrino-psychic System

Hypocorticism.

Addition's disease (adjuvant treatment).

Colibacillary meningitis (adjuvant treatment).

Colibacillary meningo encephalitis (adjuvant treatment).

Colibacillary encephalitis lethargica (adjuvant treatment).

Colibacillary myelitis of Gilbert of Lyon (adjuvant treatment).

Puerperal psychosis.

Schizophrenia, dementia precox.

Schizophrenia, catatonic stage.

Mental confusion.

Melancholia or lypomania of Esquirol.

Hypersomnia. Insomnia in the morning.

3. Digestive Apparatus

Progressive chilliness of the new-born or athrepsia of Parrot

Hepatocholitis, angiocholitis.

Chronic cholecystitis.

Chronic appendicitis ; chronic gastro-enteritis.

Entero-hepatic syndrome.

Verminosis of children.

Spasmodic colitis.

4. Cardio-hemo-vascular System

Endocrino-neurosis ; hypotension of Lean and Blondel.

Orthostatic hypotension of Lobry and Doumar.

5. Uro-genital Apparatus

Subacute puerperal fever. (Gosh)

Post-partum enteritis. (Gosh)

Colibacillary pyelo-nephritis.

Colibacillary prostato-vesicularitis.

Relapsing epydidimitis.

Acute or chronic colibacillosis.

Cystitis, prostatitis.

Salpingitis, metritis, vaginitis.

6. **Locomotor System**

Rheumatism of Poncet and Leriche.

Infective rheumatism.

Chronic degenerative rheumatism.

COMMENTARY

Colibacillinum merits neither that "excess of honour" nor that "indignity".

If according to L. Vannier this remedy shows itself to be useful in the affection having etiology of B. Coli and having impregnated moleculo-tissular espace by their endotoxin ; we should not contest the complete therapeutic action as it is done by F.-Bernoville.

But F.-Bernoville after all accepts its action in psychic manifestations. Allendy after using high dilutions have obtained good results.

We also think that Coli B. should be prescribed either in the 30 CH, or combination of 30 CH + 15 CH + 7 CH, twice a day for a long time.

In ordinary psychosis, dragging genito-urinary troubles it is surely useful.

In acute stages, it is to be replaced by *Anti-Coli-Serum*.

Finally one should not forget that a contradictional pathological totality is to be treated and that the prescription of other biotherapics will help to get back the physiological norm.

To this B. Coli may be a valuable help.

8 F

DENYS

Consult : General Bibliography.

HISTORY

It is Denys of Louvain who prepared this product in 1896.

STOCK

The filtered Bouillon of Denys was a tuberculin prepared after the separation of the microbes by filtration on bougie and non-concentrated. According to Calmette, it contains a thermolabile toxalbumine which differentiates itself from classical tuberculine.

At present this product is not available. The stocks of *Denys* is not preserved in the University of Louvin.

CLINICAL CORTICO-VISCERAL PROTOCOL
OR CLINICAL PATHOGENESIS

It results out of the observations of troubles caused by the abusive use of filtered bouillon.

1. Generalities

Sudden illness with functional troubles even lesional in persons having apparently good health.

Florid persons, with red face, congested.

Sudden depression and weakness, sometimes irregular.

Want of resistence to fatigue.

2. Nervous System

Depression with weakness which comes suddenly. There is no fixed time.

Migraine, irregular, intermittent, comes suddenly, of variable duration, 2 to 3 days or may last for 15 days, disappearing

(212)

suddenly to return suddenly at the end of 15 days even after 2 to 3 months in the same manner.

Migraine with or without fever.

3. Respiratory Apparatus

Sudden coryza that comes without any apparent reason. Discharge of liquid serous which is non-irritant and disappears suddenly.

Huskiness with the same character of suddenness.

Thoracic pains : Costal and of the nipples, especially right side.

Repeated *bronchitis*.

Asthma of plethorics.

4. Circulatory Apparatus

Precordial pains, some painful points after walking or doing some efforts.

Hypotension with the sensation of uneasiness and weakness.

5. Digestive Apparatus

Anorexia, having the character of suddenness.

Gastric uneasiness with sudden vomiting and nausea.

Diarrhoea, watery of soft stools, frothy, frequent for 2, 3, 4 days then ceasing suddenly.

Sudden appendicular inflammation, irregular.

6. Fever

Fever without any fixed time.

Pain with intense fatigue.

7. Skin

Oozing vesicular eruptions.

8. Modalities

Aggravation : By the least effort.

Amelioration : By rest.

POSITIVE DIAGNOSIS

1. Sudden pathological troubles, functional or lesional.
2. Migraine with fever.
3. Coryza with abundant acquous discharge.
4. Gastric troubles.
5. Watery diarrhoea.
6. Fever by the least effort.

DIFFERENTIAL DIAGNOSIS

Sulphur : Congestive states, auto-intoxication. Weakness at 11 a.m. Acquous diarrhoea at 5 a.m.

Sulphur-iod. : Emaciation, hypertrophy of ganglions. Cough and persisting itching eruptions.

Nux-vomica : Gastric troubles, vertigo, sneezing when walking up in the morning.

Pulsatilla : Venous congestion, changing symptoms, diarrhoea, coryza, stomach troubles after fatty food.

CLINICAL DIAGNOSIS

1. Generalities : Florid tubercular state.

Fibrous tuberculosis of plethorics.

2. Nervous system : Magraine ; depressive states.

3. Respiratory apparatus : Asthma of plethorics ; chronic bronchitis, coryza.

4. Circulatory apparatus : Hypertension ; acrocyanosis.

5. Digestive apparatus : Gastritis ; enterocolitis.

6. Skin : Eczema.

7. Locomotor system : Chronic deforming rheumatism.

POSOLOGY

At Nelson : Denys (Tuberculinum Denys) 12-1 M.

DIPHTHERINUM—DIPHTHEROTOXINUM DIPHTHERICUM

BIBLIOGRAPHY

Julian O.A. :

Materia Medica der Nosoden. Haug Verlag, Ulm/Donau 1960. Biothérapiques et Nosodes. Librairle Maloine 1962, Paris.

Zissu R. :

Pathogenesie clinique de Diphtérotoxinum. Annales homoeop·, nov,, 1964, p. 51/935.

Boericke W. :

Pocket Manual of Homoeopathic Materia Medica, 9th ed., Boericke and Tafel, Phil., 1927.

Materia Medica und Repertorium. tr. in German by, M. Harms Verlag Grundlagen und Praxis. Morgarate Harms Leer, 1972.

Romeyer :

Diphtèrie sans sérum. l'Homoeopathie Moderne, 1938, No. 16, p. 333-358.

Cartier Fr. :

Therapeutique des Voies Respiratories, 2nd. ed., Baillére and Sons, Paris 1920.

R. Schmitz-Harbauer :

Nosoden—Fälle, Zeitschrift f. Klassische Homöopathie, No. 2, p. 65, 1963, ed. 7.

Zinke :

Diphtherinum und Scarlatinum bei Tonsillen Affektionen, in Kongress berich über die 123 Jaresversammlung—Pischel. Allg. Hamöop., Ztz. No. 4, 1972, p. 123.

Chavanon P. :

La Diphtérie, 4e ed., Imprimérie St-Denis, Niort, 1932.

Allen H.C. :

The Materia Medica of the Nosodes. Boericke & Tafel. Philadelphia, 1910.

Julian O.A. :

Prevention et traitement bio-hemo-therapique des complication vaccinales 1973. Le françois, Paris 75006.

Tilitcheff :

Etude sur les syndromes chroniques post-diphtériques. L'Homoeopathie Française, 1950.

Chavanon P. :

Immunisation contre la Diphtérie. L'Homoeopathie moderne, 1934.

Desjars P. :

Commentaires a propos d'un cas de Diphterie. L'Hamoeopathie moderne, 1957.

Bernard H. :

Traitement homoeopathique de la Diphterie. L'Homoeopathie Moderne, 1937.
Nouveau traite d'Homoeopathie. t. 2, Coquemard Angouleme, 1947.

Collet J.M. :

Isopathie. Méthode Pasteur par voie interne demontrant la certitude et l'unite de Za Science Médicale, 2e ed., Vigot Fréres. 1902.

Clarke J. :

A dictionary of Practical Materia Medica, 1955, p. 665, t. 1.

HISTORY

It was on May, 1874 that Rev. Dr. T,J.M. Collet, during an epidemic in Mosul, Mesopotamia prepared an isotherapic from diphtheric membranes taken from a young girl of 20. For doing that he rolled a ribbon cloth around a stiletto so as to form a small brush. "I placed it on a coat on a tonsil and rubbed it for a moment by turning it on itself, then taking out the brush I found that some debris of false membranes are stuck to it. I cut out the end of the brush and put them in teaspoonful of water for being wet in a 150 grams long necked bottle. I shook the whole thing for about a minute and thus I obtained the 1st dilution. I did not stop there but I made several dilutions successively until I obtained the 5th centesimal dilution in alcohol. I impregnated some inactive globules of sugar of milk ; I made many packets of globules, then I crushed them for making their application more easy and I prescribed them for being dissolved according to the requirements, each in a big glass of water and to give the solution to the patient a table spoonful every 10 minutes. (p. 227-228, Isopathy).

At the end of 5 days the patient was cured. A second case of 11 June, 1874, with the same stock, then a 3rd case cured within 4 to 5 days. Then many other cases followed with the good results.

Collet named this isotherapic *Dipterine*, it is the *Diphtherinum* of Allen, Clarke, Boericke, Swan.

Boericke according to the 9th edition and the 1st German edition of 1972, maintains the indications given by Collet.

The same is the case with Clarke who mentions moreover the Diphtherio toxin contained in the membrane.

H.C. Allen in his book, "Materia Medica of Nosodes," Phila., 1910. p. 38-39, prepared Diphtherinum from diphtheric membrane in the 6th contesimal dynamised by Swan. "The Diphtheric virus" or the "Diphthero toxin" is at the base of the "Antitoxic Serum." "These dilutions have proved themselves to be efficacious, not only in diphtheria (malignant) but also in numerous cases of post-diphtheric paralysis and nervous affections after the use of the antitoxin." Having indicated the use of Diphthero toxin and antitoxic serum of Behring. Allen gives a description of the clinical pathogenesis of Diphtherinum.

This clinical pathogenesis may be summarised as follows :

Very weak subject, apathic and very much weak to make complain. State of stupor from which he comes out when he is talked to. The tonsils are swollen, red, swelling of the glands of the neck, breath and expectoration foetid, abhorring ; on the tonsils are seen thick membranes, light gray of chestnut colour ; thick tongue ; hypothermia ; weak and rapid pulse, cold extremities. The patient is prostrated, vague look, besotted, epistaxis. This state may end in collapse.

This is in fact the clinical description of Diphtheria.

But we must not forget that we have described historically the description of Diphtherinum (Nelson : Diptherium—membrane, trituration.) 6—CM.

The diphtheric nosode in conformity with french pharmaceutic legislation is no more prepared by any French laboratory, having no legislation for preparation. It is therefore not legally prescribed in France.

On the contrary we have Diphtherotoxinum and Diphthericum by Cahis of Barcelona (Spain). (Journal Belge d'homoeopathie, 1912, in Cartier, p. 112, La therapeutique des voies respiratoires).

Cahis prepares it from the filtrate of culture of the bacilli of Loeffler (see under Stock and the present method of preparation). Later on an admirable French homoeopath *Paul Chavanon* introduced it in clinical preparation. (Chavanon prepares some dynamisations according to the method of Korsakov with the dynamiser of A. Berne) in 6, 12, 30, 100, 200, 1000, 4000 and 8000 K (Korsakovin dynamisations are no more found in France). He tried the first Homoeopathic vaccin against diphtheria with 4000 and 8000 and tried to obtain the negativation of Schick's reaction. But the partial results and experiment on limited number of subjects are not conclusive. In 1953, during a study travel in Israel, O.A. Julian, after having spoken with the doctor inspector of hygiene of Tel Aviv, obtained the agreement of the latter for an experimental trial of vaccination on a group of 500 children and as much witnesses.

Returning at Paris he contacted P. Chavanon. who, being enthusiastic, began to work and after 3 weeks a packet of Diphtherotoxinum 4000 and 8000 was sent to Tel. Aviv.

Unfortunately the doctor in the meantime was on a study tour in India and the doctor who replaced him refused to do the trial.

As regards Diphthericum which is anti-diphtheric serum was introduced in the clinical practice of Nosodotherapy by Fortiei Bernoville (1935) and Barishac.

STOCK

Diphtherotoxinum

The biotherapic is prepared from Diphtheria toxin diluted for intradermal reaction of Schick described in the Codex, 1949, p. 957, obtained from Pasteur Institute.

The diluted Diphtheria toxin or *Toxinum diphthericum dilutum* is obtained by diluting with isotonic solution of Sodium chloride, the liquid of the culture of diphtheric bacilli recently prepared and filtered on a bougie of porcelain. This dilution should be such that 0.1 cm^3 of the toxin thus diluted should contain a quantity of toxin equal to the 50th of the does which, while injected sub-cutaneously, determines within 4 days the death of a cobaye of 250g. This diluted toxin serves only for the experiment of Schick, which helps to create in man a state of immunity from Diphtheria.

Diphthericum

This biotherapic is obtained from liquid anti-diphtheric serum described in the Codex, 1949, p. 737, titrated to 3000 units per ampoule of 10 cm³ obtained from the Pasteur Institute.

The anti-diphtheric serum is an antitoxic serum obtained from animals who were immunised with Diphtherio toxin elaborated by Corynebacterium diphtheriae, *i. e.*, with different transformed products of that toxin (anatoxin). This serum is endowed with specific property of neutralising the Diphthero toxin and make it inoffensive for the animals. It may be used preventively and curatively.

The anti-diphtheric serum may be used either as it is obtained from the aseptically taken blood from the numerous animals (liquid anti-diphtheric serum), or after appropriate purification in order to free it from a portion of the protein content (purified anti-diphtheric serum), or still after desication of the liquid serum or of the purified product (dried anti-diphtheric serum).

For each of these forms, the activity of the serum should be expressed in antitoxic units as they are defined hereafter according to the international convention.

In principle, the "antitoxic unit" is the quantity of antitoxin mixed with a quantity of dephtherio toxin respresenting about 100 mortal doses of (for cobaye) diphtheria toxin, which neutralises almost the totality of it, leaving only a quantity corresponding to a single mortal dose, *i.e.*, the quantity which by subcutaneous injection causes in 4 days the death of a cobaye of 250 g.

1. Liquid antidiphtheric serum : This serum is in liquid form, clear yellow, sometimes slightly opalescent. It should contain, per cm³ minimum 300 units of international anti-toxin as it is described above.

Some serums are sometimes more rich and may contain up to 400, 500 and even 1000 cm³. That strength in units should be indicated on the label of each recipient.

2. *Purified antidiphtheric serum* : This serum is obtained by submitting the liquid Antidiphtheric serum to different treatments which cause the elimination of serine and a portion of globuline (englobuline).

The purified antidiphtheric serum is generally presented either in liquid form which may be injected like liquid antidiphtheric toxin and which, like the latter should contain minimum 300 units of antitoxin per cm³ in dry form, the same as described hereafter. One may however obtain some purified liquid serums much more active containing up to 2000 antitoxic units per cm³ or more.

3. *Dry antidiphtheric serum* : It is obtained by desication at low temperature from the liquid or purificd antidiphtheric serum. This dry serum is contained in glass recipient hermetically sealed. The number of total units containing in each recipient should be indicated exactly on the lable. By dissolution in a fixed quantity of sterile water, one obtains a solution which should have the same antitoxic strength as that of the corresponding liquid serum or purified serum, *i.e.*, to say minimum 300 units per cm³.

Trial : This antidiphtheric serum should be submitted to a titration helping to control its antitoxic units. That titrating may be done either *in vivo* on the colony by inoculaing a mixture of serum and diphtherio toxin, or *in vitro* by the floculation method.

Titration on the cobaye : This titration consists in establishing the quantity of serum that is necessary to add to a determined dose of diphtheric toxin (dose L+) so that a healthy coboye of 250 g to which the mixture is injected subcutaneously succumbs only after 4 days' time.

The dose L+ represents in principle about hundred times of the lethal does for the cobaye, *i.e.* to say hundred times of the does which causes in 4 days the death of an animal having the weight of 250 g. In principle, that L+ is established experimentally for the diphtheric toxin utilised in relation to international standard of serum, taking recourse to a titration similar to that which is decribed hereafter and having the same criteria. The dose L+ is that which, mixed with an antitoxic unit causes death in 96 hours, of a cobaye of 250 g which is injected with the mixture subcutaneously.

On these conditions the antitoxic unit that neutralises almost the totality of the dose L+ of diphtherio toxin and leaves just the quantity which causes the death to the cobaye in 96 hours should have the indispensable criteria for the experimental determination of the antitoxic unit.

Technique of dosing : Prepare a series of mixtures, each containing the L+ dose of fixed toxin, and 1 cm³ of a dilution of the serum which is to be exprimented and which vary according to the titration indicated or presumed of this serum, for example 1 cm³ of a dilution by 1/250, 1/300, 1/350, etc....

Inject this serum subcutaneously to some normal cobays having the weight of 250 g (each mixture is to be injected at least to 5 cobayes). One of these mixtures, which has been injected, after a contact of at least one hour causes the death of two animals out of three, exactly in 4 days, contains, as is said above, an antitoxic unit. If, for example, the mixture in which the L+ dose has been added by 1/300 of cm³ of the serum to be examined, we may conclude that, that serum contains one antitoxin unit in 1/300 of cm³ and consequently 300 units of international antitoxins for cm³.

Titration in vitro by flocculation method : This method consists in the research of, among the variable doses of serums that are mixed in a fixed volume of toxin, the dose, in the limpid mixture thus obtained, causes which causes the flocculation to appear the earliest (initial flocculation).

To that effect one utilises a volume of toxin containing some quantity of antigen units previously determined according to the technique described above in relation to serum of internation standard, specially destined to the reaction of flocculation.

Technique of dosing : Prepare a series of tubes containing each 5 cm^3 of a diphtheric serum having for example 24 antigen units per cm^3. Thus each tube contains 120 antigen units. Introduce in these different tubes some decreasing volumes of serum for dosing : 0·5cm^3, 0·4cm^3, 0·35cm^3, 0·3cm^3 etc... Shake the mixture so as it becomes homogenious. Let it rest and examine the tubes at a fixed interval of 15 minutes, for example, and note the flocculation which begins first in one of the tubes (initial flocculation). This observation indicates that the tube contains a neutral mixture in which the toxin and the antitoxin have mutually saturated each other. If, for example, the initial floccutation appears in the mixture containing 120 antigen units and 0·4 cm^3 of serum, it is that the volume of serum contains 120 antitoxin units, which makes for centimeter cube $\frac{120}{0·4} = 30$ units.

A.—DIPHTHEROTOXINUM
CLINICAL CORTICO-VISCERAL PHARMACO-DYNAMIC PROTOCOL OR CLINICAL PATHOGENESIS

The description which follows has resulted from the consultation of the article of Allen, H.C. in his Materia Medica of Nosodes, by the study of R. Zissu in *Clinical Pathogenesis of Diphtherotoxinum* (Annales Homoeop. fr. november, 1964 ; studies of P. Chavanon and of Tilitcheff.

Finally O.A. Julian has described his own researches and his clinical experiences as a practicing doctor in the village between 1935-1939, where he had to treat cases of diphtheria.

1. Generalities

Phospho-fluoric or fiuoro-phosphoric type.
Rapid weakness.

Paleness, nonchalance, anorexia.

The child is punny, rapidly fatigued, does not like to play, has often nosebleed, repeated cold. Mediocre appetite. Is not a good student in the school.

The adult soon loses breath, coughing ; expectorates with difficulty ; breath and expectoration nauseating.

2. Neuro-endocrino-psychic System

(*a*) *Mind* : Asthenia, psycho-motor slowness (Tilitcheff) with *Paretic condition* specially of the lower limbs. (O.A. Julian)

(*b*) *Nerves* : Nasal sound, liquid discharge from the nose, difficult deglutition, because of the paralysis of the palatal vault.

Paresis of the lower limbs, steppage.

Polyneuritis, incomplete sensitivo-motrice, symmetric, flax, with distal predominance and loss of deep sensivity.

(*c*) *Endocrine* :

Thyroid : Emaciation, *chilliness*, tendency to colds and bronchitis, palpitations.

3. Digestive Apparatus

Anorexia, tongue, red and swollen.
Pain in the pregastric region.
Constipation.

4. Cardio-hemo-vascular System

Paleness, palpitations.
Hypotension, adynamia.
Tachycardia.

Thermoregulation : Vesperal fever with bad general condition.

5. Respiratory Apparatus

(*a*) *Throat* : Paralysis of the vocal chord. Bitonal voice.
Micro polyadynopathy of the two sides of the neck.
Big tonsils with false membranes.

Malignant angina from the beginning, pseudo-membranous with the state of prostration.

Thick false membranes of dark colour.

Dyspnoea, laryngitis.

(*b*) *Lungs, pleura* : Humid cough, with bad smelling, foetid expectorations, are presistent.

Difficulty to expectorate, worse at night, specially in children and old persons.

Harsh cough, voice, lost.

6. Sense Organs

(*a*) *Nose* : Bad smelling, nasal *crusts*, with foetid secretion.

Epistaxis :

Cold with bad smelling nasal secretion.

Reflux of liquids by the nose or while vomiting.

Mucous coryza, sometimes pseudo membranous or sero-sanguinolant.

(*b*) *Eyes* : Troubles of accommodation. Short sight.

7. Modalities

Aggravation by movement. *Amelioration* by heat, in bed.

8. Posology

Dynamisations : Prescribe 4 CH to 30 CH.

In subacute state : 7 CH, 30 CH.

For neurologic syndromes : 7 CH, 5 CH, 30 CH.

POSITIVE DIAGNOSIS

Paleness, fatigue, anorexia.

Throat, red, swollen ; tonsils with pseudo membranes,

Chilliness, palpitations, hypotension.

Paretic troubles, sensitive motor nerves of the lower limbs. Subfebrile state.

DIFFERENTIAL DIAGNOSIS

Nosodotherapy : See Influenzinum, Serum of Yersin, Staphylococcin.

Classical Homoeopathy : Arsenic, Lachesis, Arum triphyllum, Mercurius cyanatum, Kali bichromicum, Silicea, Thuya, Bryonia, Ferrum phos., Causticum, to mention only the more frequently used.

Renovated homoeotherapics : (in O.A. Julian ; Matiére médicate homoeopathique, Librairie Le Fransçois, Paris).

Acidum hippuricum : Weak, worn out subject, abhorring breath, thick membranous exudates on the tonsils and in the back of the throat, viscous nasal secretion, bad smelling.

Rajania subsamarata : Prostration, mouth open, swollen lips, sticky saliva, foetid breath, abhorring, hyperthermia, thready pulse ; swelling of the throat and of the region of parotids, epistaxis, contracted pupils, insensible.

CLINICAL DIAGNOSIS

1. Generalities

"Strumous diathesis in scrofulous persons, psoric or tuber-culinic, with tendency to catarrh of the throat and of the respiratory mucosa. Patient has a weak vitality for which he is suscepitble to germs of diphtheria and from the start it has the tendeney to be come malignant" (H.C. Allen).

Pseudo-suprarenalian asthenia. (Tilitcheff)
Tuberculous condition.
Demineralisation.
Preventive of winter rhino-pharyngo-trachitis. (Zissu)

Preventive of influenza (with *Influenzinum* in 5 CH or 7 CH).

Zissu specifies moreover in these preventive treatments : tissureticulo-endothelial and amygdalian tissue in 5 CH or 7 CH.

Syndrome of "patrarquerie" of Jaequelin-Bernand (O.A. Julian).

2. Neuro-endocrino-psychic System

Diphtheric paralysis.

Paralysis of vocal chord (non-diphtheric).

Myelitis (Syndrome of Guillaum Barré).

Flaccid paralysis. (O.A. Julian)

Multiple sclerosis.

Basedow's disease.

Depressive psychosis.

Anxiety neurosis.

Headache of students. (Zissu)

3. Digestive Apparatus

Cortico-gastric dysthermia. (Cl. Berger et)

Hypochlorhydric gastritis.

4. Cardio-hemo-vascular System

Myocarditis.

Cardiothyreosis.

5. Respiratory Apparatus

1. Anginas and relapsing anginas.
2. Paralysis of vocal chords (Cartier).
3. Relapsing rhinopharyngitis of children.
4. Chronic bronchitis of old men.
5. Acute or chronic bronchitis of catarrhal form of the mucouses of children and old men.
6. Trachitis and dragging tracheo-bronchitis.
7. Bronchorrhoea.
8. Spasmodic cough.

6. Sense Organs

Nose : Chronic rhinitis. Membranous rhinitis ; acute rhinitis ; epistaxis.

Eyes : False presbyopia.

COMMENTARIES

Diphtherotoxinum is an important and valuable biotherapic.

It should be considered under two aspects :

1. As a specific biotherapic for diphtheria in all its different forms.

2. As a biotherapic according to its own clinical pathogenic structure. *Its specific structure* has been valorised by the work of our great friend Paul Chavanon, who died so early.

From 1930 Chavanon started his researches on diphtheria, codified its homoeopathic treatment and of this Romeyer of Evreux made beautiful clinical and statistical study.

Chavanon published his book, *"La Diphtérie*—Traité de Thérapeutique et immunisation."* in 1932. He made a critical study about the university therapeutic and showed by the help clinical observations, the advantages and the possibilities of homoeotherapy in that affection.

He studied the clinical homoeopathic Materia Medica as well as the therapeutic of after effects due to different anti diphtheric serums.

Concerning *Diphtheroxinum* he published some clinical cases of diphtheric paralysis cured with Diphtheroxinum 30 K or 12 K and the favourable action on the carrier of the germ.

Chavanon specified the preventive vaccination with Diphtherotoxinum, 4,000 K or 8000 K at the rate of one or two doses at an interval of 4 to 8 weeks resulting in the negativation of Schick's reaction.

But the experiment was conducted on 45 subjects and the result seemed at first favourable, but was not confirmed.

The problem remained open.

As regards the clinical pathological built, Diphthericum is revealed as a polychrest nosode.

There are the tubercular states, the demineralised condition of sudden weakness and depression with fatigue, weariness of legs, the patient either young, adult or old drags on without and joy for life.

Diphtherotoxinum 30 CH (Sometimes associated with Bacillinum 30 CH) is to be advised in these cases :

Repeated colds, repeated anginas, "Influenzal states" for an "Yes" or for a "No", are to be treated by Diphtherotoxinum 30 CH and with, if necessary, Aviary 30 CH or V.A.B. 30 CH.

The same thing may be said regarding acute or chronic bronchitis, for harsh cough or for cavernous cough.

Finally O.A. Julian has advised since long time prescribing of Diphtherotoxinum 30 CH in neurological affections where predominates a motor weakness and paralysis of the soft muscles.

If the disease is recent, or if the necessity arises, this medicine may be associated with *Gelsemium, Lathyrus, Cuprum, Arsenicum, Causticum.*

The clinical results are often satisfactory, sometimes very much surprising and valuable.

On the contrary, and contrary to what was written in 1962 in *"Biotherapics and Nosodes"*, there is every reason to repeat and one should repeat the administration according to the condition of our environment, every day.

There are in Germany injectable forms of Diphtherotoxinum in 10 DH, and in 18 DH+30 DH : 200 DH (Reckeweg). The case is the same with relapsing anginas, endocarditis, pleuritis, chronic nephritis, acute or chronic polyarthritis.

As *adjuvant treatment*, it is prescribed in the cahcer of larynx, of oesophagus, of lungs.

It is also prescribed in *foetor-ore* chronic blepharitis, dyspnoea, cardiac weakness

It is after the publication of Materia Medica der Nosoden of O.A. Julian by Haug-Verlag in 1960 that the nosodotherapy took an important step in Germany and Diphtherotoxinum has gained the prestige of effective therapeutic agent.

It is regrettable however that our legislation hardly allows the injection of biotherapics.

It is great loss for the patients.

CLINICAL CASES

Case No. 1. (R. Schmitz-Harbauer, in Klassicher Homoeopathie, No. 2, 1963, p. 68).

Engineer of 28 years feels since one month nervous, anxious, with uneasiness, depressed ; sweats easily, regular stools.

Antecedants : Whooping cough, measles, repeated anginas A.T 15/9, and pulse 120.

Prescription : *Chininum Ars* D6, one tablet thrice daily.

After 14 days pulse becomes more slow, but always sweats and nervous.

Prescription : *Diphtherinum D10* brings complete cure.

Case No. 2 : (Dr. Charbaux : Revue Belge d'homoeopathie, 1949, No. 1, p. 27 to 29).

Mlle B.M....ll years.

Presonal antecedants : Chicken pox, measles, scarlatina, urticaria, sensitive throat.

Present affection : I was called to see a child who was vomiting everything except water, and has a temperature of 39·5°.

By examination, the stomach is painful but the tongue is clear. There is incessant nausea which does not cease after vomiting.

The throat is red and there is a white spot on the right tonsil with some difficulty of deglutition. The patient has thirst.

I alternated *Ipecac 6* (clear tongue with vomiting and nausea) and *Mercurius 6* (white angina).

The next day, 13th April, 1943, the situation suddenly changed. The white spot becomes a false membrane, greyish, adhering, which covers the right tonsil, and extends up to the palate and the nasal fossa.

The breath is extremely foetid, no improvement of vomiting which is bilious. The prostration is intense, the patient cannot sit up in his bed without the fear of a syncope. The temperature oscillated between 38° and 39.5°. The urine is rare and charged.

A smear of the throat reveals the presence of Loeffler bacilli.

It is a question of pharyngeal diphtheria.

The pathogenetic picture of *Mercurius cyanatus* (intense prostration, false membranes, foetid breath) is fully present. Some symptoms of *Belladonna* are also present specially the oscillating fever.

I prescribed *Belladonna* 6 and *Cyanathus* 6, alternating every two hours.

14th April : Condition ameliorates still more but the false membrane extends to nasal fossa. The patient respirates with difficulty, the nose being obstructed. There is a viscous yellowish exudate in the back of the nose. (*Kali bichromicum*).

The prescription of *Cyanathus 6* and *Kali bichromicum* 6, every two hours alternately.

16th April : The temperature is only 37.°5 ; general condition excellent. The false membrane is detached ; no prostration, the false membrane of the fossa comes off in pieces. The respiration is free. The pulse is hardly accelerated.

I prescribed *Diphtherinum* 30, one dose ; 200 a second dose, after two days (Anti-diphtheric nosode).

One day *Kali-bichromicum* 30, 2 granules, twice a day ; the other day *Cyanathus* 30, 2 granules twice a day.

19th April : The condition is absolutely normal and the patient seems to be cured. The temperature has become normal since the second dose of *Diphtherinum 200*. I stopped the prescription of *Kali-bichromicum 30* and *Cyanathus 30* and replaced it with *Pulsatilla* which suited the tubercular temperament of the patient.

29th April : The voice became nasal, foods came out through the nose. The paralysis of the palatal vault is developed, but there was neither temperature nor pain. *Gelsemium 30* followed by a new dose of *Diphtherium 200* cured very rapidly the condition.

The convalescence is rapid without incident.

Preventively *Cyanathus 6* was given to other members of the family.

Here is, therefore, an authentic case of Diphtheria with sure clinical symptoms (false membranes, paralysis of palatal vault and the laboratory proof, presence of Loeffller bacilli, found three times) cured within a few days by Homoeopathy without any intervention by serum.

This is not only one isolated case, but I have several superposable cases, while other homoeopaths also have published similar cases since the last war when there was a great recrudescence of Diphtheria cases.

B.— DIPHTHERICUM

CLINICAL CORTICO-VISCERAL PHARMACODYNAMIC PROTOCOL OR CLINICAL PATHOGENESIS

There is no pathogenesis according to experimental method of Hahnemann of Diphthericum.

F.-Bernoville prescribed as an Isotherpic in troubles resulting out of the application of anti-diphtheric serum.

Two groups of seric effects are to be kept in mind :

Local : Phlegmons.

General : 1. Paleness, anxiety, tendency to collapse, tachycardia.

One may advise, intravėnous injection of *Apis 3 DH*, 1 mlg to repeat every 30 minutes, twice and also by mouth *Diphthericum 5 CH*, 2 granules every 10 minutes.

2. Late effects beginning after 6 to 10 days with fever, urticarian eruptions, localised oedema, arthralgias, sometimes seric meningitis and still later neuritis and amyotrophies.

One may advise *Apis 3 DH*, 1 mlg by injection IV, IM or SC, every 2 to 3 days and by mouth : *Diphthericum 7 CH* with *Phenobarbital 7 CH* or *Paraphenẏlienediamine 15 CH* or *Lung histamin 7 CH.*

Diphthericum is prescribed in 4 CH to 30 CH.

D.T.—T.A.B.

BIBLIOGRAPHY

Julian O.A :
Biothérapiques et Nosodes.   Librarie Maloine, 1962.
Materia Medica der Nosoden. 2e ed, Haug Verlag, Heidelberg, 1975.
Prévention et traitement Bio-homoeo-therapiques descomplications vaccinales, 1973.   Librarie Le François, 91, Bd St-Germain, 75006 Paris.

Albahary :
Maladies médicamenteuse d'ordre thérapeutique et accidentel.   Edition Masson, 1953.

STOCK

The Biotherapic D.T.—T.A.B. is obtained from antidiphtheric, antitetanic and antitypho-paratyphoid mixed vaccin.

It is constituted by a mixture of suitable proportions of Antitoxin of Diphtheria, tetanic anatoxin and antityphoparatyphoid vaccin. 1 mlg should contain minimum 12 units of antigen diphtheric-anatoxin ; 12 units of tetanic anatoxin $+1$ milliard 50 millions of typhoid bacilli and 700 millions each of the bacilli paratyphoid A and B.

HISTORY

There does not exist any experimental pathogenesis according to the method of Hahnemann of this biotherapic.

Julian in his book *Biothérapiques et Nosodes* gives the sketch of the clinical pathogenesis in 1962.

He takes up again the clinical and therapeutic study in a pamphlet concerning the prevention and the treatment of vaccin complications.

(234)

The therapeutic and clinical use shows that this biotherapic is nearly related to the biotherapics *Paratyphoidium B*, *Enterococcinum* and *Staphylococcinum*.

CLINICAL CORTICO-VISCERAL PROTOCOL
OR CLINICAL PATHOGENESIS

1. Generalities

Fever, headaches, pains all over the body, lumbalgia.
Dysthyroid ; emotive, weak, overworked persons.

Reappearence of a latent affection or aggravation of a known affection (infectious meningitis, granulia, herpes, deficitary phenomena in the course of neurological syphilis).
Articular pains.

2. Neuro-endocrino-psychic System

Epileptiform or tetaniform convulsions.
Choreiform movements.
Hebephrenia. Catatonia.
Mental confusion with amnesia.

Deficit type of paresis or paralysis, monoplegia, hemiparasia, hemiplegia, specially of the right side.

3. Digestive Apparatus

Nausea, sensation as if he is going to vomit.
Abdominal pain.
Diarrhoea. Intestinal hemorrhage.
Pain in the right iliac fossa, appendicular region.
Hepatic congestion. Icterus.

4. Cardio-hemo-vascular System

Sudden Hypotension with lypothymia, cyanosis, dyspnoea and inversion of the blood formula.

5. Sense Organs

Eyes :
Optic neuritis, paresis of the 3rd pair. glaucoma, exopthalmia.

6. **Uro-genital Apparatus**

Acute nephritis, painful, febril, oliguria, proteinuria, hematuria.

Chronic Albuminuria.

Hypertension and uremigenous chronic albuminuria.

7. **Skin**

Different transitory eruptions (rash).

Polymorphous erythema ; nodulous erythema, erythrodermia, purpura.

Urticaria, facial herpes.

8. **Posology**

Dynamisation :

4 CH, 5 CH, 7 CH, 9 CH.

DIFFERENTIAL DIAGNOSIS

Classical homoeopathy. Think of *Acidum picricum, Phosphorus, Renovated homoeopathy, Zincum.*

Karwinskia humboldtiana. Paresis, then paralysis of the soft muscles, progressive, ascending, painless.

Hydrophis cyanocinctus : Paresis, paralysis without troubles of sensibility.

Pricking pains in the thorax and extremities.

CLINICAL DIAGNOSIS

Allergic condition — Mesenchymatosis (Psoro-sycotic conditions).

Morbid alternation.

Mental confusion.

Epilepsy, tetanus.

Paresis or wasting paralysis.

Hematuric nephritis.

Erysipelus—zona.

Pathological sequalae, after D.T.—T.A.B.

EBERTHINUM

BIBLIOGRAPHY

Julian, O.A. :

Biothérapiques et Nosodes. Librarie Maloine, 1962.

Materia Medica der Nosoden. Haug-Verlag, Heidelberg.

Paturiaux R. :

Nosodes. Revue belge d'Homoeopathie, 1953, No. 2, p. 67.

P. Valery-Radot, J. Hamburger and F. Lhermitte :

Pathologie médical. Flammarion-medicine, 1972.

Cartier F. :

Traité complet de thérapeutique Homoeopathique, t. 4, Ch. xviii, J.B. Baillére et fils, Paris, 1939.

STOCK

Eberthinum is prepared from the culture of the mixture of many stocks of typhoid bacilli, presenting themselves in lysated suspension 10 milliards per cm^3 of *Salmonella Typhi*.

TECHNIQUE OF PREPARATION

1. Stock Used

Three stocks of Salmonella typhi, Marcy 393, 424, 425.

These stocks have the classical character of the type.

They are controlled from the morphological point of view, biochemic character and antigenic character.

Very mobile rods, G— ; irregular colonies on gelose, uniform lactose— ; saccharose— ; glycerine— ; rhamnose— ; glucose + without gas ; Dulicite ~ ; mannite + ; sorbite + ; Xylose + ; H_2S + ; citrate + ; antigen som, IX, XII ; Antigen flagell. d. They are preserved in lyophilised condition.

2. Culture Media

(*a*) Maceration of chopped meat   500 g.

Water   1,000 g.

Leave in contact for 24 hours, then filter after having heated in autoclave for 30 minutes at 100° and minutes at 110°.

(*b*) *Add* :

Peptone   12 g.

Sodium chloride   5 g.

Powdered gelose   30 g.

Dissolve on autoclave at 100° for 30 minutes.

(*c*) Adjust the *p*H at 7, 2 by addition of sodium.

(*d*) Put on stove at 110° for 20 minutes.

(*e*) Distribute in tubes in Roux boxes.

(*f*) Sterilise at 110° for 20 minutes.

3. Inoculation and Culture

The three lyophilised stocks are put in solution, then inoculated in slanting tubes on media described above. After 24 hours of culture on incubator at 37°, the colonies are examined, in order to be sure of the characteristic type of these cultures and of the purity of the stocks.

The culture of each tube is washed in a volume of 5 cm³ of the Sodium chloride at 9°/°°, then taken up in dropper for inoculation on Roux boxes containing 1,200 cm³ of the same media.

The Roux boxes in their turn are put on the incubator at 37°. After 48 hours of rest on the stove, the boxes are examined individually to assure of the purity of the colonies.

Then to each one is added 25 to 30 cm³ of sterile distilled water. After suspension of the culture by manual balancing the bacterial suspension thus obtained is gathered by aspiration in a sterile recipient. This suspension is adjusted to 20 milliards of germs by cm³ by addition of sterile distilled water.

The suspension thus obtained is heated at 56° for 45 minutes then placed immediately afterwards in refrigerator at +3°, +5°.

4. Lysis and the Getting of the Endotoxins

The bacterial suspension is transferred in a recipient of resistant pyrex glass.

It is then congealed at a temperature of −30 to −40° for 24 hours. Then the suspension is left for being decongealed at +20° for 24 hours.

The total operation of congealation and decongealation is repeated 3 times, in all 4 operations.

It is then centrifuged in some sterile tubes at a speed of 6,000 t/m for a time sufficient to obtain a complete sedimentation of lysated bacterian debris. The floating suspension of endotoxin is then collected, submitted to a filtration on Seitz EKS filtre and preserved in refrigerator at −3°, +5°.

5. Detoxification

The suspension of endotoxins is added to an equal volume of sterile distilled water and heated 3 times at 75° for one hour at an interval of 24 hours.

The suspension thus obtained corresponds to an original concentration of 10 milliards of germs per cm³.

6. Distribution

The vaccinal suspension is then distributed aseptically in ampoules.

The lysate serving for homoeopathic dilution is submitted to the following controls :

(a) *Neutrality*. The pH of the lysate should be included between 7 and 7, 2.

(b) *Sterility*. Inoculation on bouillon or on nutritive gelose should not be followed by any culture.

(c) *Non-toxicity*. The injection subcutaneously of 1 ml of the lysate should not cause any accident.

(*d*) *Activity.* Three tests are to be done :

1. *Intracardiac inoculation on cobaye* : It is followed by the death of animal because of respiratory trouble and it is found after autopsy a hypertrophy of Peyer's plaques accompanied by hyperplasic endothelitis and a splenomegaly with diffused lesions.

2. *Inoculation in the mesenteric ganglion* : The same characteristic lesions are seen in weak doses.

3. *Inoculation by splanchnic contact* :   This also causes identical lesions which shows neurotropism of the endotoxin for vegetative system.

CLINICAL CORTICO VISCERAL PROTOCOL
OR CLINICAL PATHOGENESIS

There is no experimental pathogenesis according to Hahnemannian methodology.

On the other hand the clinical practice of Eberthinum has been more or less eclipsed by the biotherapic *Paratyphoidinum B.*

1. **Generalities**

Fever rising up to 40', dicrotic and dissociated pulse.

Prostrated, immobile, indifferent to persons around him.

Ochre diarrhoea, abundant, foetid.

2. **Neuro-endocrino-psychic System**

Encephalitis with intense prostration, mental confusion, acute psychosis.

Meningeal reaction.

3. **Digestive Apparatus**

Egg-shaped ulceration, superficial, painless, on the tonsil.

Hepatomegaly. Palpable spleen.

Rumbling in the right illiac fossa.

Intestinal hemorrhage.

Suppurated cholecystitis, liver abscess, suppuration of the pancreas.

Pseudo-appendicular pain ; acute peritonitis.

4. **Cardio-vascular System**

Cardio vascular collapse.

Myocardia or toxic myocarditis.

Arteritis. Phlebitis.

5. **Respiratory System**

Respiratory adynamia.

Pulmonary congestion. Pleuresy.

6. **Uro-genital Apparatus**

Rare and deep coloured urine, restlessness and burning thirst.

7. **Locomotor Apparatus**

Osteoperiostitis. Spondylitis.

8. **Skin**

Erythematous and congestive maculad on the flanks, base of the thorax, roots of the things.

9. **Posology**

Dynamisation : 4 CH, 5 CH, 7 CH, 9 CH.

DIFFERENTIAL DIAGNOSIS

Traditional Homoeopathy :

Arsenicum album, Baptisia, Iodum :

Present day homoeopathy :

Achyrantes Calea (Julian O.A. & collab. : Matiére médicale Hom., Le Franscois, 91 bd. St-Germain, 75006, Paris).

Paronichi-Illecebrum. Continuous fever, dry and burning mucosa muscular stiffness congestive headache, sensation of emptiness in the brain, double personality, acute *neuro pneumo-vascular* congestion. Involuntary loss of stool and urine.

CLINICAL DIAGNOSIS

1. **Generalities**

   Infectious conditions : Septicemia, typhoid fever, typhobacillosis, psittacosis.

   All psycho-somatic affections of which the etiological idea goes to an old typoid.

2. **Nervous System**

   Epidemic encephalitis of Cruchet and Von Economo. Curable lymphocytic meningitis.

3. **Digestive Apparatus**

   Angiocholecystitis (Acute).

   Acute hemorrhagic pancreatitis (Adjuvant treatment).

   Acute enterocolitis.

4. **Cardio-vascular Apparatus**

   Infectious myocarditis.

   Nodulous peri-arteritis.

   Pericarditis.

5. **Respiratory Apparatus**

   Pneumonia ; cortico-pleuritis.

6. **Urinary Apparatus**

   Acute glomerulo-nephritis.

7. **Locomotor System**

   Acute ostèomyelitis of adolescent.

CLINICAL OBSERVATIONS
(Revue Belge d' Homoeopathie 1953, No. 2., p. 68)

Mme R...age 55 years, was always in good health up to the age of 20 years. At that time she had a typhoid fever and since then she is never doing well. She suffers from the intestine and all the symptoms that she relates to me led me to the diagnosis of muco-membranous colitis and this was confirmed by other doctors. The least fault in diet or the least fatigue cuases great aggravation and she has burnig pains in the stomach, vomitings and cramps of the stomach. The patient is lean with ptosis and depressed.

Since 40 years all classical treatments were tried.

All the ills go no doubt up to the typhoid fever. I prescribed *Eberthinum M.*

At first she had apparent aggravation, afterwards all general and local symptoms ameliorate. Gradually all foods that were abandoned since years are tolerated. The pains of the stomach disappeared after 3 months. I prescribed a second dose of *Eberthinum M.*

Since six months, I am treating the patient and amelioration gradually continues with a hope to end by remedies selected from the Materia Medica. But the indicated nosode has very much shortened the time of cure.

ENTEROCOCCINUM

BIBLIOGRAPHY

Julian O.A. :

Biothérapiques et Nosodes. Maloine, 1962.

Materia Medica der Nosoden. 2e ed. K.F. Haug-Verlag ; Heidelberg, 1975.

Cartier Fr. :

Traité complet de Thérapeutique Homoeopathique. t. 3 ; Maladies de l' appareil digestif. Baillére et fils. Paris, 1929.

Hamburger Jean :

Petite Encyclopédie Médicale. Méd. Flammarion, 1968

Blacque-Belair A. :

Dictionnaire Médical Clinique, Pharmacologique et Thérapeutique, Maloine, Paris, 1974.

P. Vallery-Radot, J. Hamburger et F. Lhermitte :

Pathologie médicale, Méd. Flammarion, 1971.

Julian O.A. :

et collab. Matière Médical d'homeotherapie 1971, Le François, 91, bd. St-Germain, 75006, Paris.

STOCK

Enterococcinum is prepared from a mixture of many stocks of Enterococcus.

The lysated suspension corresponds to 10 milliards per cm^3 of Streptococcus faecalis for making homoeopathic dilutions.

(244)

TECHNIQUE OF PREPARATION

1. Stock Used

Three stocks of Streptococcus faecalis, Marcy 98, 428, 429 that have the classical character of the type are used.

These are controlled from the point of view of morphologic, biochemic and antigenic characters.

Diplococcus and short immobile chains Gram positive, make the bouillon turbid, coagulates milk, non-hemolytic, gelatine—; raffinose—; inuline—; mannitol+; salicine +.

They are preserved in lyophilised condition.

2. Culture Media

(a) Maceration of chopped meat   500 g.

      Water   1,000 cm^3

Leave in contact for 24 hours, then filter after having been heated in autoclave for 30 minutes at 100° and 30 minutes at at 110°.

(b) *Add* :

    Peptone   12 g.

    Sodium chloride   5 g.

    Powdered gelose   30 g.

Dissolve on autoclave at 100° for 30 minutes.

(c) Adjust pH at 7,2 by addition of sodium.

(d) Put on autoclave at 110° for 20 minutes.

(e) Distribute in Roux boxes.

(f) Sterilise at 110° for 20 minutes.

3. Inoculation and Culture

The 3 lyophilised stocks are put in solution then inoculated on slanting tubes of the media already described. After 24 hours of culture on stove at 37°, the colonies are examined to be assured of the purity of the stocks and of the characteristic type of these cultures.

The culture of each type is washed in a volume of 5 cm³ of solution of Sodium chloride at 9%, then sucked in, in droppers for inoculating on the Roux boxes containing 1,000 cm³ of the same media.

The Roux boxes are in their turn put in the incubator at 37°. After 48 hours of stay on the incubator, the boxes are examined for being assured of the purity of the colonies.

Then to each is added 25 to 30 cm³ of sterile distilled water. After suspension of the culture by balancing by hand, the bacterial suspension obtained is collected by aspiration in a sterile recipient. That suspension is adjusted to 20 milliards of germs in a centimetre cube by the addition of the sterile distilled water.

The suspension thus obtained is heated at 56° for 45 minutes, then put immediately repeated in a refrigerator at +3°, +5°.

4. Lysis and the Getting of Endotoxin

The bacterial suspension is transferred in a recipient of resistant pyrex glass, and congealed at a temperature of —30° to —40° for 24 hours. Total operation of congealation-decongealation is and heated 3 times, *i.e.*, in all 4 operations.

The sterile tubes are centrifuged at a speed of 6,000 t/m for a time sufficient to obtain a complete sedimentation of the yeasted bacteria. The floating suspension of endotoxin is then collected, put for filtration on Seitz E.K.S. filtre and preserved in refrigerator at +3°, +5°.

5. Detoxification

The suspension of endotoxin is added with an equal volume of sterile distilled water, and heated 3 times at 75° for one hour at an interval of 24 hours.

The suspension thus obtained corresponds to an original concentration of 10 millards of germs per centimetre cube.

6. Distribution

Now, one may aseptically distribute this suspension of vaccin in ampoules.

It corresponds to group D of which three different biochemic varieties are distinguished, *faecium*, *durans*, and *faecalis*. The hemolytic properties are very variable. Enterococcinum is not hemolytic.

Control of the Product

(*a*) *Neutrality* : The pH of the lysate should be between 7 and 7, 2.

(*b*) *Trial for non-toxicity* : To 5 white mice, is injected 2 ml of lysate subcutaneously ; 5 other mice get 0·75 ml intraperitonially. The mortality should be nil. If one animal dies, the experiment is done again and if the same incidence happens the lysate should be rejected.

(*c*) *Sterlity* : 20 ml of thyoglycollate media is inoculated with 2 ml of lysate. The culture is not observed even after 7 days of incubation under 37°.

CLINICAL CORTICO- VISCERAL PROTOCOL OR CLINICAL PATHOGENESIS

1. Generalities

Diarrhoea, loss of appetite, saburrhal state of the tongue.

Hypotension, slow pulse.

Diarrhoea, teething diarrhoea.

Fatigue, irritability, dimineralisation from stools with mucorrhoea.

2. Digestive Apparatus

Tongue *white as milk*, nausea and anorexia, flatulence, eructations.

Stools like "cowdung".

Morning diarrhoea with great urgency of many stools between 4 to 9 a.m.

Emotive diarrhoea.

Menstrual diarrhoea.

Pain in the colon, either transversal or lateral, left or right.

Rectal tenesmus.

Glairy mucous, bloody diarrhoea.

3. **Posology**

Dynamisation : 4 CH, 5 CH, 7 CH, 9 CH.

DIFFERENTIAL DIAGNOSIS

Consult the chapters on Proteus and the Nosodes of Bach-Paterson.

Classical homoeopathy : *Sulphur, Podophyllum, Dioscorea, Croton.*

Present-day Homoeotherapics : *Achyranthes calea, Paronichia illeceberum, Cynodon dactylon* etc.

CLINICAL DIAGNOSIS

Allegric (Psoric) condition, dominating colitis.

Colitis and enterocolitis.

Rectitis.

Hemorrnagic recto-colitis.

Dysentries, relapsing colitis.

FLAVUS

BIBLIOGRAPHY

Sevaux F :

Recherche expérimentale d'Allergie Homoeopathique. Cahiers de Biothèrapie, No. 8, decembre 1965.

Julian O.A. et collab. :

Matiére Médicale d'Homoeothérapic 1971.

Librairie Le François, Paris.

STOCK

Flavus is a bacteria called *Neisseria pharingis.* *Flava* of the family of *Neisseriacae* of Micrococcal order.

These microbes are of the form of shells disposed in pairs like coffee grains. They are Gram—.

Neisseria Flavus is an aerobic saprophyte of upper respiratory system of man. It is not considered as pathogenous. However, it has been isolated from the cephalo rachidian liquid of several children suffering from meningitis. Its name is due to the elaboration on culture media of yellow pigment.

There is no Hahnemannian pathogenesis of this remedy.

CLINICAL CORTICO-VISCERAL PROTOCOL OR CLINICIAL PATHOGENESIS

1. Generalities

Suits to phosphorics and fluorics.

Intoxination : Allergic (- psoric), mesenchymatosis (sycotic). tuberculinic.

Subject having oculo-nasal-pharyngeal irritation which may end in spasmodic rhinitis.

(249)

2. Neuro-endocrino-psychic System

(*a*) *Mind* : Bad moral, exaggerates the difficulties. *Sensitive to emotions and contradictions.*

Sensation of a ball in the throat.

(*b*) *Nervous* : *Peri orbitory headaches,* right sided (Sangunaria).

Slight tremblings localised particularly in fingers.

(*c*) *Endocrine* : Gushes of heat at night.

3. Digestive System

Dental Arthritis with loose teeth.

Bad digestion ; frequent nausea after meals.

Troubles aggravated by wine (*Zincum, Nnx vomica*).

4. Cardio-hemo-vascular Apparatus

Palpitations at night with the impression of having fever, worse after drinking wine.

5. Respiratory Apparatus

Pain in frontal and maxillary sinuses.

Discharge from the nose and eyes.

Takes cold easily, coughs and expectorates.

Sensation of a feather in the throat (*Kali bich*).

Sensative of heaviness in the larynx after talking for a long time.

Throat pain after having wet feet.
Dry throat, uneasiness at night.

Inflammation of the throat (sensation as if the palate is touching the tongue).

Wakes up between 1 to 1·30 A.M. and coughs.

Frequent loss of voice.

Dyspnoea worse at night toward 2 A.M., wakes up with suffocation.

6. Sense Organs

Nose : Dry with dry crusts. Nosebleed in the morning. Discharge of greenish pus from the nose (*Kali bich*).

Congestion of the nose at night, one nostril stops, the other opens. Better in the morning after sneezing. Easily sneezes.

Eyes : *Right-sided periorbital headache.*

Ocular fatigue; eyes swollen in the morning after waking up, heavy eyelids

Red eyes, fatigued in the evening.

Ears : Frequent otitis (one patient had otitis 25 times).

Right-sided otalgia.

7. Genital Apparatus

Menstruation irregular, in advance of variable abundance with pale blood.

Late menstruation with premenstrual syndrome.

Loss of blood during ovulation.

8. Locomotor System

Neck : Arthrosis of the vertebral column with crackings.

Back and extremities : Dorsalgia with radiation to both arms.
Arthralgias with articular cracking of the knees.

Wrists, shoulders and fingers : Pain of the left arm.

Left-sided sciatic pain.

9. Skin, Phanera

Perspiration of the palms.

Frequent ecchymosis by the slightest shock.

10. Modalities

Aggravation : By cold, by heat, in the morning when waking up.

Amelioration : By hot bath, in the spring, in autumn.

Laterality : Left.

POSOLOGY

By mouth : Granules 4 and 5 CH.

Doses : 7 and 9 CH.

Drops : 5, 7, 9 CH in the evening when going to bed, then 5, 7, 9, 15 CH, then drops 5, 7, 9, 15 and 30 CH.

DIFFERENTIAL DIAGNOSIS

Kali bichromicum : Coryza and sinusitis with the sensation of obstruction of the nose, and tickling in the nostrils.

Yellowish or greenish discharges, viscous or thready, forming some elastic greenish plugs, adherent, which leave the mucous burning and inflamed.

Otitis with yellowish, viscous and thready discharge.

Arthralgias, but the pains of *Kali bichromicum* are localised on small spots, which may be covered by finger tips. They are throbbing and burning, very much localised and disappears suddenly.

Zincum : Aggravation by wine, but the depressive condition is very much accentuated.

General weakness.

Cannot keep the legs in place.

Among the modern homoeotherapics, let us mention :

Galphimia glauca : With its hypersensitiveness to change of weather.

Hypersecretion of nasal and ocular mucosa.

Sneezing, and vesicular eruptions.

Luffa operculata With fronto-occipital headache, acute or chronic inflammation of the nasal mucosa formation of crusts and the falling of hairs.

CLINICAL DIAGNOSIS

1. **Generalities**

   Depressive states.

2. **Neuro-endocrino-psychic System**

   Headache ; disthyroidia. (O.A. Julian)

3. **Digestive System**

   Dental arthritis ; dysphagia ; digestive troubles after meals.

4. **Respiratory Apparatus**

   Red anginas ; dry cough, aggravation in the morning.

5. **Sense Organs**

   (a) *Nose* : Spasmodic coryza ; sinusitis.

   (b) *Eyes* : Conjunctivitis ; repeated otitis.

6. **Uro-genital Apparatus**

   Dysmenorrhoea ; endometritis ; pollako menorrhoea.

7. **Loco-motor Apparatus**

   Arthrosis. Rheumatic arthritis.

   Cervicalgia.

   Cervico-brachial neuralgia.

   Sciatica.

8. **Skin, Phanera**

   Dehydrosis of the palms of Tilbury Fox.

   Ecchymosis.

FRAMBOESINUM

This product was used by Dr. De Baudre of Maison-Laffite (L'Hom. françoise 1936, p. 387).

De Baudre also got prepared another nosode *Leprum* from a pustule of a leper but had not proved result.

PREPARATION

It was the serosity of *Pianoma* taken from a non-syphilitic subject.

CLINICAL PATHOGENESIS

No homoeopathie experiment exists.

For Baudre it is specific for Pian (Framboisia). As homoeopathic indication it has some common points with *Psorinum* : chilliness often accompanied by lowering of temperature, like *Carbo-veg*.

Is no more sold in France.

GONOTOXINUM
(Antigonococcic Vaccin)

BIBLIOGRAPHY

Julian O.A. :

Biothérapiques et nosodes. Librairie Maloine, 1962, Paris.

Materia Medica der Nosoden. Haug-Verlag, Heidelberg.

Cartier F. :

Traité complet de therapeutique homoeopathiqne, t. 2. Librairie Baillére et fils, Paris, 1929.

L'Homoeopathie moderne :

Numéro spècial consacre aux remedes biochimiques. Voi articles : H. Boiron : Nosodes, Isopathie, Opotherapie, Biochimie. L'Hom. moderne, No. 10, 15 mai. 1936.

Fasquelle Robert :

Eléménts de bactèriologie médicale. Méd. Flammarion, 1957, Paris.

Ferron Azéle :

Bactériologie, 1970.

STOCK

It is prepared from anti-gonococcic vaccin described in codex 1949, p. 965, supplied by Pasteur Institute.

PREPARATION

It is a suspension of gonococcus entered in a dropsical media, killed by heating at 58° and titriating 4 milliards of germs per milimetre.

CONTROL

(a) *Sterility* : Inoculation on bouillon or better on gelose should not be followed by any culture.

(b) *Non-toxicity* : By subcutaneous injection of 1 ml to mice weighing 20 g no accident should be caused. The rabbit should undergo the injection of 5 ml of the product without any incident.

HISTORY

The biotherapic *Gonotoxinum* is of recent use. It is as a result of the disappearance of *Medorrhinum* in 1955 (see article) that this biotherapic is introduced in homoeotherapy.

Cartier mentions in his treaty (II. 167) the use of *Gonotoxinum* which is the same *Gonococcus* treated in glycerine and attenuated in high dilutions The clinical cases are less numerous tnan *Medorrhinum*.

Fortier-Bernoville devoted two issues of L'Homoeopathie moderne (see Bibliography) to the study of nosodes where *Gonotoxinum* is not mentioned.

Gonotoxinum has only replaced *Medorrhinum* for some time but it was neither the object of clinical researches nor of a pathological experiment according to the Hahnemannian methodology.

CLINICAL CORTICO-VISCERAL PROTOCOL
OR CLINICAL PATHOGENESIS

Yellow, greenish urethral discharge.
Burning during micturition, turbid urine.
Flocculent urine.
Prostatic congestion
Narrowing of the urethra.

Tumefaction of the urinary meatus of women, congestion of pseudo glands, skin around the meatus.
Congestion of bartholin glands.

Inflammation of the col uteri.

Cystitis, metritis, salpingitis.

Conjunctivitis.

Articular rheumatism.

POSOLOGY

Dynamisation : 4 CH, 5 CH, 7 CH, 9 CH.

DIFFERENTIAL DIAGNOSIS

Thymol : (Julian O.A. Matiére médicale d'homoeopathie, 1971). Frequent micturition with imperius urging, turbid urine with proteinuria, brown bloody leucorrhoea, bad smelling.

CLINICAL DIAGNOSIS

Chronic mesenchymatosis (sycosis).

Complementary to *Medorrhinum*

Dragging urethritis.

Relapsing cystitis.

Prostatitis. Metritis of the neck.

Orchitis. Bartholinites.

Priapism. Epidydimitis.

Conjunctivitis. Opthalmia.

Nasal polypus.

Adenoid vegetations.

Cryptic chronic tonsilitis.

Chronic laryngitis. Ozena.

Articular rheumatism.

HAFFKINE

HISTORY

It is an anti-pest vaccine specified by Folley, a non-homoeo-path and introduced by Barishac in clinical Homoeotherapy and also by F.-Bernoville. Prieur has also made a clinico-therapeutic study (Bulletin du C.H.F., 1958, p. 257).

PREPARATION

There are two anti-pest vaccines. The one is from Pasteur Institute constituted by a suspension of bacilli killed by formol and contaning two milliards of germs per millimetre, the other is the vaccine of Haffkine the culture of which is killed by heat-ing at 55°. The product does not exist at present in any pharmacy of France. (Nelson—Pestinum 30—200).

PATHOGENESIS

No Hahnemannian experiment exists.

CLINICAL DIAGNOSIS

Barishac specified it for influenza, in the disease of Folley and by Prieur in epidemic meso-encephalitis.

COMMENTARY

It seems that in the place of Haffkine *Serum of Yersin* may be easily used (See Serum of Yersin).

HIPPOMANES

BIBLIOGRAPHY

Allen T.F. :

Encyclopaedia of Pure Materia Medica, v. 4, p. 589.

Clarke J.H. :

A Dictionary of Practical Materia Medica, v. 1, p. 905. London, 1955.

Boericke W. :

Pocket Manual of Homoeopathic Materia Medica, 9th ed., 1927.

Hering :

Guiding Symptoms 1879, New ed., 1966, v. 6, p. 43.

STOCK

It is a substance, mucoid, sticky, whitish or dark, having the smell of urine which floats in the aminotic liquid or is found attached to the membrane of the foetal organ of the mare, towards the last month of pregnancy.

A trituration is prepared with the dried substance taken out of the tongue of a filly which has just born.

This first preparation was made by the veterinary doctor John Heiffrich, a member of the Academy of Allentown.

HISTORY

Hering reports an experiment in *Arzneiprufungen*.

Some clinical trials were made by Helffrich, Floto, Reichhelm, Deidhard. F. Hasmann made a proving on himself and on others. But we do not know the results of the proving. He has used the medicine in 3 DH and 30 CH alternately.

(259)

This nosode has not received any great trial clinically.

Let us also mention here that in the antiquity, according to the Greek writers, this was advised as aphrodisiac.

In France this nosode cannot be prescribed at present.

Nelson of London has Hippomane (Horse serum), in 8-200.

CLINICAL CORTICO-VISCERAL PROTOCOL
OR CLINICAL PATHOGENESIS

1. Generalities

Great weakness of hands and feet.

Fingers benumbed.

Indifference to the entourage.

Nonchalant.

Subject with pale face as if suffering from a great weakness, numbness of the body and the mind.

Icy coldness in the stomach.

Violent pain in the wrists.

Benumbed wrists as if paralysed, morning in the bed.

Weakness of fingers and hands, cannot hold anything.

2. Neuro endocrino-psychic System

Deep melancholic state.

Remains alone in a corner, does not like to know anything.

Cataleptiform condition.

Restless sleep, tosses constantly in the bed.

Takes long time to sleep, insomnia in the second part of the night.

Headache with vertigo, somnambulism, yawning, gushes of heat in the head. Sensation of being thirsty.

Pain within the head ; sensation of pressure on the temples.

Violent headache, sensation of heavy weight on the skull worse in the sun.

Need for lying down but does not ameliorate.

Choreiform Movement :

Strange sensation as if the head will fall off.

Sensation of a knot in the throat.

Headache, better lying on the painful side, aggravated by walk and in the sun.

Paresia of hands and feet.

Weakness of the knees and the feet.

Acroparesthesia.

In the evening, painful cramps of fingers and feet and the palatal vault is insensitive.

Arms seem to be paralysed.

Weakness of hands and fingers.

Involuntary contractions of the lower lip.

3. **Digestive Apparatus**

Bitter taste in mouth, white tongue, the tip is red.

Salivation increased with headache and sore throat.

Desire for acids and horror for sweet things.

Icy coldness in the stomach.

Sensation of emptiness in the stomach and in the head.

Nausea in air currents, vomiting.

Stools, soft or hard as marbles.

Sensation of spasmodic constriction in anal sphincter.

4. **Respiratory Apparatus**

Irritation of larynx, as if burning.

Pricking in the throat while deeply breathing.

Dry cough during sleep.

5. **Sense Organs**

Eyes : Visual troubles, candle light seems to be bluish.

Movement of eyes painful.

Nose : Sensation of coldness in the nose while breathing.

Morning nosebleed.

6. Uro-genital Apparatus

Urinary : Frequent micturition in thin jets with effort. Sensation of swelling of the lower abdomen ; sensation of uneasiness during urination and drawing pain from anus to urethra.

After urination, loss of spermatic fluid.

Genital : Male : Prostatic heaviness.

Testicular pain.

Increased desire.

Female : Menses before time.

7. Locomotor System

Upper extremities : Left arm as if paralysed.

Violent pains in the wrist.

When waking up wrist, specially left, seems to be paralysed, lets fall objects.

Sensation of sprain in the wrist.

Formication in the right hand.

Lower extremities : Weakness of the whole leg, sensation of sprain.

Articular rigidity of feet.

Sensation of weakness and dryness of the soles.

Cold feet.

Cramps of fingers specially towards the end of the day.

8. Skin, Phanera

Hairs dry, fall out.

Pruritis on the torso and between shoulders.

9. Thermoregulation

Chill along the back.

Aggravation being hotly covered and in bed.

Fever in the evening, persistent headache.

10. **Modality**

Aggravation : In the sun, in the evening.

Amelioration : In bed.

Laterality : Left.

CLINICAL DIAGNOSIS

Chorea ; melancholia ; paralysis of the wrist ; rheumatism. Impotency.

HYDROPHOBINUM

(Lyssin)

Consult : General Bibliography.

HISTORY

In the 15th century *Athanasius Kircher* (*Magnus de Arte magnetica*) had, we may say, the intention of using this nosode. He administered in rabbies the compress of the hairs of a rabid dog.

Lux suggested the use of vesicules of *Marochettin* which form under the tongue of the individual who is suffering from rabbies.

But the merit is due to Hering who, in 1833 experimented this nosode and proposed it for therapeutic use. He took the saliva of a rabid dog in a picturesque situation which is described in his Materia Medica and made of it first three dilutions and triturations, then pushed it up to 30th. Hering made a complete pathogenesis of this nosode in 60 pages of his guiding symptoms. This author indicates the curious fact that some of the symptoms of the pathogenesis were felt by himself and his collaborators while preparing the trituration, and so by simple inhalation of the triturated product. The product was then experimented between 1833 and 1869 by *Schmidt, Behlert, Redmond Cox* and *Knerr*. Clarke devotes equally numerous pages for this nosode. By the side of *Hydrophobinum* of Hering, Clarke used *Hydrophobinum Pasteurianum i.e.* to say some anti-rabic dilutions of anti-rabbic vaccins of the Pasteur Institute, which according to the author has produced towards 1886 some grave accidents, even mortal. In his Materia Medica he gives the symptoms observed in rabbies, some symptoms

(264)

observed in some cases of antirabic treatment by the vaccine of Pasteur Institute, and finally some extracts of the pathogenetic experiment of Hering.

The works of Hering are therefore of a date earliar than the discovery of the vaccine by Pasteur. It is not also astonishing that at the time when the idea of microbe had ¡hardly began to dawn, the first experimentator homoeopath had thought that the saliva of rabid dog contained the venom and not a virus. H.C. Allen (Materia Medica of the Nosodes) describes it in 34 pages and even asks if the poison of the saliva of the dog was not the *Thyocyanate* which, one knows, is always present in the normal saliva which would be transformed into cyanide. This hypothesis may at present make one smile but there is no doubt that the pathogenesis of the Nosode *Hydrophobinum* offers some analogies to those of the serpent poison and particularly to that of *Lachesis.*

It is to be regretted that this Nosode used with success by generations of homoeopathic doctors is no more in pharmacetical market of France.

PREPARATION

Lysate of saliva taken from a rabid dog.

PHARMACODYNAMIC CORTICO-VISCERAL PROTOCOL OR CLINICAL PATHOGENESIS

1. Generalities

General depression, impatience, irritability, gay and smiling, then taciturn and melancholic.

Fear of becoming mad, fear of rabbies, bizarre apprehensions during pregnancy.

2. Neuro-psychic System

Mind : Generalised hyperesthesia, caused or aggravated by the sight of water or thinking of it.

Fear of bad news.

Fear of becoming angry.

Cannot bear the heat of the sun.

Fear of water, cannot bear the sound of water flowing from a tap.

Nervous System : Chronic headache, worse by bright light or by the sight of the flowing water.

Convulsions coming at the sight or by the noise of flowing water or while thinking of it or by sudden flash of light.

3. Digestive System

Hypersalivation of a viscous, frothy saliva. Forced to spit constantly. Spasms of the oesophagus while swallowing liquids.

Spasm of the stomach with nausea and vomiting.

Urgent need for running to stools, hearing or seeing flowing water.

Acquous, abundant stools with abdominal pains, worse in the evening.

Desire for salt, for chocolate.

Aversion to water.

4. Respiratory Apparatus

Throat painful, constant desire for deglutition inspite of the difficulty.

Constriction of the neck in the course of a sore throat, while drinking.

Respiratory spasms.

Barking cough, cough by swallowing water.

5. Uro-genital Apparatus

Need for urination seeing flowing water.

Rare, smoky urine containing sugar.

Hypersensitiveness of the vagina, causing difficulty of coition.

Uterine sensitiveness with prolapsus.

Sexual excitement.

6. **Loco-motor System**

Spasmodic pains in the hips.

7. **Skin**

Bluish colour of wounds.

8, **Modalities**

Aggravation : By the sight or noise of flowing water, by brilliant light, radiating sun, going in a carriage, while bending down.

Amelioration : By cold.

POSOLOGY

With Nelson : Hydrophobinum (Lyssin) 6-10M-CM.

POSITIVE DIAGNOSIS

1. Hydrophobia. Irritability. Rapid eiocution.

2. Male sexual excitement and aphrodisia with uterine prolapsus in women.

3. Spasms of organs—nervous, digestive, urinary.

4. All the uneasiness increase by looking at flowing water or by the sight of it by a bright light.

DIFFERENTIAL DIAGNOSIS

Lachesis : Loquacity, phobia of constriction ; nervous hypersensitiveness.

Cantharis : Great irritability, hydrophobia, burning in stomach and urethara. Priapism with exaggerated sexual desire.

Hyoscyamus : Spasmodic norvous troubles, weakness, hallucinations and tendeney to erotic mania.

Stramonium : Convulsions at the sight of water, by bright

light, nocturnal fears, spasmodic constriction of the throat and of the oesophagus.

Belladonna : Hypersensitiveness and hyperexcitability of all the senses. Dilated pupils, photophobia. The look of the water makes him furious.

CLINICAL DIAGNOSIS

1. Generalities

Sunstroke ; convulsion during pregnancy, hydrophobia.

2. Neuro-psychic System

Erotomania ; somnambulism, chronic headache, tetaniform convulsions.

Epilepsy ; general paralysis.

Delirium tremens.

3. Digestive Apparatus

Toothache. Sialorrhoea.

Spasmodic dysphagia.

Dysentery. Involuntary stools.

Dysuria, enuresis.

4. Respiratory Apparatus

Spasmodic cough ; respiratory paralysis (asthma, paralytic lungs of children).

5. Genito-urinary Organs

Satyriasis, vaginismus. Prolapsus of the uterus.

Dysuria, enuresis.

6. Loco-motor System

Sacro-lumbar ; coxarthosis.

INFLUENZINUM

BIBLIOGRAPHY

Fortier-Bernoville :

L'Homoeopathie Moderne, No. 6, 15 mars, 1936, 2e numéro spécial consacré à l'Isopathie et aux Nosodes.

Julian O.A. :

Biotherapiques et Nosodes. Maloine, 1962.

Demageat :

Influenzinum. Les Annales Homeop, franç., Mai, 1968, p. 63-403.

Braun A :

Essais de dèmonstration des réactions sérologiques par l'action des Nosodes de la grippe. Allgemeine Hom. Zeitung, 1972.

Cartier F. :

Thérapeutique des voies respiratoires. Baillére et fils. 1020.

Nebel :

Communication sur la grippe. Le Propagateur de l'Homoeopathie, 1934, No. 1.

Cartier F.

Traité complet de Thérapeutique Homoeopathique. Baillére, 1929. t. 4., Ch. XVIII : Les Nosones Homoeopathiques, p. 95—105, grippe, p. 122—125.

STOCK

At present the biotherapic Influenzinum is a specific preparation The stock is prepared by Pasteur Institute. It is anti-grippe vaccin prepared from 2 varietles of viruses, the one being that of ordinary influenza A.P.R.—8 and the other

A-Singapore-1, 1957, which is called Asiatic influenza. The preparation of this mixture is, 3 parts of Asiatic virus and one part of European virus. These viruses are cultured on chicken embryo, and titrated by the reaction of Hemagglutination of Hirst, after purification, and concentration by formol. The stock contains *Influenza titrated* 500 units of hemagglutinant per millilitre.

It is interesting to note that Pasteur Institute prepare specially this vaccine mixture for Homoeopathic uses.

In fact the antigrippe vaccine sold to the public by this organization is absorbed on Alumina freezing. The presence of these "freeze" is not justified in Homoeopathy. It is therefore a pure product specially prepared that we use in Homoeopathy.

The present-day Influenzinum has therefore the advantage over the old of a great security in the sense that the presence of virus is absolutely guaranteed. But on the one hand we may regret that a single group of virus, the group A, is represented while 3 groups are actually known A, B and F, M, and on the other hand the stock is exempted from all the traces of mucosity and of associated microbes. It therefore loses in polyvalence that which is acquired in security.

In fact the stock furnished very every year according to the epidemology and its data, only the character remains constant (Nelson prepares a great variety of stocks.

HISTORY

Following the famous "Spanish Influenza" of 1918, some nosodes of Influenza appeared.

Thus Pierre Schmidt of Geneva prepared the Nosode Influenzinum-Spanish, but he neither specified the composition of the stock nor the origin.

In the year 1938 appeared an article of Dr. Beeby in Homoeopathic Recorder concerning this Nosode and made a comparative study with Influenzinum of Dr. Nebel.

Nebel of Lausanne prepared towards 1938 a series of Nosodes but they are not found at present.

For the sake of history we mention here the different Nosodes of Nebel.

1. *Common Influenzinum.*

2. *Influenzinum* of A. Nebel 1933, constituted by a great variety of products obtained from the expectorations with many stocks of *B-Coli* and several homoeopathic remedies.

3. *Influenzinum I.C.E.* composed of Influenza, B-Coli, Encephalitis, Staphilococcus.

4. *Inflnenzinum I.C.E.S.* a mixture of Influenza, B-Coli, Encephalitis.

5. *Vaccin E* : Injectable.

6. *Encephalitis Lethergica* 100,000.

O.A. Jullian had the possibility for a few years of using the last one in different neurological affections and the results seemed encouraging.

The disappearance of this stock is regretted.

In the case of a paralysis of the type of Aran-Duchesne a favourable result was obtained.

According to Demageat there exists an Influenzinum 1918, prepared by Bach and Dichington but the stock is not known

There even exists an Influenzinum 1918, prepared by Nelson Laboratory in 30 CH and an Influenzinum with *China* used in Influenza sequalae of Spain.

All these nosodes exist no more in pharmacy.

At Nelson are found at present the different types of Influenza and Influenzinum. Consult Documentary No. 5, pt. 1.

As regards Influenzinum of Dr. Nebel here is what writes Cartier "......our confrére of Switzerland considers this remedy as preventive and curative of Influenza".

Clarke attributes to it an abortive value. Wheeler was successful with it in Influenza in the 30th.

It is necessary to try the polyvalent Nosodes. Polyvalent at 6, 20, or 30 of Streptococcinum, Staphylococcinum, Pneumococcinum, Pyocyanicum (Cartier IV, p. 124).

There exist also several stocks of "Grippen Nosoden" in dynamizations D 6 to D 400, prepared by the Laboratory Mueller, Goepingen in Germany and utilised by Voll according to Electro-acupuncture-orgenometry and tested therapeutically with his apparatus.

Reckeweg has prepared the "Grippe-Nosode-Injeel-forte D6, D10), D30, D200, which are to be used as injections.

Our present day Influenzinum, as has been remarked by Demagent, does not correspond to the old stock.

The English and the German preparations are clearly efficacious.

The preparation of our Influenzinum is scientifically more correct but the reverse of the medal is sure loss of its theraputic power.

There exists no pathogenetic experiment according to the method of Hahnemann.

CLINICAL CORTICO-VISCERAL PROTOCOL
OR CLINICAL PATHOGENESIS

1. Generalities

General ill feeling with chill, headache, diffused pains.
General stiffness.
Hyperthermia at 39°-40°C.
Asthenia and anorexia.
Neurotic. depressive person.
Chronic mesenchymatosis (sycosis).

Predisposition to hydrolipopexia by disthyroidia with the tendency to hypotension.

2. Neuro-endocrino-psychic System

Meningitic syndrome.

Encephalitic syndrome with vomiting.

Headache of influenza : Eyes are heavy and sensitive to movements, stiffness.

3. Digestive System

Pharyngitis.

Gastro-intestinal pain.

Weakening diarrhoea.

Weakness of the anal sphincter.

4. Cardio-hemo-vascular System

Lipothymia – Hypotension.

Weakness of the myocardia.

Cardiac neurosis.

Leucopenia with mononucleosis.

Venous and arterial congestion of the lower limbs.

5. Respiratory Apparatus

(*a*) *Throat* : Pharyngo-laryngitis.

Nasal voice.

Stridulous laryngitis of children.

Chronic laryngitis.

(*b*) *Lungs, Pleura* :
Dry painful cough.

Bronchitis, broncho-alveolitis.

Broncho-pneumonia of influenza.

Subacute oedema of babies.

Bronchial asthma.

6. Sense Organs

(*a*) *Nose* : Oculo-nasal catarrh.

Coryza of influenza.

Polysinusitis.

(*b*) *Eyes* : Conjunctivitis of influenza.

(*c*) *Ears* : Otitis of influenza.

7. Loco-motor System

Rheumatoid pains during humid and cold weather.

POSOLOGY

Dynamisation : 4 CH and 5 CH in granules, 7 CH and 9 CH in globules. The injectable forms that are found in Germany are very active.

DIFFERENTIAL DIAGNOSIS

Mimosa pudica : Inflammation of the oculo-nasal mucosa. Suborbitary headache, worse by movement, better while closing eyes. Diarrhoea with colic and irritating stools..

Galphimia glauca : Hypersensitiveness to change of weather, Hypersecretion of nasal and ocular mucous.

Luffa operculata : Fronto-occipital headache. Acute or chronic inflammation of the nasal mucosa.

CLINICAL DIAGNOSIS

1. Generalities

Influenza, measles.

State of Jacquelin-Burnand (extreme weakness).

Mesenchymatosis with hydrolipopexia, oliguria, disthyroidia in hypo.

Stimulating action in the case of weakness and fatigue. (Reckeweg)

2. Neuro-endocrino-psychic System

Influenza encephalitis.

Syndrome of meningitis.

Post-grippal depressive neurosis.

3. **Digestive System**

   Entero-colitis of influenza.

   Diarrhoea of influenza.

4· **Cardio-hemo-vascular System**

   Varicose ulcer (think of Oscilococcinum).

   Venous stasis of lower limbs.

   Intermittent lameness.

5. **Respiratory System**

   Acute and chronic rhino-pharyngitis.

   Laryngitis of influenza.

   Chronic atrophic rhitinis.

   Bronchial asthma.

6. **Sense Organs**

   Nose-Eyes-Ears :

   Nasal polypus.

   Sinusitis, otitis.

   Acute coryza, chronic coryza, blepharitis, conjunctivitis.

7. **Loco-motor System**

   Infectious rheumatism.

COMMENTARY

Influenzinum, because of its preparation and modalities, its administration by mouth only is legal in granules and in doses which have limited its theraputic utility.

The stock of Nelson seems to me very active.

And, moreover, the injectable variety in different dilutions and mixture according to the method of Reckeweg, allows to say that the indications given in this monograph are not only a reflection of the mind only.

LEPTOSPIRA
(Ictero—Hemorragiae)

BIBLIOGRAPHY

Schmitz-Harbauer R :

Traitement par Nosodes. Klassische Homöeopathie, No. 2, mars, avril 1963.

Askenasi J. :

Revue de Presse Homoeopathique de langue . allemande. Cahiers de biothèrapie, No. 4, sept. 1975.

Gellot G. :

Un cas de leptospirose. Annales Homeop. Fr., 14e année, No. 7, juillet 1972.

Carbon Cl. :

Leptospirose. G.M. de France, t. 80, No. 26, du 14 sept., 1973.

Ballery P. Radot, Hamburger J. et Lhermitte F. :

Pathologie médicale.

Fasquelle R :

Eléments de Bactériologie Médicale. Flammarion, 1959.

Ferron Azéle

Bacteriologie, 1970

STOCK

The Leptospiras are of the order of spirochaetales.

There are two types of Leptospira ictero-hemorragiae of *Inado* and *Ido*, 1914 and the varieties of Leptospira bataviae, *canicola* (*of dogs*), pomona (diseases of porchers) etc.

The clinical description has been given by Larrey during the campaigne of Egypt, by Mathieu under the name of relapsing icterus, by Weil in Germany, whence the name Disease of Mathieu and Weil comes.

Man is contaminated by infected animals directly or indirectly, specially the *rat* which is the carrier of the germs, but porcs and dogs may also be infected. The contamination may results out of a bath in ponds or in rivers.

It is a real professional disease of sewer men, road sweepers and workers of slaughter houses, of butchers etc....

The stock is obtained from a lysate of Leptospira icterohemorrhagiae, diluted and dynamised according to Homoeopathic Pharmacological Practice (Consult : Documentary 5 and 7).

HISTORY

Introduced by R. Voll and his school.

Testing by Diatherapuncture may reveal the Leptospira which is different from hepato-vesicular, cardio-vascular and other affections. It was then understood that the origin of diseases in the patients came from a known or unknown infection by this spirochetiae. In France, it is O.A. Julian who first made the patho-genetic study with the grace of Mme. Binsard, head pharmacist and Mlle. Noyer, the deputy pharmacist of the Laboratoires of Dolisos who prepared the stock. At present the legal prescription of the isopathic is allowed.

CLINICAL CORTICO-VISCERAL PROTOCOL
OR CLINICAL PATHOGENESIS

1. Generalities

Pseudo-grippal state with chill, headache, diffused pains and asthenia. *Morbiliform eruption in erethematous patches.*

2. Neuro-endocrino-psychic System

Syndrome of meningitis with headache and vomiting, myalgia, rachialgia and fever.

3. Digestive Apparatus

Relapsing infections. Icterus with fever of Garnier and Reilly. Intense jaundice (cuteno-mucous), stool normal, very deep coloured urine.

4. Sense Organs

(a) *Nose* : Epistaxis.

(b) *Eyes* : *Infection* ; *Conjunctivitis* with photophobia. Photophobia.

5. Uro-genital Apparatus

(a) *Urinary* : *Oliguria, azotemia, albuminuria.*

6. Loco-motor System

Musculo-articular pains.

7. Skin

Naso labial herpes ; petechiae.

8. Biological Characteristics

Polyneuclear hyperleucocytosis.

Hyperbilirubinemia with transaminesis, normal or moderately increased.

Hyperazotemia, albuminuria, cylindruria.

R.L.C. is equal to clear liquid, lymphocytary ; albumin slightly increased.

POSOLOGY

Dynamisation : Used in France as *Isotherapic* in 4 CH, 5 CH, 7 CH, 9 CH. Is used in Germany : With Mueller, Goeppingen for testing with Diatherapuncture of Voll and in therapeutic as *Leptospirasis* 60 DH, 100 DH. 400 DH, in injectable ampoules.

POSITIVE DIAGNOSIS

Asthenia with pseudo-grippe state.

Jaundice.

Musculo-articulo pains.

Naso-labial herpes.

Syndrome of meningitis.

DIFFERENTIAL DIAGNOSIS

Achyranthes calea : Muscular pains, congestive headache, thirst for cold water, dryness of mucouses, medium fever.

Mandragora officinalis : Alternate euphoria and depression, hepatovesicular troubles, musculo-articular pains, herpetiform eruptions.

Guatteria Guameria : A remedy of liver, of biliary ducts, of kidney, of pancreas. Billious vomiting ; yellow or greenish stools, with nauseating smell.

Agave tequilana : Sad, asthenic persons with hyperacidity, complete anorexia, takes drinks only.

CLINICAL DIAGNOSIS

1. Generalities

Epidemic encephalitis.

Curable lymphocytary meningitis.

Acute angiocholecystitis.

Acute hemorrhagic pancreatitis.

Muscular rheumatism.

COMMENTARY

Leptospira seems to be of great therapeutic value in acute or subacute hepato-biliary affections.

It is very near to *Phosphorus, Chloropromazine*, seems to hold the first place in importance.

The clinical pathogenesis brings out a physiognomy which clearly shows its value in the degenerative processes of the hepatic function and of the hepatic gland.

LUESINUM OR SYPHILINUM

BIBLIOGRAPHY

Allen T.F. :

The encyclopedia of Pure Materia Medica. NY., 1877, New edition : 1964, Gregg Press. Incorporated New Jersey, U.S.A. v. 10, p. 636.

Allen H.C. :

The Materia Medica of the Nosodes, with provings of the X-ray, Boericke and Tafel Phila., 1980.

Clarke J :

A dictionary of Practical Materia Medica, London, 1955, v. 3.

Kent J.F. :

Arzneimittelbilder. Tr. en allemand par le Dr. Edward Heits. Karl F. Haug-Verlag. Ulm/Donau, 1958.

Julian O.A. :

Biothérapiques et Nosodes. Maloine, Paris, 1962. Materia Medica der Nosoden. 2e ed., Haug, Heidelberg, 1975

Sananes R. :

Luesinum. Cours du Sèminaire de 2e année de l, Insitut de recherche et d'enseignement de la Societé Médicale de Bio-thérapie, 1972.

Vannier L. :

Syphilinum. Cours du C.H.F., mars, 1948.

Tyler M.L. :

Homoeopathic Drug Pictures. The Homoeopathic Pubg.
Co., Limited. 152 Landor Road, London. S.W.9, Revised
ed., 1952.

Baur J. :

Notes sur syphilinum. Cahiers du Groupement Hahnemannien de Lyon. Dixiéme ser., No. 5, 1973, p. 182-192.

Johin J.P. :

Syphilinum. Cahiers du Groupement Hahnemannien de
Lyon. Onziéme ser. No. 1., 1974, p. 27-31.

Dorcsi (Vienna) :

Kongressbericht über die 123 Jahrversammlung (Report of
Dr. Pischel). A.H. Zeitung 1972, No. 4, p. 176.

Paturiaux : Luesinum dans l'Epilépsie :

Revue Belge d'Homeop., 1953, No. 1, p. 41

STOCK

The biotherapic *Luesinum* is prepared from the serosity of
treponema of syphilitic chancres.

COMPOSITION

It is a lysate corresponding to 0,001 cc per cm^3 of treponemic serous fluid without any stabilising or preserving agent.

1. Technique of Preparation, Collection of the Scrous Fluids

The collection is done in the conditions required by para 1
of the letter of 26 January, 1936 (ref. Ph. 3 B/S and V/J 166).

1. These collections are presented in sealed capillary tubes.
They are the objects of different controls.

(*a*) *Examination under ultra-microscope* : Reveals the presence of abundant thin, rigid, immobile spirochets. The very
regular pires are 6 to 12 in number. The length of these elements is 6 to 12 μ, their thickness is about 0·5μ. These characters help them to be classified as *treponema pallidum.*

(b) Examination after colouring by the Fontana Tribondeau method. The brown coloured treponema are revealed on a yellow background.

(c) *Cytological etiology* : Shows sufficiently numerous lematies, more or less weakened leucocytes, some epethelial cells.

2. Initial Dilution of the Serous Fluid

The serosities are diluted in 100 times their volume of sterile water.

3. Lysis of Treponemic Bodies

The initial dilution by 1/100 is congealed at—20°, then decongealed at ordinary temperature, which is to be done four times.

4. Sterilisation and Distribution of the Initial Dilution

The lysate thus obtained is sterilised by filtre EKS, then distributed in fractions of 10 ml in sterile phials.

5. Stocking of the Initial Dilution

The fractions of 10 ml of initial dilution are lyophilised so as to be preserved without the fear of any change. Each phial contains a quantity of lyophilised product corresponding to 0·10 ml of serous fluid. This lysate is characterised by its technique of preparation and by their control test.

6. Dilution

The content of the phial is taken up again in 100 ml of sterile distilled water so as to bring the concentration of the final product to 0·001 ml per ml of treponemic fluid.

7. Filtration and Distribution of the Final Dilution

The final dilution is filtered on EKS filter and distributed aseptically in sterile ampoules of 1 ml.

8. Non-toxicity

By subcutaneous injection of 1 ml to some rats weighing 20g each, there will be no accident. A rabbit should bear without any damage the injection of 5 ml of the product.

Let us note here for memory that some *Hepato-Luesinum* (Liver of heredo-syphilitic) and *Rachi-Luesinum* (Cephalorachidian liquid of syphilitics) were used. These nosodes are no more prepared. The first was preferably used in syphilitic hepatitis and the second in the nervous diseases of syphilitic origin. (It is available at Nelson. See-Documentary No. 5.)

HISTORY

From 1830 Lux suggested the therapeutic use of the secretion of a syphilitic chancre as an etiologic nosode.

But it is Swan who published the first pathogenesis in the Medical Adventis, 1880, v. 21, p. 123—142.

According to H.C. Allen the experiment conducted by Swan was done on 5 persons (2 women and 3 men) whose identity is given and on five others who remained anonymous.

Similarly, Dr. Marisson experimented on one person. Dr. Berridge also on one person ; finally Dr. H.H. Carr on 3 persons.

Allen, T.F. refers to H.T. Ostrom, *Organon*, v. II, 1879, p. 262 with an experiment on one person.

A clinico-therapeutic study was done by Th. Wildes and was published in the Homoepathic Physician, 1891.

CORTICO-VISCERAL EXPERIMENTAL PROTOCOL PHARMACODYNAMICS OR PATHOGENESIS

1. Generalities

Typology : Persons of neuro-psychic *unstability*.

Changing humour, stereotype, rigidness because of tendinous osseous pains, specially of *long bones* and worse at night.

Adult : From baby to young boy has the look of an "young old" with wrinkles on the forehead and face ; eyes slightly sunken in the sockets, protruding frontal eminence, dented teeth, tibias are like sword blades, sickly, punny, more or less apathetic.

General action : The action of *Luesinum* is manifested on the nervous system, cortico-medullar system, on visceras, arterial visceras, arterial vessels, on mucouses and skin, on long bones.

Finally its action is more particularly seen in persons having syphilitic intoxication, acquired, old or hereditary. Some morphological structures are marked : *Macrocephale*, dislocated structure, rigid gestures, angulation of the elbow in an obtuse angle, flexible hands with slender fingers. Hutchinson type of caries which is known by the name of *fluoric luetism*, the *fluoric phenotype*. To be added to the classical syphilitic etiology :

—Alcoholism.

—Viral toxi-infection.

—Therapeutic damage in young (iatrogenic diseases).

2. Neuro-psychic System

(*a*) *Psychic* : Morning prostration ; indecisive, disordered, unstable. Need for different activities, intuitive subject but has no sense of descipline.

The adult has perturbation of memory, forgets the name of films or theatres, name of the square of his own town. Difficulty to concentrate his thought and to calculate.

Becomes nervous, indifferent, apathetic ; trembling of hands, some gestures are awkward, which exasperate him.

All these troubles are aggravated at night, and the patient wakes up in the morning completely worn out.

Fear of becoming mad, of paralysis, of becoming incurable.

Depressed, fear of being ruined.

Obsessional state ; should wash his hands constantly for the fear of microbes ; should see whether the door is well closed under lock and key.

Delayed growth of the child, static troubles of the spine. Retarded intellect with difficulty in Mathematics and also in grammar. Seaside aggravates ; on hills he is better. Nightly aggravation.

(*b*) *Nerves* : *Headache* of linear type, going from one frontal eminence to the other, persistent, deep seated.

Occipital pain as if the skull is lifted.

Bone pains, *lancinating*, aggravated at night, increasing and decreasing gradually.

Facial naturalgia, specially *right sided.*

Insomnia between midnight and 6 A.M., with restlessness and bone pains.

3. Digestive System

(*a*) *Mouth-Tongue-Pharynx* :

Deformed dented teeth, often caried and irregularly arranged.

Sensation of a worm moving in the teeth.

Cupuliform teeth (Kent) of children.

Tongue covered with white patch, thick, with the imprint of teeth.

Cracked, fissured, painfnl, burning tongue.

Foetid breath, excessive salivation, specially at night (drains on the pillow).

Burning pain in the pharynx along the oesophagus.

(*b*) *Stomach-Intestines-Abdomen* :

Great desire for alcohol, dislikes meat.

Acid and burning stomach, nausea and vomiting.

Abdominal flatulence.

Ano-rectal *stricture*, ulceration, anal fissures.

The patient dislikes washing.

Bleeding hemorrhoids with burning and pricking pains.

Chronic, stubborn constipation in an emaciated subject, earthy colour ; foetid breath.

Sudden diarrhoea, coming towards the end of night at 5 A.M., aggravated on the seaside.

Rectal paresis, peri-anal ulceration with painful fissures, bleeding easily and discharge of pus.

4. Cardio-hemo-vascular System

Nightly lancinating precordialgias from the base of the point of the heart.

Pressive pain above the sternum.

Pulsation of "hot" blood flowing in the arteries.

5. Respiratory System

(*a*) *Throat* : Hypertrophy of the tonsils.

Dragging inflammation of tonsils.

Ulceration of the vocal chord.

Painful sensitiveness of larynx by touch.

Acute laryngeal pain, comes at night, which forces the patient out of bed and walk in the room.

Aphonia, specially in women before menses.

(*b*) *Lungs, Pleura* : *Night cough*, dry tearing cough, the patient wakes up between 1 to 4 A.M., cannot lie on the right side ; clear aggravation before storm.

Chronic asthma, in summer, in hot and humid weather.

6. Sense Organs

(*a*) *Nose* : Burning and itching of nose.

Burning coryza with yellowish, greenish, irritating dis-charge.

Repeated formation of crusts in the nostrils which are dry and adherent.

(*a*) *Anosmia* : Caries of the nasal bone ; perforation of the palate.

(*b*) *Eyes* : Ptosis, unilateral or bilateral, the patient seems sleepy.

Ocular pains, violent, linear, from one eye to the other, worse at night, with photophobia and lachrymation.

Vertical *diplopia.*

Redness and swelling of eyelids with the sensation of sand in the morning, agglutination of eyelids.

Phlyctenary inflammation, chronic, relapsing, of the cornea.

Unequal pupils, strabismus.

Ears : Chronic otalgia, specially right-sided with purulent otorrhoea.

Caries of the bones of the inner ear.

Progressive deafness, also recessive.

7. Uro genital Apparatus

(*a*) *Urinary* : Slow micturition, difficult micturition, must press with the impression that the meatus is choked in the morning.

Pollakuria. Nocturnal enuresis.

(*b*) *Genital* : *Male* : Induration of the spermatic chords and of the testicles.

Chronic inguinal adenopathy.

Woman : Induration of the neck of the uterus.

Narrowing of the vagina.

Chronic vaginitis, vaginal touch is painful. Abundant leucorrhoea, may flow along the thigh, thick, irritating, greenish, worse at night with lumbar pain.

Pruritis and ulceration of the vulva.

Algo-menorrhoea, oligomenorrhoea, spaniomenorrhoea.

8. Locomotor System

Cranial exostosis, sensitive, painful.

Occipital pain with insomnia.

Pain and rigidness of dorsal muscles.

Cervico-dorsal pain, worse at night by movement, better by heat.

Scapulo-humeral pain, pain of the deltoid aggravated at night, by raising the hand, better after walking during the day.

Bone pains of the tibias at night.

Painful contractions of tendons and muscles of the legs, drawing specially at night, obliging the patient to go out of the bed and walk in the room.

Rigidness and coldness of the extremities.

9. Skin, Phanera

Hairs fall out, hairs on the body fall out.

Early greyness of the hairs.

Copper coloured papulo-pustular eruptions of the integument.

Pustular eruptions of the skin, brown, reddish, with coppery spots.

Abcess with foetid discharge.

Maculae, ulceration, induration of skin.

10. Modalities

Aggravation : At night ; by touch, seaside, during storm.

Amelioration : During the day ; by slow walk, on mountains.

Laterality : Right.

POSOLOGY

From 4 CH to 30 CH.

May be prescribed : 5 CH+7 CH+30 CH, 2 to 5 granules morning and evening.

POSITIVE DIAGNOSIS

Nervous subjects with obsessional ideas, stereotyped.

Amnesia of proper names.

Intellectual paresis with particular difficulty in Mathematics and language.

Nocturnal linear bone pains, cutaneo-mucous induration.

Nightly aggravation of all symptoms.

DIFFERENTIAL DIAGNOSIS

Classical homoeopathy indicates : *Phytolacca, Aurum, Lycopodium, Sepia, Ignatia* and *Lachesis.*

Renovated homoeotherapy : *Astragallus excapus*—Nervous subjects, anxious with tendency to depression and obsession. Cortico-visceral lability and dystonia. Motor incoordination.

Argentum metallicum : Paretic subjects with muscular cramps ; chronic laryngitis and pharyngitis.

Hypogenital, hypochondriac, hyposthenic.

Cobaltum nitricum : Fatigue, paleness, frontal headache, vertigo, bone pains, alternate excitation and inhibition.

CLINICAL DIAGNOSIS

1. Generalities

In children : Psycho-motor retardation.

Particular difficulty for learning Mathematics and also language ; characterial instability with aggressiveness, anger, association in band (delinquent children).

In adult : : Cortico-visceral perturbation in tertiary heredi-tary syphilis. The pathological symptoms appear in a "fluoric" type or in "phospho-fluoric" type having the dominating characteristic of aggravation at night, linear bone pains ; stereotyped. The syphilis has irreductible serology (O.A. Julian : Etudes Hahnemanniennes, cliniques et thérapeutiques, v. 2., p. 183, Le François, Paris), ethylism, toxicomania, old before age.

2. Neuro-endocrino-psychic System

Obsessional anxiety neurosis : Of incurable diseases, of being ruined, at night.

Stereotyped individuals : Continual repetition of the same gestures. same tics, same words (washed hands frequently, always verifies whether the doors are locked, indefatigably repeats the same thing).

Aprosexia : Loss of memory, difficult to fix attention, inaptitude to work, intellectual slowness.

Insomnia from midnight to 4 A.M.

Headache, occipital or temporal.

Tabes : Trigeminal neuralgia.

Facial paralysis : Ethylic polyneuritis.

Syndrome of Dejerine-Sottas or progressive hypertrophic neuritis.

Romberg symptoms ; fulgurating pains, ataxia, nystagmus, generalised muscular atrophy.

3. Digestive Apparatus

Dental caries, sialorrhoea.

Marginal exfoliative glossitis.

Hypertrophy of tonsils.

Hemorrhoids, anal fissures, chronic constipation.

Rectal stenosis.

Diseases of Nicolas and Favre.

Rectitis, recto-colitis, hemorrhagic.

4. Cardio-hemo-vascular System

Syphilitic aortitis.

Vascular sclerosis and hypertonia.

Angina pectoris.

Nocturnal heartaches.

Hodgson's disease.

Arterial aneurism (adjuvant treatment).

Mitral contraction.

5. Respiratory Apparatus

Aphonia ; chronic laryngitis.

Dry cough, dyspnoea at night.

6. Sense Organs

Nose : Ozena.

Ethmoiditis.

Sphenoiditis.

Ears : Otosclerosis of Bezold.

Chronic suppurated otitis.

Vertigo with cicatricial otitis.

Menier's disease.

Laryngeal syphilis.

Laryngeal polypus and papillomae.

Eyes : Pustulous conjunctivitis.

Parenchymatous keratitis.

Irido cystitis.

Strabismus.

7. Uro-genital Apparatus

Enuresis ; testicular ectopia.

Impotency, sclero-gamnous syphilis of testicles.

Atrophic vaginitis, cervicitis, cystic ovaritis.

Fibroma ; induration of the neck of the uterus.

Algomenorrhoea, frigidity, sterility.

8. Locomotor Apparatus

In children : Rachitis, juvenile osteochondritis, osteopsa-tyrosis, *i.e.*, Lobstein's disease, Sicheurmann's disease ; Parrot's disease (syphilitic osteitis of the new-born), dissecting osteo-chondritis or Koenig's disease ; idiopathic osteonecrosis of the posterior epiphysis of the calcanum or Sever's syndrome (O.A. Julian : Recherehes théoriques et pratiques en Homeopathie, v. 1, p. 347—354, 1965.   Le François, Paris).

In adult : Ulceration and necrosis of bones, vertebral caries, cysts of bones (O. A. Julian. See above).   Paget's disease ; fibrosic rheumatism.

9. Skin Phanera

Neurodermitis ; ichthyosis ; psoriasis.

Alopecia ; pelade.

Herpes, lichen planus ; keratodermia, pemphigus.

Syphilitic onyxis ; onychorrhexia.

Lenticular erythema or post erosive papulous erythema.

COMMENTARY

Luesinum is a useful remedy of rapid action, of inestimable value.   It is a "royal" remedy.

It should not be prescribed only on etiological basis.

It is of no importance whether syphilis is a hereditary element, but it is essential that one should think of it whenever there are the essential characteristics of this remedy.

It is the remedy of children, of the 1st and 2nd infancy.

The characteristic troubles with their noisy manifestations which are violent and fleeting, perpetual contests, the refusal to all elementary discipline and associability.

It is the "Cancer" child, who lags behind in the class, whose results in orthography, grammar, language and specially in mathematics make their teacher and parents hopeless.

It is a child who always cries, one cannot understand by which end to catch him because mildness or scolding has no effect on them.

Prescribe *Luesinum* 30 CH, 15 CH, in espaced doses, at an interval of 10 days and *Luesinum* 6 CH or 9 CH in granules, 3 granules morning and evening except on days of the doses of 30 and 15 CH.

With it may be added *Cresol* 30 CH, *Ambra grisea* 7 CH, *Anacardium* 30 CH according to the modalities selected on simillimum or similima. See also D.N.A. and R.N.A. in 30 CH (Ibid).

Regarding the adolescents *Luesinum* will be welcomed when higher studies or integration in manual work creates some behaviorial conflicts or difficulty of adaptation.

Finally the adult persons from the 50th year, will be largely benefited by *Luesinum* when there is the manifestation of symptoms of sclerosis, specially cortico-vascular with weakness of memory, exaggerated auto-satisfaction, stubborn insomnia of the second half of the night with lancinating pains of bones (*Asafoetida* : Coldness in bones). There also is prescribed *Luesinum* 30 CH +15 CH +7 CH, 2 granules each morning and evening daily. Of course in such a case *Cresol, Cobalt nitricum, Argentum metallicum*, etc., may help to cure these morbid troubles.

Finally whatever may be the age, *bone affections*, specially affections of long bones require frequent prescription of *Luesinum*. Similarly in old syphilis, having irreductible serology, *Luesinum* should be thought of.

Let us conclude that *Luesinum* like *Medorrhinum*, like *Tuberculins*, and V.A.B. (ex-B.C.G.) is a very important biotherapic in the daily practice of a doctor.

Before finishing here are two cases :

Case 1

On the 1st July, the year 1958, the mother teacher of De Fr......François consulted us for this child of difficult character since sometime. François is 6½ years' old but his behaviour is changed since 3 years. As a consequence of a strong emotion (fear), this boy becomes nervous, irritable, angry, aggressive. Does not sleep the whole night or has very restless sleep with dreams and cries. He remains somnolent in the day and sleeps during recreation.

When wakes up, complains of headache, has nausea and sometimes vomits badly digested food.

Was treated by a pediatrist who recommended a separation from the family for 3 months which caused a temporary amelioration.

At present all psycho-somatic symptoms have appeared.

The examination shows that the child seems to become nervous and tuberculino-luetic.

Cervical micropolyadenopathy, sub-maxillary and of the groins. The thorax is keel-shaped, lever going beyond the border of the false ribs, tongue charged with a yellow white coating. Hutchinson type of teeth, reflexes are normal.

The first treatment was as follows :

Every Sunday one dose in the following order :

Luesinum 9 CH, *Ambra gresia* 7 CH, *Luesinum* 6 CH, *Rana bufo* 7 CH.

During the week while waking up 15 gtts of following complex : *Anacardium* 4 CH + *Lycopodium* 9 CH + *Senna* 4 CH.

While going to sleep : 15 gtts of *Ignatia* 5 CH and before midnight 15 drops of *Cina* compound.

Comes on the 19th August, 1958, *i.e.*, 6 weeks after with clear amelioration. He has grown up 1·17 mm, weight 22 kg, no headache while waking up, vomited 4 times during the 1st week, two nosebleeds. Still nervous, restless.

We saw the child many times up to the 31st October, 1959 and we may conclude : Characterial stability, remained nervous but neither aggressive nor angry, doing clearly better in the school ; normal social behavior, friendly relation with his schoolmates. Somatic side : Body 1·23 m., weight 25 kg ; liver normal, tongue clear.

The series of medicines are those mentioned above with some modifications according to the evolution of the condition are *Anacardium, Lycopodium, Senna, Strammonium* and the biotherapic *Luesinum*.

Case 2

Dess.... Philippe, 10 years, is a terrible boy, of a very difficult character, screaming, angry, incites his brother and sisters to do wrongs, works very badly in the school, has always bad marks. Capricious, eats bad, irregularly, hold himself vaulted, works up at night, dreams, and wakes up the whole family. Sudden cries of wickedness, cannot remain still, talkative, chews his nails throughout the day.

After the 1st examination it was noted :

When 7 weeks old had toxicosis, then between 2 to 5 years had measles, rubeola. chicken pox, bronchitis, and appendicular pains. At 7 vaccinated B.C.G., had local becegitis with dragging suppurations. Had chronic vaccinosis (oxyuris).

It is a fluoric, nervous, hectic child, bad dentition, holds himself vaulted, with a clear beginning of cypho-scoliosis, flatness of the vaults of the soles, ogival palatal vault, medial fissure of the upper lip, narrow shoulders, the thyroid glands are slightly big, the liver is big, sensitive, goes beyond the ribs and the Mac-Burney point is clearly painful ; body 1·40 m, W-30 kg, A.T. 12/8.

Treatment : Every Sunday evening, while going to sleep one dose in the following order : *Calcarea fluorica 7 CH, Luesinum 9 CH, Agaricus 7 CH.*

During the week : When waking up 15 drops of *Lycopodium 9 XH* ; when going to sleep *Colocynthis 7 CH*, 15 drops ; before noon meals 15 drops of Organo-drainol and after 3 meals one teaspoonful of Genoverian coffee.

Two months later very clear amelioration and the boy was treated up to the 3rd June, 1959 and received as other remedies: *Natrum muriaticum 7 CH* : *Hepar sulphur 30 CH*, *Gl. Thymus 4 XH*, *Levisticum 3 XH*, *Ambra gresia* 5 and *7 CH*, *Bio-mag* tablets and *Luesinum*.

The balance-sheet is as follows : The child is nervous but social behaviour is normal, very clear characterial improvement and better results in the school.

I have seen the mother on the 6th March, 1964 and she said :

"Stabilisation of character, working as an apprentice of a pastry maker very correctly. His relations with his brothers and sisters and friends are quite normal. Somatic side : Body 1·23 m, w. 25 kg, liver normal, tongue clear.

In 1959 his psychosomatic condition was better because this boy wrote to his doctor to tell him, "I am on leave. I am well, sleep well, and I think that you are glad ; after sometime we will meet in Paris".

From an ex-bad boy this post card sounds agreeable.

Case 3

Dr. R. Paturiaux: *Luesinum* in epilepsy. (Revue Belge d'Homoeopathie, 1953, No. 1., p. 41.)

On March 1938, M.D. came to consult me and asked me if I have any medicine, which may cure him from his epilepsy.

He was a young man (30) whose family antecedants and personal antecedants, gave me no information. Present affection has begun from the age of 15.

The patient has a swollen face, full of acne and seems depressed. He replies hasitatingly to my question ; seems to bring back his thought from far away. Is it his pathological condition ? I think that at least this condition should be due to 40g of *Luminal* which he takes daily since 4 to 5 years ; he has arrived to this high dose without any result ; only he has become deeply intoxicated. He has great troubles of memory and abundant salivation specially at night. Besides that there were very few symptoms. As regards the disease, every night since 15 years, without any exception, 4 to 6 attacks of epilepsy, violent attacks during sleep, trismus without any aura noticed by his entourage (the patient is married) ; congested face, trismus, terrible jerkings. In the morning the patient wakes up and does not remember anything. His whole body is painful, and often he bites his tongue. Never an attack during the day not even during the siesta after meals.

Basing on the symptom, aggravation at night and no few other symptoms mentioned above I prescribed *Luesinum 200* and I advised to stop all tranquilisers.

After one month, I saw the patient again. No change. Suppression of *Luminal* did not aggravate. I prescribed *Luesinum 30* followed after 8 days by *Luesinum M*. After one month no amelioration.

I abandoned *Luesinum* to replace with *Rana bufo 30*. No result. I prescribed a dose of *Ignatia M* because of the changing temperament which has begun since sometime ago. That dose was taken one day in the morning. In the evening they called me urgently. He has become furiously mad, he breaks everything, beats his wife and his father and causes some injuries. He recognised me and I happened to get rid of him and told them to send him in a hospital for maniacs.

For eight months he was interned, but he had no epileptic attack during this period. His nights were prefectly calm. Finally one night the attack reappeared and on the next day he woke up perfectly healthy of mind. The attacks became regular, 4 to 6 at night. I had no desire of having a new experience but he insisted.

I found no other remedy but *Luesinum* and I prescribed *Luesinum* 10,000. It was taken at 7 P.M. The night was worse than ever. The attacks came at an interval of half an hour and for the first time instead of ceasing in the morning, it increased to the point of subintrant. Between attacks the patient was not conscious. This condition lasted for 21 hours.

Finally after an entire day, the attacks stopped. The patient slept for 3 days almost a comatose sleey and he woke up cured, completely cured and he never had an attack.

MALANDRINUM

BIBLIOGRAPHY

Clarke John H. :

A dictionary of practical Materia Medica, v. 2., p. 390, 1955.

Allen H.C. :

The Materia Medica of Nosodes : B.T., Phila, 1910.

Julian O.A. :

Biotherapiques et nosodes. Maloine, 1962.
Materia Medica der Nosoden, 2e ed. K. Haug-Verlag. Heidelberg, 1975.

Consult : General Bibliography.

HISTORY

According to Jenner the cow-pox of bovides would be caused by the contacts of the udder with the grass which have been grazed by horses suffering from Malandra. The link between these two and affections attaching some species of other animals, is proved by Homoeopathy. Malandrinum, the nosode of disappearance of which is regretted, has proved to be a good preventive of small-pox and a desensiblising agent for affections sequalae of vaccination.

The term Malandra designates the hollow of the fold of the knee of the horse while Solandra indicates the hollow of the fold of the hoof. By extension Malandra is called as a kind of eczema, dry or weeping, affecting that part and one may think that, that disease has a viral origin identical to the vaccin, although we have no proof of this fact.

(299)

The nosode Malandrinum was first used by Bosokwitz of Brooklyn and then studied by : Straube, Raue, Burnett, Clarke, Carlton-Smith Jefforson, Guernesey. A very wide experiment was carried out by Wesselhoeft, Allen, Steere, Holcombe and the students of "Hering College" towards 1900-1901.

Boskowitz triturated the serous fluid of Malandra then prepared 30 HC, while Wesselhoeft and his collaborators used 30 K, 35 K, and 200 K.

A.L. Marcey (Homoeopathic Recorder, v. 14, p. 530) says that during an epidemic of small-pox he got prepared the vaccin at the same time, day took two doses of 30 K, the vaccin did not take up. Called in a family of 4 children for vaccinating them. He gave at the same time *Malandrinum* 30 K to 3 of the boys. The vaccin took up only on the 4th who tolerated it badly and was cured by a dose of *Malandrinum*. In another family the elder who was vaccinated had small-pox while his four brothers not vaccinated but who took *Malandrinum*, were safe.

Cannot be prescribed in France.

STOCK

The lysate is obtained, without addition of antiseptic, from exudates of the horse malandra.

CORTICO-VISCERAL-PHARMACODYNAMIC
PROTOCOL OR PATHOGENESIS

1. **General symptomatology**
   Occipital headache with pale colour of the face.
   General malaise.
   Foetid respiration
   Lumbar pains.
   Turbid urine containing acetone and uric acid.

2. Skin-Phanera

Dry skin, scaly with itching.

Rhagades of hands and feet, specially from washing or during cold weather.

Intense itching and cracks in the toes.

Crust on the upper lip with stinging pain.

Pustulous eruption of the integument with itching, specially in the evening.

Tendency to chronic suppuration ; wounds are late to cicatrise.

Sub-dermic growth of bony hardness.

POSITIVE DIAGNOSIS

Dry skin, pruriginous with crusts and cracks.
Occipital headache with pale colour of the face.
Urine, turbid, acetonomic and uric.

DIFFERENTIAL DIAGNOSIS

Thuya : Action on post-gonococcic or vaccinal manifestations with tumors.

Hydrogenoid type, fatty aspect of the face with varicocities on the wings of nostrils, violet lips, trophic troubles of nails, cold hands as if dead, intestinal fermentation, fixed ideas and insomnia between 3 to 5 A.M.

Silicea : Sycotic type, post-vaccinal troubles. Demineralisation, headaches, sweats, tendency to suppurations and slow cicatrisation, chilliness.

Graphites : Carbo-nitrogenoid type, apathetic, chilly, venous and circulatory stasis, lymphatism, chronic constipation without motion. Skin dry, rough, vesicular weeping eruptions ; thick yellow secretions, cheloids.

Petroleum : Psoro-tuberculinic type, chilly, fearing cold, dry skin, fissures, vertigo with nausea ; intestinal fermentation.

CLINICAL DIAGNOSIS

1. Preventive of small-pox. To be prescribed during epidemic.
2. Desensibilising the bad effects of anti-pox vaccin.
3. Malignant pustules.
4. Furoncles. Anthrax.
5. Chronic oozing eczema, after vaccination. Impetigo.
6. According to Cooper, it is of use in the last traces of cancer.

POSOLOGY

At Nelson : 30 CM.

MALARIA

BIBLIOGRAPHY

Clarke J.H. :

A Dictionary of Practical Materia Madica, London, 1955, v. 2., p. 302.

Allen H.C. :

Materia Medica of Nosodes. B & T, 1910.

Julian O.A. :

Biothérapiques et nosodes. Maloine, Paris.
Materia Medica der Nosoden. 2nd ed. Haug-Verlag, Heidelberg, 1975.

HISTORY

The nosodes relating to Malaria are badly defined.

The ideal would have been to use the dilutions of different plasmodia. Such products were not experimented.

Towards the middle of the last century Bowen experimented a curious product which he called "Vegetable nosode" and of which one finds in the "Materia Medica of Nosodes" by Allen a complete pothogenesis.

STOCK

The product was prepared from the mire, taken during dryness of a malarial marsh. This slime is introdcced with some water in some glass bowls which are stoppered and left for a week for being decomposed. It is a kind of vegetable Pyrogenium. The pathogenesis scatched by Bowen by absorbing the 1st decimal of the liquid filtered after two weeks, taking 10 drops in 90 drops of alcohol and by inhaling the gas produced by the decomposition of the slime. This product was not long ago somewhat current, until it was completely used up. In reality it was not a nosode. B.T. have prepared a 30th dilution of the mass decomposed for two or three weeks.

Allendy in 1936, clinically experimented *Malarianum* which was prepared from malarial blood and was proved to be a specific in patients suffering from chronic malaria.

None of these nosodes are now found in France and cannot be prescribed.

CORTICO-VISCERAL PHARMACODYNAMIC PROTOCOL OR PATHOGENESIS

1. Generalities

Sensation of great fatigue, general weekness.

Weakness as if from a long disease with loss of appetite.

Feels very weak and languishing, no desire to move, abulia.

Stupor, as if paralysed with sensation of pricking in the whole body.

Headaches and gastric troubles in a closed room and amelioration in a room with open windows and in open air.

After a short walk fatigue and pain in the sacro-pelvic region.

2. Neuro-psychic System

Mind : Feels stupid, asleep.

Hypochondria.

Fear of becoming mad.

Often sighs, restless, nervous.

Nervous : Occipital pain, worse at night, by lying down on he back or on the left side.

Pain on forehead and on cheek bones.

Sleep not resposing, wakes up fatigued, indisposed, with vertigo, which causes sleeplessness.

Sleeps while reading, somnolence during the day. Frequent yawning and stretching.

Restless at night, cannot find a cosy position for rest, worse in the morning.

Vertigo when standing up, must make effort for walking.

3. Sense Organs

Eyes : Heavy and sleepy.

Sight weak, hazy, difficulty for reading.

Burning in the eyes as if from live charcoal.

Pain in the internal corner of the right eye.

Ears : Drawing pain in the pavilion of the ear.

Nose : Sensation in the root of the nose.

Yellow nasal secretion, falling in the back of the throat, specially in the morning.

4. Respiratory Apparatus

Weak respiration, slow, superficial.

Sometimes need for deep inspiration.

Constant cough, hacking, explosive, while speaking and turning in the bed.

Sensation of burning pain on the left side of the chest extending to the shoulder blade.

Sensation of burning pain in the chest from 10 A.M. continuing throughout the day.

5. Circulatory Apparatus

Sensation of beatings of the heart radiating in the chest, while resting the face on the left hand.

Circulatory troubles : Sensation of coldness starting from the legs extending to the whole body.

6. Digestive System

Pain of the teeth of the upper jaw.

Sensation of pepper on the tongue.

Tongue white with a median brown streak.

Sensation of dryness in the mouth but really the mouth is humid with pasty saliva.

Lips are dry.

Desire for cold drinks, lemonade, acid things, potatoes, beefsteak.

Bitter taste, nausea, disgust for food ; does not eat for the fear of becoming ill.

Frequent pyrosis.

Nausea, tries to vomit.

Burning and rumbling in the stomach and in the belly.

Peri-umbilical pains with sensation of heat and heaviness in the abdomen.

False urgency for stools.

Constipation.

Diarrhoea, painless, with intestinal weakness.

Morning diarrhoea with soft, yellow, dirty stool.

Frequent stools, 4 to 5 times a day with liquid mucus, streaked with blood.

Bleeding hemorrhoids, not painful but cause uneasiness.

Liver, drawing sensation, cramps, after urinating.

Dull pain, beating pain in the region of liver and under the scapula (right) aggravated while lying down, better by strong pressure.

Pain in the left hypochondria, worse sleeping and ameliorated by slow walk.

7. Uro-genital Apparatus

Coloured urine, like coffee with the smell of ammonia.

Rare urine, difficult expulsion, with frequent ineffectual urges.

8. Loco-motor System

Weakness of the neck and pain in moving the head.

Lumbar pain and weakness, aggravated while lying on the back or by walk, better by lying on the belly.

Painful sensation in the back, as if going to burst and the pain reaches up to the hips.

Sensation of coldness in the left forearm, reaching upto hand and fingers.

Sensation of paralysis in arms but can move them if he wished.

Hands cold during the day, hands and feet cold at night.

Pain and weakness of the arms.

Pain above right iliac region.

Coldness of feet, which rises towards the knees and to the whole body.

Dull pain of the muscles of the back, of the lumbar region, of muscles of the left hip and thighs.

Sensation of fatigue and bruise of the upper extremities, extending to the lower limbs and to the whole body.

Pain in the knees, by standing and bending.

Dull pain of the external sciatic nerve of the left hip.

Flushes of heat starting from knee, rising upto the throat ; no sweat, amelioration while lying down.

9. Skin

Dry, yellow skin.

Eyes and face are yellow.

Pruritus of cheeks and of the face, then of limbs, better by slight rubbing and scratching.

11 F

10. Thermoregulation

Sensation of having cold or of becoming feverish

Coldness for an hour, fever at 6 P.M.

Coldness with flushes of heat, desire for fresh air.

Coldness begins at noon, every 2nd day ; icy coldness on hips, which spreads over the body, followed by fever, general perspiration, worse drinking.

Wakes up as if frozen, when perspiration stops.

Pain of the legs, of the body with sensation of coldness followed by persipiration.

High fever at night, and in the morning with rapid pulse ; skin hot and dry, drawing pain in muscles and in bones, and a marked weakness of the arms.

Face hot as if from a rush of blood spreading on the whole body and the head.

Delirium at night, talks and signs, finds no rest.

Abundant and profuse sweat at the least effort.

Fatigue in the morning, heavy eyes, vertigo and nausea.

Wakes up at midnight, feet hot, palms burning, followed by abundant sweat on the lower part of the body, more marked on the flexional folds and on the back.

Lancinating pain of the left hypochondria extending to the left leg.

Modalities

Aggrvation : By the least effort, in a closed room.

Amelioration : By rest, by fresh air, by strong pressure.

POSOLOGY

In the list of Nosodes of Stauffen, Goeppingen (Federal Germany) are found : Malaria 60, 100, 200, 400 and Malaria tropica 60, 100, 200, 300, 400 in injectable ampoules.

POSITIVE DIAGNOSIS

1. Sensation of general weakness. Paleness.

2. Occipital headache with vertigo and nausea.

3. Troubled sleep with the sensation of rollings as if on waves.

4. Weak respiration with hacking cough, explosive.

5. Sensation of pepper on the tip of the tongue and desire for cold drinks, acid foods, potatoes, beefsteak.

6. Morning diarrhoea, bloody. Liver painful. Spleen painful.

7. Pains of the limbs and of the back.

8. Fever, coldness, then heat and abundant perspiration.

DIFFERENTIAL DIAGNOSIS

Arsenicum : Thirst for small quantity of cold water, physical and mental restlessness from 1 to 3 A.M.

Vomiting after having taken a small quantity of food, diarrhoea with brown stools, bloody stools.

Eupatorium perfoliatum : Periodical attacks of fever, with the sensation of general bruised pain ; deep pains in bones.

Natrum muriaticum : Chill between 10 to 11 A.M. with beating headache, herpes of lips, amelioration by sweat and tendency of periodicity.

China : Periodic attack of fever ; with a stage of restlessness and of chill and great cold followed by a stage of heat and the need to uncover, then sweat.

Restlessness ; hepato-and spleno-megaly.

Chininum sulphuricum : General weakness with pain and sensitiveness of the cervico-dorsal region. Periodic fever. Periodic neuralgia.

Ipecac : Periodicity of troubles, irritation of the respiratory mucouses, nausea, hemorrhage.

Pulsatilla : Mouth dry, absence of thirst ; vertigo while walking up, erratic pains ; shiverings ; palpitations, watery diarrhoea.

Acidum aceticum : Intense thirst during fever ; weakness and emaciation, dyspnoea, bloody stools, oedema of feet and of legs.

CLINICAL DIAGNOSIS

1. **Generalities**

   Post-infectious asthenia.   Anemia.   Paludism.
   Addison's disease.   Infectious rheumatism.
   Malta fever.

2. **Neuro-psychic System**

   Hypochondria.   Cerebral anemia.

   Insomnia. Neuritis. Sciatica.

3. **Respiratory System**

   Cough. Bronchitis.

   Pretubercular state.   Beginning of tuberculosis.

4. **Digestive System**

   Entero-colitis.

   Toxicosis of babies.

   Hepato-cholitis.   Cholecystitis.

   Splenomegaly.

MALLEINUM OR HIPPOZAENINUM

BIBLIOGRAPHY

Clarke J. :

A Dictionary of Practical Materia Medica.

Julian O.A. :

Biothérapiques et nosodes.   Maloine, Paris, 1962.

Materia Medica der Nosoden, 2nd. ea.   1975, Haug-Verlag, Heidelberg.

Boericke O.E. :

Pocket   Manual of Homoeopathic Materia Medica, p.   421, Boericke & Runyon, New York, 1927.

Homoeopathische Mittel und ihre   Wirkungen, Materia Medica und Repertorium, 1st German ed., Verlag Grundlagen & Praxis.M. Harms, Leer, 1972.

Consult : General Bibliography.

HISTORY

Origin of the Nosode is full of confusion.   *Lux* prepared towards 1820 some dilutions of nasal mucus of a horse suffering from glanders which is called *Ozenine.*

According to Hering this nosode was introduced in Isopathy by Drysdale and the first preparations were done by *J.J.Wilkinson, Spinola, Bollinger* and *Virchow.*

These authors used some triturations and dilutions of the "secretion" of glander of horses.

They called this nosode *Hippozaeninum.*

Quite recently this badly defined nosode is replaced by *Maleine*, a kind of toxin used in veterinary medicine to cure glander of horses.

The experiment of Hering being exclusively clinical there is no real pathogenesis of this medicine which is no more mentioned among the products obtainable in France.

At Nelson, London it is found by the name of Hippozaeninum 6—200—10 M.

STOCK

Lysate obtained from the glander of horse.

CLINICAL CORTICO VISCERAL PROTOCOL
OR CLINICAL PATHOGENESIS

1. General Symptomatology

Consumptive state in grave diseases, like cancer, syphilis, tuberculosis.

Painful swelling of parotids and maxillary glands.

2. Ear-Nose-Throat

Red swollen nose with congestion and ulceration of the mucouses.

Frontal sinusitis.

Nasal secretion corresive, bloody, abhorring.

Formation of nodosities on the wings of the nose.

3. Respiratory System

Nasal voice : short irreggular, noisy respiration.

Suffocating attacks following abundant expectoration.

Spasmodic cough.

4. Skin

Swelling of glands ; nodules of the muscles of arms.

DIFFERENTIAL DIAGNOSIS

Psorinum :   See monography.

Bacillinum :   See monography.

Kali bichromicum :   Viscous secretions, adhering, thready, with pseudo-formation and ulceration.

Aurum :   Caries of bones with foetid suppurations.

CLINICAL DIAGNOSIS

Scrofulous state.

Ozena.

Chronic rhinitis.

Bronchial asthma.

POSOLOGY

At Nelson : 6, 20, 10 M.

MARMOREK
(Serum of Marmorek)

BIBLIOGRAPHY

Vannier Léon :

Le serum dilué de Marmorek. l'Homoeopathic franç., Mai 1912, p. 324-335.

Le traitement des tuberculiniques. —Serum de Marmorek, l'Homoeopathie Franç., 5th year, 1925, feb., No. 2.

Les tuberculines diluées Marmorek, Spengler, Denys. Cours d'Homoeopathie du C.H.F., 21, jan., 1947.

Les tuberculiniques et leur traitement homoeopathique Doin, 1958.

Consult : General Bibliography.

HISTORY

It was in 1903 that Marmorek (Acad. of Méd. of Paris, 1903) exposed the encouraging results obtained with his serum. The serum of Marmorek was obtained from horses, vaccinated by the filtrates of young cultures of tubercular bacilli called "primitive", *i.e.*, having not yet acquired their viro-greasy shell and have developed within fine veils without having the Ziehl.

STOCK

The culture media of these primitive bacillies is constituted by the serous of leucotoxic "calf" mixed in a glycerine bouillon. The "calf" serum is made leucotoxic by previous injection to the animal of a sufficient quantity of peritonial exudate (rich in mono-neuclear leucoytes) and of emulsion of the liver of cobaye. The tubercular bacilli cultured in the media will produce a toxin of weak action of which 8 to 10 ml kills a cobaye of 400 g in about a week but against which the animals may be immunised by injecting them at regular intervals 6 or 9 times a dose of 5 ml. The animals thus treated will sustain, without any damage, the inoculation of a suspension of virulent B.K., or at least will live longer. It is this toxin which is used to immunise the horses. According to Dr. Leon Vannier, besides the toxin, the horses were treated by some cultures of streptococcus collected from the expectoration of tuberculous patients and by some suspension of "dead and sensibilised dead bodies of bacilli".

Marmorek thought that his serum neutralised the real B.K. toxin which are impossible to be produced artificially outside a living organism and which would be according to him different from the tuberculin.

This serum is inoffensive. It causes less anaphylactic accidents. Marmorek recommended its use by rectum but Hamburger criticised strongly that technique thinking that the antitoxin cannot cross the healthy anal mucouses.

Calmette thought that the serum of Marmorek does in no way neutralise the tuberculin and that it is very poor in antibodies (according to Calmette it does not contain sometimes any). Gruner after having assessed the value of the serum of Marmorek thought that there is no difference between this and the serum of an ordinary horse.

However, between 1903 and 1913, some spectacular clinical ameliorations were observed and never was an accident caused.

In Isopathy serum of Marmorek was never an object of real pathogenetic study. Nebel of Lausanne was the first to consider this serum in dilution, in medium dilutions. Its use was described by Léon Vannier (*Loc. cit*).

This nosode is not found at present in France and there does not exist any equivalent. However we may think of using

V.A.B. in its place (see article).. It is still found with Nelson, London in 12 and 1 M.

CLINICAL CORTICO-VISCERAL PROTOCOL
OR CLINICAL PATHOGENESIS

1. Generalities

According to the first observation of Dr. L. Vannier, *Marmorek* may be used in two categories of diseases. The tuberculinics and tuberculars.

According to this author the clinical aspects of tuberculins are as follows :

1. Fever without precise etiology.
2. Repeated coryza.
3. Dental troubles.
4. The constipated.
5. Cardiac neurosis.

All these intoxicated types may benefit by the use of one or many doses of *Marmorek.*

As regards the real *Tubercular patients*, the prescription of the nosode is indicated in tubercular patients having deficient reticulo-endothelial reactions, in fibro-caseous forms, in tuberculosis of bones, tubercular peritonitis and renal tuberculosis.

General Symptomatology

Emaciation.
Febrile condition.
Stubborn constipation.

The subject is *lean, pale, nervous, anxious, restless, hypersensitive.*

2. Neuro-psychic System

Irritability ; insomnia.
Neuritis and toothache ; neuralgias of upper extremities, of thorax, erratic pains.

Pain at the apex of the lungs.

Axillary pains which change places.

Intercostal pains, variable seats.

Asthenia.

3. Digestive System

Dry lips, deep-red colour in the middle of the lips, crusts in the corners.

4. Respiratory Apparatus

Diffused thoracic pains ; revealed by percussion of the thorax.

Pain in the apex of the lungs.

Axillary pains with adenopathy of sub-maxillary glands.

5. Loco-motor-System

Muscular cramps ; arthralgic pains.

Suppurating osteitis with fistula.

Pains of the limbs, erratic, acute, sudden, with muscular pains, sub-febrile state coming after a walk of fatigue.

6. Skin

Miliary eruptions, some red points, more or less pruriginous.

Dryness of the skin.

Granite like look of the skin.

7. Circulatory System

Erethysm of the heart.

Arterial hypertension.

Modalities

Aggravation : Before menses, by cerebral overwork, by walk, by prolonged exercise.

Amelioration : By rest.

POSOLOGY

With Nelson : 12 CH, 1 M.

POSITIVE DIAGNOSIS

1. Adenopathies of ganglions.
2. Anorexia with hypotension and emaciation.
3. Dryness of the skin and of mucouses.

DIFFERENTIAL DIAGNOSIS

Calcarea phos : Marmorek is a complementary.

Pains of growth, headache of students.   Desire for smoked or salted meat.

Diarrhoea after cold drinks.

Sulphur iod : Adenopathies ; emaciation ; hypertrophy of tonsils.

Trachitis with fatiguing cough.

Pruriginous erruptions.

Natrum muriaticum : Emaciation, headaches, depression, median fissure of the lower lip.

Thirst, dry mouth, mapped tongue, oily skin.

CLINICAL DIAGNOSIS

1. **Generalities**

   Tuberculinic condition, emaciation. anorexia.

   First stage of tuberculosis.

   Gougerot-Sjogren Syndrome.

2. **Nervous System**

   Insomnia of school children ; takes much time to fall as leep.

   Headaches, neuralgic type of arnold.

   Dental pains because of demineralisation.

   Thoracic pains of pluritics or bronchitics.

3. Respiratory Apparatus

Laryngitis. Bronchitis.
Broncho-pneumonia.
Pulmonary congestion.
Pleuritis and pleuresy.

4. Digestive Apparatus

Nervous dyspepsia.
Tubercular peritonitis.
Spasmodic constipation.

5. Loco-motor Apparatus

Tubercular rheumatism of Poncet-Leriche.
Arthralgias ; tubercular osteitis with fistula.

6. Skin

Impetigo ; erythematous lupus ; Above-maleoral symetric cyanosis of young girls.
Acrocyanosis.
Rosy pytiriasis of Gibert.
Bernier-Boeck-Schaumann's disease.
Acne rosacea.
Chillblains.

COMMENTARY

We should repeat, as in the case of other nosodes that the prescription of Marmorek requires first of all a drainage of the patient. *Natrum muriaticum, Sulphur iod., Calcarea phos, Crataegus, Solidago. Bryonia, Aurum.*will often be the most appropriate medicines.

Marmorek is a valuable remedy for clinical prescription ; it is a faithful and active remedy but it should be regretted that it can no more be prescribed in France.

One may certainly use V.A.B. as substitute (ex-B.C.G.) as much as a *simile.* We advise our readers to read attentively the article on *Toxoplasma Gondii* which seems to have the first place in the evolution of modern pathology.

MEDORRHINUM

BIBLIOGRAPHY

Hering C. :

The guiding symptoms of our Materia Medica, v. 7, p. 292-324, Gregg Press, 1967, Philia., 1888.

Allen H. C. :

The Materia Medica of Nosodes. **B.T.,** Phila., p. 295-344.

Clarke J :

Dictionary of Practical Materia Medica, London, 1955, v. 2., p. 400.

Loos-Julius :

Propagateur de l'homoeopathie, 1909.

Sieffert :

Revue homoeopathique françoise, 1909.

Kent J.T. :

Arzneimittelbilder. German tr. of Dr. Ed. Heits, Haug-Verlag. Ulm/Donau, 1958.

Vannier L. :

Medorrhinum. Cours d'Homoeopathie du C.H.F., 1946-47.

Kent J.T. :

Medorrhinum, French tr. by Dr. Perichon-Bastaire, Annales Homoeop. fr. No. 7, Juillet, 1972.

Tyler M.L.

Medorrhinum. French tr. of Perichon-Bastaire, Annales Homoeop. fr., mai 1972 and No. 7, July 1972.

Lefort E.F. :

Medorrhinum. Aspects de l'Homoeopathie, Ed. Farnese, 1963.

Sananes R. :

Medorrhinum. Cours au Séminaire de 2e année de l'Institut de Recherche et d'Enseignement de la Société Médicale de Biothérapie, 1972.

Julian O.A. :

Biothérapiques et Nosodes. Librairie Maloine, Paris, 1962.

Julian O.A. :

Materia Medica der Nosoden, 2e ed. Haug-Verlag, Heidelberg, 1975.

Donner F. :

Quellenverzeichnis der Arzneiprüfungen (1937). Medorrhinum : Transactions of the International Hahnemannian Assoc., 1889.

Kunzli (St. Gallen) :

Indikations syndrome von Medorrhinum. Compte rendu de la communication à la 123e Reunion de la D.Z.H.A. du 19 au 22 mai, 1971.

Mouezy-Eon. :

Medorrhinum. Le Propagateur de l'Homoeopathie No. 9., Nov., 1932.

STOCK

The stock is obtained from purulent urethral secretion taken during the period of discharge from several patients, otherwise healthy and have not yet been treated by antibiotics or sulfanilamide.

This secretion is examined under microscope.

(*a*) *Cytological examination* showing very numerous polynuclear and epithelial cells.

(*b*) *Examination according to Gram*, putting in evidence the presence of Neisseria Gonorrheae, as well as epithelial cells.

This examination proves the complexity of the stock of Medorrhinum which is not like Gonotoxinum which is a simple culture of Gonococcus but well at the same time a complex bringing the germs in the media of reactional morbid elements.

The material taken is then homogenised, diluted and lysated.

The biotherapic Medorrhinum is prepared from a lysate obtained without the addition of antiseptic, from purulert ure- thral secretion of blenorrhagia of several patients during free discharge.

COLLECTION OF THE SEROSITIES

The collections have been done under the conditions required in the para 1 of the letter of the 26th January, 1956 (ref. Ph 3 B/S and V/J 166) of the Central Services of the Pharmacy (3e Bureau-Serums and Vaccins.)

TECHNIQUE OF PREPARATION

1. Recep tion of the Collection

The collections are sent in sealed capillary tubes. They are subjected to different controls.

(*a*) *Cytological examination* : The examination between lamellas shows very numerous weakened polynuclear and some epithelial cells.

(*b*) *Examination after colouring by Gram method* : Puts in evidence some Gram negative diplococcus, intra and extra- cellular, and some very numerous, very weakened polynuclear and some epithelial cells. These characters added to the clinical examination help to classify the germs as Neisseri Gonorrhoeae.

2. Dilution of Serosities

The serosities are diluted in 100 times of their volume of sterile distilled water.

3. Lysis of the Cells and of the Microbian Matters

The initial dilution of 1/100 is congealed in 20°, then decongealed in ordinary temperature four times successively.

4. Sterilisation and Distribution of the Initial Dilution

The lysate obtained previously is sterilised by filtration on EKS filters and divided in fractions of 10 ml in sterie phials.

5. Stocking of the Initial Dilution

The fractions of 10 ml of the initial dilutions are lyophylised so as to be able to be preserved without modification. Each phial contains a quantity of lyophilised product by the technique of preparation and by its tests of control.

6. Dilution

The contents of each phail is taken up again in 10 ml of distilled water so as to bring the concentration of the final product to 0,001 per millimetre of urethral secretion.

Filtration and Distribution of the Final Dilution

The final dilution is filtered on E.K.S. filter, then aseptically distributed in 1 cm³ ampouls.

8. Control

(a) *Steriality* :

Inoculation on bouillon or better on gelose should not be followed by any culture.

(b) *Non-toxicity* :

By subcutaneous injection of 1 ml to rats, weighing 20 g each, no accident happens. The rabbit should bear without damage the injection of 15 ml of the product.

HISTORY

First pathogenesis has been done by Swan.

According to H.C. Allen the pathogenesis of Medorrhinum was done by Ren Dell, C.H. Allen, Fincke, Norton, Frost, Farrington, Cleveland, Laure, Morgan, Berridge, Wilder, Huggins, Ostrom, Nichols, Peace, Sawyer, Carr, Rigler.

MacDonald in England, Noegerath and Lydston in America have published some case reports of this remedy. Some observations of clinical and pathological symptoms have also been published in Berrige's Mss, while the "Materia Medica" by Swan contains symptoms observed by him.

Let us note that Burnett prescribed *Glinium* 1000 which is no other than *Medorrhinum*, as he has stated that, 'because I obtained its stock myself from a typical case".

We have given here this information from a historical view only. In the present practice, however, the name Medorrhinum only is current.

CORTICO-VISCERAL PHARMACODYNAMIC EXPERIMENTAL PROTOCOL OF PATHOGENESIS

1. Generalities

Typology : Weak subjects or who has become weak ; *busy hasty* ; time seems to him pass very slowly.

Irritated in the morning, cannot remain in place, legs are restless, feet are restless, feels better by the end of afternoon and *almost frequently gay*, even *joyful* in the evening.

Passes a good part of the night in night clubs or in other places of enjoyment.

Exhausted ; lies down during the dawn and wakes up morose.

It is a complete portrait and does not warrant a necessity of all of its elements being present in a patient to base your prescription.

General Symptomatology

A remedy of chronic stage , it will be indicated in the general morbid condition known as chronic reticulo-endotheliosis (H. Bernard) or chronic Mesenchymatosis (H. Bernard) or *Connectivosis* (Julian) and what is more classic in homoeopathy the *sycosis* of Hahnemann.

It is the consequence of metabolic and toxic metabolism with hydric retention by catabolic slowness.

It is the hydrogenoid condition of Grouvogl with corticovisceral inhibition more or less intense or differential.

Sensitivity to barometric modification or hygrometric modification ; *better by seaside after a bath.*

Fear of air current and coldness.

If his condition develops, he has an *amnesia of recent facts, of proper names, of figures.*

In a high degree, premature silliness. Cannot speak without tears, afraid of catastrophies, remains constantly morose, sad, restless and hasty.

In *pediatry*, the following characteristics are found : Child anemic, polyadenopathic, big head, face often in sweats and frequent catarrh of the respiratory tract.

The babies have red buttocks, irritation around anus, and this may be found in children, adults or in old persons.

Pathognomic characteristic : The patient, whatever, may be his age, likes to lie down in knee-elbow position, on his belly, buttock in the air. face pushed into pillow.

When this key symptom is absent the medicine may be prescribed but when present it is very valuable.

The woman who, having a chronic gonorrhoea which is neglected, has a pale sickly face, has muscular or articular rheumatic pains, always in a suffering condition and a total absence of libido.

The men are "old", intellectually and physically.

These are advanced sycotic conditions, which are neglected.

2. Neuro-endocrino-psychic System

(a) *Psychic* :

Very nervous, feeling of a general worn out condition, worse in the morning.

Starts at the slightest noise.
Irriated for nothing, weeps easily.

Difficulty of remembering proper names, initial letters of words ; forgets letters while writing.

Difficulty to carry on a conversation, ideas do not follow each other.

Mental confusion, "As if what is done to day has been done a week ago".

When thinks of mental trouble, the mental troubles are aggravated.

Cortico-visceral dystonia.

Adult is worn out, hasty in the morning, restless, tries to finish everything during the day in order to live his life at night.

Child, irritable, angry, hasty, does homework hastily with many mistakes. In the evening feels well, gay, no fatigue and refuses to lie down early.

(b) *Nervous* ·

Frontal headache, permanent, with the sensation of a band around the skull ; nausea aggravated by bending forward.

Neuralgia, specially of the head, coming and going suddenly, worse, specially in the morning and ameliorated by moist weather and at seaside.

Vertigo, worse by movement, better by lying down.

Sleep difficult after midnight and after 4 A.M.

Dreams of drinks.

Hallucinations, hears some one speaking in a whisper behind him.

Sees figures looking at him from behind some furnitures.

(c) *Glands* :

Dysfunction.

Hypophisary : Impotency or amenorrhoea, asthenia.

Hypothalamus : *Thyroid* : Troubles of basal metabolism, troubles of sleep.

Ovary : Troubles.

Testicular : Hypertrophy.

3. Digestive System

(a) *Mouth - Tongue - Pharynx* :

Yellowish teeth even after eating.

Mouth dry, burning, bad breath.

Charged tongue, whitish at the base, with aphthae.

Coppery taste in the mouth.

(b) *Stomach - Intestines - Pharynx* :

Wolf's hunger, even after eating.

Intense thirst ; desire for beer, for liquor.

Desire for stimulants, sweets, green fruits, ice, acid foods, salt.

Need for tobacco.

Nausea after eating or drinking water.

Vomits of glairy substances, of bile.

Pain in the stomach, like cramps, not better by eating.

Plexalgia, with agony.

Hepatic and splenic pain with nausea, vomitings, and whitish foetid stools.

Constipation with difficulty of expulsion of the stool, and the evacuation becomes easy by bending backward.

Pricking pains in the anus with redness and foetid oozing, having the smell of fish brine.

Rectal prolapsus of children.

4. **Cardio-hemo-vascular System**

Tendency to *collapse* with the need of being fanned ; to uncover inspite of cold sweat.

Dyspnoea, beating of the heart.

Precordial pains, cutting, pricking, agg. by movement.

Precordical pain radiating to the left hand.

5. **Respiratory Apparatus**

Throat :

(*a*) Pharynx loaded with mucus falling from the retronasal region.

Spasm of glottis, dryness of the throat causing cough when lying down.

(*b*) *Lungs-Pleura* :

Dry, painful cough, worse at night, better lying down on the belly, aggravation in hot room.

Asthmatic dyspnoea in children, better lying on the belly protruding the tongue.

Asthma with difficult expiration ; partially better in knee-elbow position.

Difficult, viscous, small greyish glairy substances are expectorated.

Ameliaration of the respiratory troubles by the seaside.

6. Sense Organs

(a) Nose :

Dryness of nasal mucus. Stopped nose.

Anosmia.

Nasal secretions, white, yellowish, bloody.

Epistaxis ; pricking and tickling in the nose, sensibility by inspirating and aspirating air.

Acquous coryza with frontal pain worse towards 10 A.M.

(b) Eyes :

Eyelids glued in the morning.

Sensation of sand under the eyelids.

Troubles of vision, black or brown spots in the visual field.

Objects look double or very small.

The subject seems not to see what is before him.

Lashes fall ; pockets under the lids.

Sensation of protrusion of eyes with pains in eyeballs.

Induration of the borders of the upper eyelids.

(c) Ears :

Itching of the auditive conduit (external).

Hypoacousia, even complete deafness.

Thinks hearing voices.

Pains along the eustachian tube, Irradiating to the ears.

7. Uro-gental Apparatus

(a) Urinary :

Incontinence of urine at night.

Deep yellow urine, having, the strong smell of ammonia, covered with a greasy layer.

Albuminuria, hyalin cylinders in urine.

Oedema of the feet and ankles.

Inflammation of the kidneys, bladder, prostate.

Weakness of the bladder, pollakuria and very weak flow of urine, often broken.

(*b*) *Genital* :

Man : Seminal loss at night followed by great weakness and impotence.
Impotence, following dragging gonorrhoea.

Testicular pains, pains of spermatic chords, specially of the left side with concomittant pain of the left sciatic nerve, aggravated by the least air current.

Wart formation on the scrotum.

Woman : Dysmenorrhoea with pains of sacro-coccygian and anterior face of the thighs, better by folding the thighs on the belly.

Breast cold as marble, sensitive to touch.

Abundant leucorrhoea, greenish with the smell of *brine water* and intense vulvo vaginal itching.

Augmentation of sexual desire after menses and gushes of heat and sweats. Metritis (exo-endo-cervicitis), dragging.

Chronic pain of the ovaries.

Warts of labia majora and of the perineum.

8. Loco-motor System

Great pain of the heels and soles.

Restlessness and burning pains of the feet, better by cold air and cold sweats of the soles.

Shoulder pains and pains of the small joints.

Neuralgic type of pains coming and going suddenly, worse *in humid weather or before a storm.*

Deformation of finger joints with rigidness.

Acute or chronic rheumatic pains.

Acute rheumatism, aggravated by movement.

The chronic rheumatism is better by movement.

Burning pain of the vertebral column, hands and feet.

Lumbar pain, lumbo-sacral pain, pain of the hips and thighs left sided sciatica.

9. Skin, Phanera

Cold skin, clammy, shining, with abundant cold sweats having foetid smell.

Coldness of some localised regions : Tip of the nose, tip of the breasts, end of the phallus, palm and feet.

Yellow spots on the back and hands.

General puritus, aggr. while thinking of it.

Broken, deformed nails with transversal streaks.

Mucous and skin growths ; peduncular warts, pointed warts, flat warts, seborrhie soft warts. Polypus : Nose, os uteri, vagina, peritoneal region.

Herpetic eruptions on integuments with intense itching. Abundant dandruffs.

Dry hairs.
Relapsing herpes of lips.
Sweat by the least effort.

10. Modalities

Aggravation : By thinking, by touch ; on mountains, by current of air.

During the day ; by dry cold.
Worse on Saturdays and Sundays.
Amelioration : By seaside, in humid wheather.
Lying on the belly ; at night.

Laterality
Left, not absolute.

POSOLOGY

Prescribed from 4 CH to 30 CH. We prescribe 5 CH, 7 CH and 30 CH.

POSITIVE DIAGNOSIS

Subject, hasty, amnesia of recent facts.

Amelioration of all the symptoms by the seaside.

Better by knee-elbow position.

Impatient legs, hasty.

Musculo-articular pains, burning of the small joints and of the backbone.

Wolf hunger, need for alcoholic drinks ; defecation easy while bending backwards.

Itching. Dermo-mucous growth ; with smell of brine.

Growths, warts, polyps.

Tip of the nose, phallus, breasts are cold.

DIFFERENTIAL DIAGNOSIS

Classical homoeopathy : *Psorinum, Thuya, Natrum sulphuricum.*

Renovated Homoeopathy

Argentum metallicum : Hypochondria with greyish face, emaciated, prematurely old, loss of memory, weeps for nothing, left sided hemicrania, terrifying dreams, importency with polution at night, frigidity, leucorrhoea.

Melia-azadirachta indica : Loss of memory, forgets proper names, depressed, forgetful, sensation of ebriety, dreams of rowdy crowd, bitter taste in the mouth, trembling and weakness of the legs, rheumatic pain of the lower limbs, perturbation of libido, abundant leucorrhoea.

Venus merceneria : Loss of coordination of ideas, psychomotor incoordination when writing, headache, vertigo, dreams of spiders, of violence and death ; cardialgia, arthralgia, itching of limbs, of the back, of integument.

CLINICAL DIAGNOSIS

1. Generalities

Degenerative tendency of reticulo-endothelial system.

Cancer condition.

2. Neuro-endocrino-psychic System

Cerebro-medullar degeneration.

Enuresis.

Characterial troubles, specially of children.

Early senescence with amnesic troubles.

Plexalgia ; left sided sciatica.

Crepuscular state with hallucinations.

3. Digestive Apparatus

Stomatitis ; aerophagia.

Chronic tonsilitis.

Alcoholic hepato-gastritis.

Toxicosis ; verminosis with anal itching.

Atonic constipation with earthy stools.

4. Respiratory Apparatus

Epistaxis ; rhinitis.

Spasmodic laryngitis.

Asthma with nocturnal cough ; cough, dry, ameliorated by knee-pectoral position or on "four feet".

5. Sense Organs

Blepharitis : ophthalmia.

Diplopia.

Otosclerose , hard of hearing.

Nasal polypus.

Frontal sinusitis.

6. Uro-genital Apparatus

Chronic urethritis : Urine "by drops".

Impotence, prostatitis, prostatic adenoma.

Salpingitis ; vaginismus, pruritus vulvae.

Condyloma of vulva ; warts, polyps of the neck of the uterns.

Masturbation ; enuresis.

7. Loco-motor Apparatus

Gonorrheal rheumatism.

Scapulo-humeral periarthrosis.

Gout, pain in the heels, left sided sciatica.

Polyarthrosis, chronic and developing.

8. Skin-Phanera

Onychosis, onychophagia.

Warts, condylomas, peduncular benign tumors.

Peri-anal eczema of children.

Senile pruritus ; dehydrosis.

Impetigo ; eczema of the integument.

CLINICAL STUDY

We have the good luck to find in the work of De Lefort : "Aspects of Homoeopathy", the two romantic portraits, feminine and masculine Medorrhinum. Here are the long extracts :

"The traits, of which the contour is only a far away memory of the beauty of a sixteen years' old girl, are lost under that skin, which has lost its appearance of freshness and health. The colour is yellow, not marked by the regular patches of *Sepia* but of faded tone, waxy, almost green and uniform, more marked around the eyes and on the borders of hairs which become grey very soon (Dr. Bernard) and make the blonde hopeless (men become very soon bald, which is still more grave). The eyes are damaged with blepharitis. The lashes are not enough to mask the crusty and oozing borders of the eyelids, and the tears are often there which recall it seems, the "tears of Priape", the price the unfortunate woman has to pay for her first contamination without taking into account the tears that she has caused somany others to shed, unforgettable memories of impure and disordered contacts. The mouth is not much better than the eyelids : crusts, labial herpes, which do not invite kisses. It attracts much less if the ingenious lover knows what is behind the mouth—yellow teeth, loaded tongue, which is thick in the morning (sadness of a livid awaking after the night badly used), white at the base, otherwise red, aphtae everywhere, a pharynx loaded with greyish or bloody mucus. Is there not what will discourage the least delicate partner ? But how to know ? It would be however the case of the saying—"before loving one should know what he loves".

The voice, inspite of the marks impressed on the face, alone is symptomatic. It is the voice of a woman who has smoked too much, drunk too much, who likes beer and liqueur, the costly drinks, so much costly for the pockets of the students of old, the crooking voice of drunkard, of the girl whose existence aggravates the rhinopharyngitis and the laryngitis of which the diagnosis is very easy to make.

"This is all for the face. And the body ! can it compensate the imperfections. ?"

"One would so desire ; but alas ! it is not so. That will not prevent our Venus with her prominent buttocks, because her hips are very strong, to become nacked".

"She is not very hot, but she requires to be fanned. That nudity displayed willingly in her favourite position, on her belly, which ameliorates all her uneasiness by offering the view of her skins that are marked than her face (the legs are almost opal white with slight disquamation), but strewn with pointed small warts, corny, disseminated growths. The unfortunate woman scratches, scratches like Chaplin, the nose which irresistibly pricks her and when she undresses she scratches everywhere on the body even the place where it is not elegant to do so and which may cause dangerous doubts. Her skin is cold and humid, the more cold on the tips of the breasts. If they have not always the cold breasts, the breasts are of marble hardness. They have the characteristic coldness which is of the marble hardness the characteristic coldness which recalls the verse of Baudelairs :

"Separate us from the world, let the screen close.
And let the lassitude bring repose.
I want to lose myself in your deep throat.
To find on your breasts the coldness of grave".
    "The love of Medorrhina is a dangerous play".

In the most secret corners of her anatomy are concealed, as it is known, some dangers which are expressed by some signs which snould give warnings beforehand to the lover. Let us no more speak of the look as we have said enough, but let us speak of the smell because this smell attracts us. The sweats of her armpits have not the attraction of a perfume. However, it is nothing in comparison with other secretions. An albuminous irritating leucorrhoea, which causes pruitus of which we have already spoken, has more repelling musty smell. One may like the fish but there are some places where one whould not like to find them ; specially where it is not the question of the smell of fish, fresh sea-fishes preserved in salt. We have said enough. Love makes one blind. And let it be said that if it blindfolds, it stops also the nose because there are some lovers who do not care for these informations.

"But the test is not yet at an end. Hardly the male who is satisfied and who begins to take the needed repose by the side of his love, in a _Nirvani_ of beatitude and silence, when he feels himself to come out and finds that Medorrhina is not satisfied.

It is the time, let us recall, of Musset when 'on her embalmed bed the swooned Vanina, presses still her lover while sleeping'. But alas ! our Medorrhina, is not sleeping, quite the contrary, she disturbes her partner in his sleep. *"Lassata sed non satiata"* ; her desires, not calmed down, is increased and there she is maltreating the unfortunate to force him to begin again the exercises, which were soon interrupted at his will. It is as much dangerous for the latter, as being awaken from his slumbering repose; he understands the imperfections which were masked before because of his impatience. Becoming clear in his mind, he discerns the defects of this demanding body, that minute patches on the skin, the foetid sweat, and the smell... in short let us no more insist. He should begin again however he can. He must have some courage and when he is successful to repeat, let us give him some credit, though we do not like it. Such is the last trait, lest flattering, yet helps to situate her on which we will leave Medorrhina in the hope that she will not take too longtime to appease her desire which is, more than ever intempestuous.

Here is the Masculine Type

"The individual, who has been in his youth favoured by a gonorrhoea or his ancestors were unfortunate to have it before him, is a curious person. Such a being is frequently met with, although less common, sufficiently different, capricious, full of tics and manias; comic, picturesque, sometimes amusing, often troublesome, interesting to look at but difficult to live with.

"Full of contradictions and burst of humors, perpetually restless, even unbalanced, his activity is more apparent than real, more noisy than active, is goaded by a secret desire which is difficult to understand. It is necessary to be in his existence in order to know him well, admitting that it is possible to do so. The best way to know him is to pass one day in his company. Let us see how he uses his time.

"He wakes up late because he has lied down late and he has not slept well. He took long time to fall asleep even when he has put himself to bed at a reasonable time. He woke up at 3 A.M. (like his neighbour Thuya and Arsenicum). His dreams were less rejoicing, peopled with sad things. He sees incongruous persons and places where he had been before but found there remorses and dead bodies. He has tossed on his bed many times. Sometimes he has put his hands crossed above his head (like *Pulsatilla, Nux vomica,* or *Lac caninum*). Very often he will draw up his legs and push his head into his pillow, a very unreposing posture.

His waking under these conditions is naturally bad. His night has not relaxed him ; on the contrary, he does not love the morning. The dawn seems to him disheartening even if it is 10 A.M.

"He becomes angry, irritated. On his armchair, he displa ces objects unnecessarily. His legs constantly move. It is often compared with the flies on a bell. But it is worse, because his restlessness is of no use ; it often disturbs others in their work.

"His fatigue which is not dissipated since he is awake, is aggravated by all contradictions that he himself creates. He questions his collaborators, becomes breathless, indignant, becomes suffocated, becomes still more worse.

"In his feverish undertakings he loses himself. He becomes irritated, thinking that he is not well understood by his collaborators. He becomes angry and curses ; he speaks, but utters only half of the words. He is losing his memory, he loses the sequence of what he wishes to say. He wishes that others should follow up his thoughts but the unfortunate does not see clearly his own thoughts and expresses himself badly. Incapable to fix his attention in course of conversation he is distracted. He has no attention to what others say, but thinks of other things. He begins again, puts some questions which have already been replied. He has not heard them. If he is the master he cries out : Oh ! how badly helped I am ! If he is an assistant he sighs : The master does nothing understand ! If he is a supplier : The clients do not know what they want !

"And thus the morning passes away in delirious 'kohu-bohu." However, in the evening he begins to calm down and it is then that he becomes conscious that the clock goes very slow. If he has to wait at the house for someone, he becomes fretful. Minutes seem to him hours. If he has a ren dez vous for business, he thinks that he is retained for too long a time and that all is nothing but some time lost during which he could have undertaken so-many new projects with which his brain is crowded.

"He goes to his letters, but the secretary is slow."

"She does not even understand him. How can she" ?

"At first, over and above his hasty words, he soon becomes hazy, begins again, and can no more follow what he has dictated. If he finds the words he pronounces only half of them, the beginning being swallowed up. It is not at all astonishing that the importunate, who hangs himself, is a *Medorrhinum*."

"And then, he forgets everything. First of all, and it is most dangerous in the daily life and in business, he forgets the most recent facts. He cannot remember proper names, even his own. Most common things escape him. He may take notes himself but that does not improve things. He forgets words while writing (like *Lycopodium*), he writes half of what he aimed to write, let alone his spelling mistakes. He does not use capital letters and omits the first letters.

He becomes exasperated for all the obstacles that are put on his way by the *Medorrinum* and the more he becomes nervous the more it goes bad to worse because all those he resents aggravate when he thinks of them.

The hours thus pass feverishly but while this condition

increases in his brother *Luesinum*, he becomes appeased when the night comes. He is typically a man of the evening.

"He loves the outings, the theatres and night clubs and it is only in that way the night is pleasing to him becuase if he likes the night he is afraid of the darkness, It is in the light his life is dear to him. Very often his dinner does not satisfy him. He will take his supper in a cabaret. He is of those who do not disdain the rounds of the Grands Ducs and impenitent night birds. Thus he will drag himself up to the dawn, before returning home sadly when the day breaks.

> Already on the footpath sound my nightly steps,
> O Paris ! you hear me walk.
> When I see pass in the taciturn dawn
> The Cart of the gardner folk.

CLINICAL CASES

Here is a case report by Dr. Sananes from lecture mentioned above on *Medorrhinum*.

On February 1971, we undertook the treatment of M.K... a Spanish painter, age 42. He came for his trouble of micturition which was not well diagnosed. Physically he had a chronic blepharitis which aggravated regularly in the morning since 15 years. He believed that his urine troubles were due to a Gonorrhoea badly treated in his youth, of which he remembered well because his troubles being at that period of life. By anal palpation a big prostate was found. There was great sensitiveness of his rectum and a humid itching which irritated the patient as well as his blepharitis. His spermogram was insufficient, the survival after one hour is 30% of the spermatozoas. His troubles ameliorated very much on the sea-side, without anxiety or restlessness—the characteristics of the remedy. He admitted of a morose temperament with obsession related to his urethra which made him more hopeless when he was not painting or when he was on leave.

The administration of *Medorrhinum* cured him of his blepharitis and troubles of the urethra, the volume of the prostate diminished making him greatly free from his pessimism during leisure.

Here are now some cases of Dr. Schepens : Medorrhinum, in Revue Belge d'Homoeopathie, 1950, No. 1., p. 170-186 :

(1) The 25th March, 1943 : A man of 52 years, mechanic in profession complained of losing his heart in case of need, felt and tired the least effort bathed him with sweats, he woke up sweating at night.

Since one year he has been feeling a pain in his chest ; sensation of constriction as if the heart is squeezed in a vice, accompnaied by anxiety. This pain may come spontaneously, even at night, but came on regularly after muscular strain or after walking fast.

Auscultation of the heart revealed dilation of the left heart with a clear mitral sound.

He was suffering since the age of 20 from lumbar pains followed by turbid urine.

He admitted of having gonorrhoea at the same age; constipation complicated by orchitis and right sided epididymitis. At present the testicle and epididymus are slightly swollen and painful by palpation. Sometimes a mucus discharge, free of gonococcus, was seen in the morning. The sexual desire was completely lost, the patient had become completely frigid.

Blood pressure 12. 5/23. 5.

Blood analysis : 10500 poly. Neutro 84%, Lymphs 15%, Sediment 2 mm per-hour, Urea 22%, B.W. Kahn : negative.

The patient had consulted many heart specialists who treated him symptomatically, having for the result intoxication and no amelioration of his symptoms that he had.

Face to face with the failure of the treatment aimed at ameliorating the circulation and the function of the heart, I have made a careful examination of the patient trying to find out the cause of his present condition. Basing on Gonorrhoea that he had 32 years ago, I was able to ameliorate and to make disappear the circulatory and cardiac troubles and correct the blood formula.

Here is the detail of the treatment :

31st March, 1943 : The patient received *Medorrhinum* 30, 200, 1000. One dose a day for three days. Since that time, the tension comes down regularly ; 19/00, 14th May ; 17/9, 18th June ; 16/8, 3rd July, 15/9 28th Sept.

The heart was becoming better, the sound became less and less perceptible and the precordial pain completely disappeared. He had almost every month one dose of high dilution of *Medorrhinum*, 1000 or 10,000.

10th August, 1943 : Following the first dose of *Medorrhinum* 10,000 he was attacked on the following day by a kind of syncope which was very temporary and incomplete followed by a painful irritation of the urethral passage with doubtful abundant and sterile discharge.

28th September, 1943 : Generally he felt very well.

Followed the patient up to the 5th July, 1944, he still had a slight swelling of the right epididymus. Virility completety restored. He had taken up again his profession of motor mechanic and felt himself to do great efforts for his work.

He received some doses of *Clematis* and *Thuya* for complete cure of the chronic epididymitis.

Blood analysis : 31st July, 1943 has some results . R.B.C. 41,60,000 ; hemoglobin 99% ; white B.C. 3. 500 ; poly : 78%, Mono 22%.

I had news in 1950. He was well.

(2) A young girl of 23 years, suffering from chronic blepharitis since the age of 10.

She suffered much from her eyes, specially in artificial light, intolerable pains which prevented her from going to clubs. It became impossible for her to read in the evening. In the morning the eyelids were stuck together and were very painful to detatch, much secretion.

Dr. Diochers who undertook her treatment said that the father of the girl was treated by him for Gonorrhoea before his marriage. Taking for granted that it was a case of hereditary form of Gonorrhoea he gave her high dilutions of *Medorrhinum* at long intervals, repeated only when the preceding dose ceased to act. The young girl was entirely cured.

(3) Dr. Laren (extract from Clarke's Dictionary) :

It was the case of a French Canadian of delicate constitution who after having worked the whole winter in a mill began to cough in the spring with considerable deterioration of his general health ; got back home and went for treatment to Dr. Laren. He was suffering from a persistent cough and his prostate was enlarged.

Inspite of carefully selected medicines, the patient took to his bed, and Dr. Laren noticed that the patient coughs less when lying down with his head turned on a side on his pillow. The persistent cough and this peculiar position suggested him *Medorrhinum.*

After taking the medicine an abundant gonorrhoeal discharge from the urethra appeared and immediately the cough with all its symptoms ameliorated.

In fact the young person was contaminated a few weeks ago, but because of want of vitality the disease could not make its appearance in the natural way and took the shape of a respiratory trouble.

Dr. Thomas Wilde thinks that favus, the tenia of the head, the Tharsi opthalmic with scaly borders of eyelids, crusty, irritated and red with the fall of eye-lashes are the cases of suppressed Gonorrhoea in one or the other parent.

The irritation of the skin may extend upto the perineum and to genital organs.

He cites the case of a young girl of 11 years, whose face was marble white with profuse crusty eruptions in patches, the eyelids also were affected and almost devoid of hairs, the skull covered with a thick crusty mass from which flowed an ichorus liquid of bad smell. That eruption was descending to the neck and back to reach to the perineum ; the vulva was covered with a deep red eruption which secreted a pale yellowish serum which hardened the linen and stuck dresses to the body. Wilde said to the mother that he can cure her daughter but at first there will be a serious aggravation of the disease for several months.

The mother made no objection.

The child got a dose of *Medorrhinum C.M.* (Swan), the eruption aggravated rapidly, but the appetite, the general condition and the sleep were better. The child was completely cured in 9 months.

Burnett reports the following cases :

1. He has cured with *Medorrhinum 1000* a person who was suffering from epileptic fits at each menstrual period. The attack began late morning.

2. Some polyps, which appeared after chronic purulent discharges.

3. A case of rheumatism of the left wrist.

4. Masturbation in a child.

5. Albumin in the urine containing mucus.

6. A man who had chronic spasms ; the leg rising above the bed.

7. Sycotic asthma aggravated from 2 to 4 A.M.

8. Psoriasis of the palms.

9. Rickets in children having hypertrophy of glands, which were better on the seaside.

5. Clinical Case

Diagnosis : Chronic adenitis : Extract : Case of the month : British Homoeopathic hospital.

J.B.......2 years and a half, had swollen glands at the age of 12 months. Radiography showed nothing. The throat was very often infected. He began to have the fit of coughing by a cold which lasted for months and coughed incessantly at night.

He had no appetite, loved fruits, fats and sweets. He had an optimistic temperament.

Took too much time to fall asleep, restless ; he took off his dresses and had dreams. He took strange positions in bed, lied on his belly, legs drawn up under the body, the face on the pillow. The mother thought that he was going to be suffocated, so she turned him up but he used to take again the same position. He was easily afraid and wanted to be caressed. His cervical glands on the left side were bigger than those on the right. His tonsils were not hypertrophied and did not seem to be infected. The chain of glands thaet wre related to the tonsils could not be felt.

He did not seem to be tubercular and he had no history of T.B. in the family.

A dose of *Medorrhinum 200* was given.

During the following visit much improvement. He had a cold which lasted for a short time.

The last report : Amelioration was remarkable as regards health. The glands were hardly palpable.

COMMENTARY

Medorrhinum, the biotherapic of hydrogenoid constitution, of sycosis chronic mesenchymatosis according to the terminology and according to the studies of H. Bernard, is an active and faithful remedy and helps an amelioration or a cure, of course when it is correctly prescribed.

In babies it is *particularly useful*, specially in eczema of the buttocks.

In children, asthma having nightly aggravation accompanied with the key symptom that the child lies on the belly with the buttocks up in the air and do not keep any dress on the body.

In women, in chronic and difficult infectious disease. It is not a remedy of post-gonorrhœal sterility, but it helps to raze the barrier of toxins.

In all post-vaccinal cases (with encephalitic troubles), its action becomes more efficacious if alternated with *Vaccinotoxinum 15 CH* or *Corticotrophine 7 CH or 30 CH*. Similarly in exudative dermatosis, the *pulmonary affections* (asthmatiform) and migrain.

In *allergic conditions*, following an antibiotic treatment.

In *chronic uretheritis*, gonorrheal or not, it is very actively associated with *Argentum metallicum*.

Finally with *Thuya*, *Natrum sulphuricum*, and *Vaccinotoxinum* used alternately, it becomes a marvellous remedy of cancer.

Contrary to *Psorinum*, which seems to have less rapid action, *Medorrhinum* is a biotherapic useful and efficacious in practice and of which the therapeutic result is rapid and evident.

Like *Luesinum* it is an important remedy of daily prescription.

MENINGOCOCCINUM

BIBLIOGRAPHY

Lefort (de Tours) :

Les hypersomnias. Les Annales Hom. Franc., No. 2, Nov., 1959, p. 14-26 (or 94-106).

Julian O.A :

Biothérapiques et Nosodes, Maloine. Paris, 1962.

David Castro, George Washington and Galvas Nogueria :

Prophylaxis del Meningite pelo Meningococcinum, Similia, No. 13, 1975 (fr. tr. by M.H. Carette).

Roberta Andrade da Costa :

Pharmacopoea Homoeopathica Brasilia, Meningococcinum : Revista de Homoeopathica. Ano 39, No. 2, Julio a Dec de 1974.

STOCK

Neisseria Meningotides was discovered by Weichselbaum in the year 1887 in the cephalo-rachidian serum of patients having acute meningitis.

It is a Gram negative diplococcus arranged in the form of "Coffee grains".

The culture is done on gelose enriched with blood and the principal biochemical characteristics are fermentation without gas of glucose or of maltose and has no action on *Saccharose* or on *Levulose*.

In the bacterial wall, some polyside antigens of the type of A.B.C.D. were recognised by agglutination with saturated serum.

(347)

Thermostable endotoxin of the superficial layer of the wall is put in evidence by its *dermonecortigenous* power.

The meningococcus is the host of the rhinopharynx hence its pathogenetic power in the Rhino-pharyngitis, cerebro-spinal meningitis, septicemia with purpura and eventually in the syndrome of Waterhouse Friderichsen.

CLINICAL CORTICO VISCERAL PROTOCOL OR CLINICAL PATHOGENESIS

Its use in Nosodotherapy is very limited.

It is Lefort de Tours, who while studying hypersomnias told the therapeutic use of this Nosode (Annales Homoeop. Franç, No. 2, 1959).

The stock is a lysate obtained from the culture of a mixture of many stocks of *Meningococcinum*.

According to Lefort, when "the indication of *Helleborous* includes the attack of the brain, it is then the picture of acute meniningitis which is the field of *Meningococcinum*, an infinitely valuable remedy which gives very often unexpected results" (loc cit., p. 26-106). Further on Lefort says : "In an attack of extreme gravity, *Opium, Helleborous, Nux moschata* and above all *Meningococcinum* cause real resurrection" (Loc cit. p. 27-127).

According to Lefort grave hypersomnia and meningitis requires *Meningococcinum*.

It is to be prescribed in high dilutions 7 CH, 9 CH and 30 CH.

It is evident that in acute meningitis, this remedy is the only help by the side of auto-infective allopathic treatment.

The present day importance of *Meningococcinum* is proved in vaccinal prophylaxis thanks to the works of D. Castro and De Nogueira done in the month of August, 1974.

It has been done during an epidemic of cerebrospinal meningitis in the State of san-Paulo, Brazil in the town of Guaratingueta.

STOCK

Doctoress Helena Minin homoeopath pharmacist has prepared the *Nosode Meningococcinum 10 CH* from the stocks of *Neisseria Meningitidis*, type A and C inactivated by heat (autoclave 120).

Administration : A single drop dose, directly dropped in the mouth, on the tongue of each person who is present in the ambulance whese the preventive vaccination is given.

The total population of the town of Guarantiguta was estimated at 78,136 persons. There were about 30,455 persons aged less than 15 years, and 18,000 of these were vaccinated. And 640, aged more than 15 years, who were the most disinherited persons of the town were vaccinated. This vaccination was given between 2 and 4 August, 1974.

The statistics gathered by the authors were subjected to a comparative control which revealed the value of Nosodotherapic vaccination.

It was thus established that the "least frequency of meningitis in the group of population studied should be attributed to the use of the nosode...and the difference between the immunissed and non-immunised groups is highly significative."

According to the authors the duration of the immunity would be 3 months. It is , as such, advised that the dose should be repeated.

In the group vaccinated, there were seven cases of meningitis of whom : one fell ill after two days of vaccination which shows that they were already infected : two others, fell ill in the year

1975, therefore after the period of immunisation, in 3 months, the time attributed by the authors to the resistence caused by the Nosode in 10 CH.

Only 4 cases were proved to be failure.

It is desirable that such experiment should be carried on in cases of other contagious diseases also.

Thus a well conducted Nosodotherapy may take the place of Pasteurian vaccination which is not always free of iatrogenic dangers.

MONILIA-ALBICANS

or

CANDIDA-ALBICANS

BIBLIOGRAPRY

Fallex Jean :

Antibiotiques fongiques et Sycose. Courrier des Medicins Homoeopaths français No. 22, avril, 1959, p. 14.

Julian, O.A. :

Biothérapiques et Nosodes Maloine, Paris 1962.

STOCK

Candida albicans or Monila albicans is a mushroom which appears in culture like oval or round yeasts, budding, with thin walls, accompanied by mycelian filaments formed of articles of variable lengths and have round endings. It is characterised by special spores (Chlarnydospores) of 6 to 12 μ diameter with thick separating wall.

Its identification is done by the physiological character of assimilation and and fermentation of sugar.

A saprophyte of the human and animal digective tract, which may under some conditions (antibiotherapy, diabetis) prolifer and provoke some pathological manifestations of the skin, of mucouses and of visceras.

Its homoeopathic preparation is made from M.T. (alcoholic) 1/10 of a lysate of culture of Monila Albicans supplied by Pasteur Institute.

The clinical pathogenesis is the work of Jean Fallex.

(351)

CLINICAL CORTICO-VISCERAL PROTOCOL
OR CLINICAL PATHOGENESIS

1. General

Allergoso-mesenchymatous subjects (Psoro sychotic), with pathological reactions on the skin, mucouses and on organs (digestive, genital).

2. Digestive Apparatus

(*a*) *Mouth, tongue, pharynx* :

Tongue, thick, dry, cracked, red, scrotal.

Tongue white on its posterior part, like soft brush.

. *Aphthous*, stomatitis with vesicles, white deposit and foetid breath.

Gingivitis. Bleeding.

Dryness of the mouth and of the tongue.

Dry lips, cracked, scorched, crusty.

(*b*) *Stomach, intestines, abdomen* :
Painful spasmodic enterocolitis.

Constipation.

3. Respiratory Apparatus

Allergic asthma.

4. Genital Apparatus

Vulvitis and lichenoid vaginitis with vesicles and pustules ; intense itching and oozing which may end in keratinisation.

Kraurosis of vulva.

Utero-ovarian congestion.

5. Locomotor System

Polyarticular arthritis.

6. Skin

Eczema with the characteristic of linear fissure localised in the folds of the skin and mucouses.

Interdigital eczema of feet with maceration of the skin under which is formed a fine crack, linear and red more or less deep and painful.

Vesicles on the back of the feet.

Peri-ungual inflammation and attack on the keratine of the nails with less thick furrows.

Interdigital eruption vesiculous and itching, onyxitis.

Linear form of eczema, localised at the back of the knee joints, peri-anal, inguino peri-anal, under the breasts, axillas, folds of elbows.

Symmetric eczema of the thorax, arms, forearms.

POSOLOGY

J. Fallax recommends 15 CH.

DIFFERENTIAL DIAGNOSIS

Thuya, Medorrhinum.

CLINICAL DIAGNOSIS

Aphthae ; aphthous fever ; gingivitis ; painful, spasmodic enterocolitis ; constipation after antibiotics ; allergic asthma, vulvitis and vulvovaginitis, kraurosis of the vulva, fissured, linear eczema of the folds of the skin and mucouses.

Interdigital eczema of hands and feet.

Dermatosis after antibiotics.

MORBILLINUM

BIBLIOGRAPHY

Julian O.A.

Biothérapiques et Nosodes. Maloine, 1962, Paris.

Materia Medica der Nosoden, 2e ed., Haug-Verlag, Heidelberg, 1975.

Valette, A.A.M.

Homoeopathie infantile. Maisonneuve, 1974.

Imhauser, Hedwig

Homoeopathic in der Kinderheilkunde. Haug-Verlag, Heidelberg, 1970.

Jousse R.

Protegez vos enfants par l'Homoeopathie, Peyronnet, Paris, 1953.

P. Vallery-Radot, J. Hamburger et F. Lhermitte

Pathologie médicale. Flammarion médecine, Paris 1971.

C. E. D. H.

Pratique homoeopathique en médecine infantile. Centre d'études et de Documentation homoeopathique. Imprimérie du Sud-Est, Lyon, 1975.

STOCK

The biotherapic *Morbillium* is prepared from the exudate of the mouth and pharynx of patients suffering from measles and not yet treated.

The lysate is presented in the form of ampuls of 1 ml. Lysate corresponding by cm^3 to 0.001 cm^3 of bucco-pharingeal exudates and do not contain any stabilising or preserving materials. It is to be used in homoeopathic dilutions.

COLLECTION OF THE EXUDATES

The collections have been done under the conditions requi-red in the paragraph one of the letter of the 26th January, 1956 (Ref. Ph. 313/S & V/J 166) addressed by the Central Services of Pharmacy (3e Bureau : Serums & Vaccins) to the President of the syndicate of pharmacists and special homoeopathic laboratories.

1. Technique of Preparation

The first collections were done in May 1957 and put in Petri Boxes. When they arrived they were subjected to the following examinations :

(*a*) *Cytological examination* : Examination between lamellas shows same epithelial cells and mucus in abundance.

(*b*) *Examination after staining* : According to the method of May Gründwald Giemsa shows a microbian flora, abundant polymorphous, some polynuclears and some monocytes.

2. Initial Dilution of the Exudates

The exudates are diluted in 100 times their volume of distil-led water.

3. Lysis of Cells and Microbian Elements

The initial dilution at 1/100 is congealed at 20°, then decon-gealed in ordinary temperature, 4 times successively.

4. Sterilisation and Distribution of the Initial Dilution

The lysate previously obtained is sterilised on EKS filter, then distributed in fractions of 10 cm^3 in sterile phials.

5. Stockage of the Initial Dilution

The fractions of 10 cm^3 of the initial dilution are lyophilised so as to be fit for being preserved without deterioration. Each phial contains a quantity of lyophilised product corresponding to 001 cm³ of exudate. This lysate is characterised by its technique of preparation and by its control tests.

6. Filtration and Distribution of the Final Dilution

The final dilution is filtered on EKS filters and distributed aseptically in ampuls of 1 cm³.

It is the ribovirus, isolated and cultivated at first by Enders and Peebles in 1954 on monocellular culture.

HISTORY

It appears that this nosode was prepared by Gross, a contemporary of Hering (Bibliothéque Homoeopathique de Genéve, 1835, p. 370). Gross used to soak some globules by the blood of the patient suffering from measles, dynamised and used by olfaction. According to another version he used to give some natural gloubles to the patient suffering from measles who used to keep him in his hands firmly closed and afterwards he used to make dilutions from these globules.

Gallavardin (Propagateur de l'Homoepathie, 1921, p. 271) says that he used in 1912 some granules of *Morbillinum* which he got from the medicine bag of *Des Guidi* who introduced Homoeopathy in France. Inspite of the fact that the granules were some 70 years old, they were quite active.

There is no experimental pathogenesis.

CLINICAL CORTICO VISCERAL PROTOCOL
OR CLINICAL PATHOGENESIS

1. Generalities

Hyperthermia up to 38°--39°. Nasal and ocular catarrh. Nasal voice, rough cough, lachrymation.

Grumbling child ; koptik symptom.
Diffused bronchitic rales.

Followed by an exanthema : macular exanthema, beginning on the face and behind the ears thence extending to the whole body from above downwards, which disappears in 4 to 5 days.

Fine scaly disquamation.

Aggravation of a first infection.

2. Neuro-endocrino-psychic System

Obnubilation, troubles of perception.

Generalised convulsions.

Meningism.

3. Digestive System

Mouth, tongue, pharynx :

Small white patches ; surrounded by a red areola, slightly raised seen on the internal walls of the cheeks and on the mucosa of the gums (Koptic symptoms).

Stomach, intestine, abdomen :

Abdominal pain, localised at the appendicular region.

Acute mesenteric adenolymphitis.

Adenosplenomegaly.

4. Cardio-hemo-vascular System

Tachycardia.

5. Respiratory Apparatus

Hypertrophy of the superficial glands of the neck; throat red, irritated.

Feline cough.

Radiograph shows accentuation of hilifuge opacitis.

Paroxysmal respiratory bradypnoea (stridulous laryngitis).

Polypnea ; flapping of the nasal wings, snoring.

Diffused branchial rales and densified murmurs.

Purulent pleurisy.

6. Sense Organs

Nose : Catarrh of the nose.

Eyes : Lachrymation ; photophobia.

Optic neuritis.

Ears : Acute otitis.

7. Genito-urinary Organs

Spontaneous abortion.

8. Skin-Phanera

Rosy maculae, round and oval, of different shapes separated by healthy skin disappearing by pressure.

Papulous eruption.

Miliary, confluent, scarlatiniform eruptions.

Ecchymotic spots.

POSOLOGY

Dynamisations : 4 CH, 5 CH, 7 CH, 9 CH.

CLINICAL DIAGNOSIS

1. Measles.
2. Primary infection tbc.
3. Phlyctenular conjunctivitis.
4. Acute coryza.
5. Acute otitis.
6. Dermo-epidermitis.
7. Erythematous lupus.
8. Spontaneous abortion.

MUCOR-MUCEDO

BIBLIOGRAPHY

Pommier de Santi :

Mucor Mucedo in E.N.T. : Bulletin de la Société francaise d'Homoeopathie, 1955, p. 153-165 (Special number).

Julian, O.A :

Biothérapiques et Nosodes ; Maloine, Paris, 1962.

Deroche et Vannier, H. :

Asthme et mycose. Communication a la Soc. fr. d'homoeopathie, ler juillet, 1948.

STOCK

Lysate obtained by isolating and transplanting the mushroom Mucor-Mucedo from the medium of culture at 25°.

CLINICAL CORTICO VISCERAL PROTOCOL
OR CLINICAL PATHOGESIS

1. **Generalised**

   State of mycosycosis of Jean Fallax.

   Asthenia, emaciation, anemia.

   Decalcification with phosphaturia.

   Neuro-vegetative dystonia.

   Dryness of phaneras.

2. **Respiratory System**

   Humid asthma, dyspnoea and expectoration.

   Rhinitis. Chronic sinusitis.

(359)

3. **Sense Organs**

Ears : *Chronic otitis dragging supporting.*

Nose : Vegetative adenoids.

Spasmodic coryza.

4. **Digestive Apparatus**

Tonsillitis. Phlegmonous.

Adenoiditis during the pushing of the teeth.

Enteritis of babies.

Hypertrophy of tonsils.

Dental arthritis.

5. **Uro-genital Apparatus**

Hyperfolliculinism.

Catamenia sinusitis and anginas with leucorrhoea.

6. **Modalities**

Aggravation : In spring and autumn.

Amelioration : Prolonged stay at seaside but a slight aggravation at the beginning.

DIFFERENTIAL DIAGNOSIS

Arsenicum album, Niccolum, Nuphar luteum, Gonotoxinum.

According to Pommier de Santi Mucuo-mucedo may replace Strepto-entero-coccinum.

POSOLOGY

Dynamisation : According to Pommier de Santi : 11 DH 8 CH, 30 CH.

MUCOTOXINE

History : Communicated towards 1934, by Cahis of Barcelona.

Preparation : Lysate of culture of Micrococcus catarrhalis, of Pneumo-bacilli of Friedlander and the titragenous Micrococcus.

At present, not found in France.

CLINICAL INDICATIONS

Acute or chronic bronchitis of the muco-catarrhal form in children and in olds.

POSOLOGY

Dynamisations : 4 CH, 5 CH, 7 CH, 9 CH.

An isopatherapic may easily replace this Nosode.

May be had of Nelson, London : Micrococcus catarrhalis 12-200 and Friedlander (Bacillus Friedlander) 6-30.

INTESTINAL NOSODES
OF
BACH-PATERSON

CHAPTER I
BIBLIOGRAPHY-HISTORY-STOCK

BIBLIOGRAPHY

Bach, Ed :

The rediscovery of Psora : and effective method of combating intestinal toxemia. *The Medical World, March, 1928* B.H.J., March, 1929.

Bach, Ed. :

Chronic disease : an effective method of combating intestinal toxemia. *The Medical World, March, 1928.*

Paterson, Elizabath :

A survey of nosodes. B.H.J., July, 1960.

Paterson, John :

Lecture demonstration showing the technique of the preparation of the non-lactose fermenting nosodes of the bowel and the clinical indications for their use.—The Congress of Liga Homoeop. Intern. Glasgow, August, 1936.—The transactions of the congress, p. 214—244.

Sycosis and Sycotic-Co (Paterson)—B.H.J., April, 1938. Psora and sycosis in relation to modern bacteriology. Liga Hom. Int. August, 1936, Glasgow, p. 206 - 213.

Indication for the use of the intestinal nosodes in diseases of children. B.H.J., October, 1937.

Clinical notes and observations of 22 cases from which a diplococcus was isolated in stool culture. Paper read before the Scottish branch in November, 1932.

Julian, O.A. :

Biothérapiques et Nosodes. Libralrie Maloine, Paris, 1962.

Wheepler, C.E. :

Bach Edward and J. Dishington : The problem of chronic disease. Intern. Homoeop. Congress, 1927.

J. Hui-Bon Hoa :

Les Nosodes intestinaux. Ed. Coquemard, Angouleme, 1966.

J. Paris :

La Flore intestinale. Ed. Laboratoire Cassenne, Paris.

Paterson, John :

The Bowel Nosodes. B.H.J., v. II, No. 3, July, 1950.

Up-to-date with Nosodes. B.H.J., v. 43. No. 3, July, 1953.

Homoeopathic Study Group, Oakland, U.S.A. :
Indications for the Nosodes Dys. Co. (Bach). **B.H.J.**, v. 64, No. 4, October, 1975, p. 210.
Consult also General Bibliography.

HISTORY

Hahnemann has always tried to fight Psora. For him, skin manifestations of which the Psora is only an aspect, are the effects of an internal morbid condition which he calls latent Psora. This concept led Hering to the preparation of some first Nosodes, *e.g. Psorinum*. Towards 1925, the British doctor Bach, an eminent bacteriologist prepared some vaccins from many stocks of intestinal saprophyte bacilli. Being attaracted by the Homoeopathic doctrine, Bach communicated with other British doctors : *Wheeler, Dishington*, then with *Paterson, Ross* and *Gordon*. The works of these authors were presented at the International Homoeopathic Congress, London, 1927, while *Dishington* communicated at the same time the therapeutics by the intestinal nosodes in the British Homoeopathic Journal, 1929 (see also l'Homoeopathie française, 1930, p. 798 and 1931, p. 74, 157, 306).

For Bach-Paterson and their collaborators, the Psoric diathesis has, for its foundation, a deep trouble of the intestinal apparatus. They made experiments of about a hundred of stocks taken from selected patients which we are enumerated below conforming to the list supplied by the Pharmoceutical Laboratory, Nelson, London.

Bach Nomenclature		Bacteriological Nomenclature
B. Morgan	← ——— →	Proteus Morgani
B. Dysentriae	← ——— →	Shigella dysentriae
B. Gaertner	← ——— →	Salmonella Enteridis
B. Proteus	← ——— →	(*a*) Proteus vulgaris
	← ——— →	(*b*) Proteus mirabilis
B. Mutabile	← ——— →	B. Coli Mutabile
B. Faecalis	← ——— →	Faecalis Alkaligenes
B. No.7	← ——— →	(*a*) B. Asiaticus
	← ——— →	(*b*) B. Cloacae
	← ——— →	(*c*) B. Freundi
Sycoccus	← ——— →	Streptococcus faecalis
B. Coli	← ——— →	Escheria Coli.

The list of Nosodes having no equivalent in the bacteriological nomenclature : B. Morgan-Gaertner ; B. No. 15 ; Cocal Co.

We are going to sketch the clinical pathogenic picture of these nosodes according to the English authors and to those of J. Hui-Bon-Hoa.

We will speak separately of Proteus and Esch. Coli.*

The common character of these nosodes is that they do not ferment the lactose. They distinguish themselves according to their effects on fermentation on other sugars.

Although these nosodes are not now prepared in France, we will indicate the method of preparation which the authors used, specially that of *Mme. Paterson* who still continues the works of her husband.

---

*A new nomenclature with the reoperative dynamisations has just been communicated to us by the Lab. Nelson, London which is as, follows :

Bac. n°≪7≫(Paterson) 6 c, 9 c, 30 e, 200 c, 1 m, 10 m, 50 m, cm.

Bach, n°≪10≫(Paterson) 6 c, 9 c, 12 c, 30 c, 200 c, 1 m, 10 m, 50m, cm.

Coccal-Co (Paterson) 12 c, 30 c, 200 c, 1 m, 10 m, 50 m, cm.

Dys-Co (Bach) 12 c, 30 c, 200 c, 1 m, 10 m, 50 m, cm.

Faecalis (Bach) 12 c, 30 c, 1 m, 10 m, 50 m, cm.

Gaertner (Bach) 12 c, 30 c, 200 c, 1 m, 10 m, 50 m, cm.

Morgan (Bach) 12 c, 30 c, 200 c, 1 m, 10 m, 50 m, cm.

Morgan-pure (Paterson) 6 c, 9 c, 12 c, 30 c, 200 c, 1 m, 10 m, 50 m. cm.

Morgan-Gaertner (Paterson) 6 c, 9 c, 12 c, 30 c, 200 c, 1 m, 10 m 50 m, cm.

Mutabile (Paterson) 6 c, 9 c, 19 c, 30 c, 200 c, 1 m, 10 m, 50 m, cm.

Poly-bowel (Bach) 12 c, 30 c, 200 c, 1 m, 10 m, 56 m, cm.

Proteus (Bach) 12 c, 30 c, 200 c, 1 m, 10 m, 50 m, cm.

Sycotic Co (Paterson) 6 c, 9 c, 12 c, 30 c, 200 c, 1 m, 10 m, 50 m, cm.

C—Centesimal Hahnemannian.

STOCK

The preparation of these nosodes is as follows :

1. An emulsion of the fecal matter is done by pouring 5 mlg of sterile water in the tube which was used for the collection with the *Porte-coton* (cotton-holder, charged with germs).

2. A petri box is smeared with a drop of that emulsion by means of a glass rod (the surface of the medium should be quite dry and soft).

3. Then it is put in the incubator @ 37° of temperature for 18 hours.

4. The box is examined in sunlight.

5. A colony is taken out with a sterilised platignum spatula and then it is transplanted on gelatine.

6. The transplanted culture is put in incubator for 18 hours.

7. *Identification* : With tne culture are cultivated some well selected sugars : Glucose, lactose, saccharose, dulcite. Then it is verified of which the sugars is fermented.

8. *Preparation of vaccin* : The surface of the gelatine is covered with sterile water for 18 hours, then the solution is sealed in tubes and heated in a *Bain-Marie* (a water bath used by a chemist) for 30 minutes at 60°.

These nosodes are not found at present in French pharmaceutical commerce.

Now-a-days the Bach-Paterson nosodes are replaced by several biotherapics of which *Enterococcinum* and *Proteus* are of first importance, the other being *Colibacillinum, Parathyroidinum B* and to a certain extent *Eberthinum.*

Isotherapics of stools of patients may also be prepared and also of the culture of isolated bacterias.

All these nosodes may be had of Nelson, London.

CHAPTER II

B. MORGAN OR PROTEUS-MORGANI

None of these intestinal nosodes was the object of Hahnemannian experiment.

It is Elizabeth Paterson who has given a list of symptoms that she has collected from the patient cured by the different nosodes from about 300 clinical cases.

STOCK

Gram negative bacilli, short, isolated, facultatively anaerobic, isolated from fecal matters of children suffering from summer diarrhoea. The diarrhoea is caused by these bacilli.

1. Generalities

It is often the question of a patient having blooming face, but in whom dominates a key-symptom : *The congestion*, cutaneous, pulmonary, hepatic, intestinal, cerebral, present or in his pathological antecedants.

2. Neuro-endocrino-psychic System

(*a*) *Psychic* :

Anxious, unstable, depressed, weeping or tense, active.

Tormented by his health.

Cannot remain alone.

Depression : Tendency to suicide.

Fear of unknown persons.

Fear of the crowd.

(*b*) *Nervous* :

Headache with red face, worse during *storm*, *heat*, by journey, by contrariety.

(369)

Migraine at the beginning of the menstruation.

Sensation of vertigo after strong nervous tension.

Periodic migraine, every week.

Congestive frontal headache, sometimes situated on the vertex or occiput specially in the morning.

(c) *Endocrines* :

Congestion of thyroid.

3. Digestive Apparatus

(a) *Mouth, tongue, pharynx* :

Dryness of the mouth, bad breath, salivation.

Lips very red.

Fissures of the joints of lips.

Tongue burning ; pain in the root of the tongue.
Ulcers and aphthae of the mouth.

(b) *Stomach, intestines, abdomen* :

Desire for fat, sweets, eggs, butter.

Pyrosis, acidity.
Burning of the stomach and of the throat.

Acidity and gastric pain, amel. by eating.
Painful sensation in the epigastrium.
Borborygmi.
Pain on hepato-vesicular region.
Redness and humidness of the naval region.
Constipation with anal pruritus.
Diarrhoea in the morning and after meals.

Anal fissure.

4. Cardio-hemo-vascular System

General arterial congestion, specially cerebral.   High blood-pressure.
Venous congestion with hemorrhoids and varices.
Venous stasis of extremities, of legs and feet.

5. Respiratory System

(a) *Throat* :

Dry, burning and red.
Sensation of an apple seed, easily suffocated.

Inflammation of the tonsils which are covered with cheesy substances.

Cervical adenopathy.

(b) *Lungs, pleura* :
Congestive rales.
Dry, suffocating cough.
Hoarse cough in the morning, difficult to hack up the phlegm.

Short respiration.
Pleurodynia.

6. Sense Organs

(a) *Nose* :

Anosmia.
Nasal fissure.
Congestion of the frontal and maxillar sinuses.
Epistaxis.
Dryness of the nasal mucous membrane.

(b) *Eyes* :
Granular inflammation of the cornea.
Chalazions.

(c) *Ears* :
Noises in the ears.
Otorrhoea.
Catarrhal inflammation.
Diminution of hearing.
Furuncle of the meatus.

7. Uro-genital Apparatus

(a) Urinary :

Frequent painful micturitions.
Strong and corrosive urines.
Glycosuria.

(b) Genital :

Feminine

Intense vagino-vulvar pruritus.
Corrosive leucorrhoea, fetid, yellow, brownish or greenish.
Congestion of Bartholin gland.
Furuncle of the vulva.
Dyspareunia.
Menorrhagia and metrorrhagia.
Masculine
Eruption on the scrotum : Vesicular, desquamous, oozing.
bright red, pruriginous.

Eruptions on the perineum and on the groins.

8. Loco-motor System

Rigidity of the back and shoulders ; scapular pains.
Painful swelling of the articulations of hands.
Nodosity of fingers.
Painful swelling of the knees.
Soles painful.
Aggravation of pains at night, by heat, at the beginning of movement.

Feels hot at night.

9 Skin, Phanera

Papulo-pustular eruptions on the face.
Eruptions aggravated by heat, by washing.
Cannot bear the touch of linen on the skin.

Skin sensitive in the sun.

Erythrocyanosis of legs and feet.

Eczema of babies during teething.

Erythemotous aura around ulcers of legs.

Fetid sweat of the feet.

Fissure of heels.

Hairs fall out.

10. Modalities

Aggravation : By heat, at night, and by washing.

Ameoliration : While eating, by prolonged movement.

POSOLOGY

Dynamisation : 12 c, 30 c, 200 c, 1 m, 10 m, 50 m, CM.

According to Hui-Bon-Hoa, a high dilution 30 c is prescribed in acute stage. In chronic cases, says the author, "during exacerbation of a miasm, it is necessary to prescribe a high dilution (1 m, CM) and the doses should be repeated ; during the chronic phase, it is necessary to use a lower dilution and to repeat.

In cases of lesions, a lower dilution is to be used in 12 c, which should be repeated until the patient feels well.

In mental cases, a high dilution is to be prescribed (50 m, CM) and should not be repeated.

POSITIVE DIAGNOSIS

Key symptoms : Congestion of organs and mucouses.

Irritable, depressed persons.

Congestive headache with vertigo.

Hepato-gastric congestion.

Articular congestion.

Congestive, oozing, pruriginous eruptions on the skin.

Eczema of babies during dentition.

DIFFERENTIAL DIAGNOSIS

Sulphur : Morbid metastasis. Burning sensation in the organs and of the mucous membrane ; burning pruriginous eruptions. Red orifices.

Patient busy, restless. Contrariety.

Sensation of weakness at 11 a.m.

Psorinum : See the article on Psorinum.

According to Mme Paterson : *Sulphur, Pulsatilla, Graphites, Sepia, Calc. carb., Kali carb., Calc. fluor., Nux vomica., Natrum carb., Causticum, Petroleum, Lycopodium, Psorinum, Thuya, Tuberculinum, Rhus-tox., Kali biochromaticum, Silicea, S.S.C. (Sulf+Sil+Carbo. veg.)* ; *Kali sulph., Hep. sulph., Natrum sulph., Calc. sulph., Medorrhinum, Calc. silicate.*

CLINICAL DIAGNOSIS

1. Generalities

To be prescribed when "there is a history of repeated congestion of the lungs or of a broncho-pheumonia in children, or biliary diskinesia of women during menopause. (J. Hui-Bon-Hon).

2. Neuro-endocrino-psychic System

Depressive psychosis.

Menace of cerebral congestion.
Menstrual migraine.

Hepatic migraine.

Congestive headache.

Menier's syndrome.

Agoraphobia.

3. Digestive Apparatus

Chronic cholecystitis.
Biliary lithiasis.

Constipation.

Anal pruritis.

Warts on the tongue.

Glossodynia. Apthae.

Fissures of the joints of lips.

Anal fissures.

4. **Cardio-hemo-vascular System**
Varices.

Hemorrhoids.

Erythrocyanosis of young girls.

Hypertension.

Cerebral thrombosis.

5. **Respiratory Apparatus**
Broncho-pneumonia.

Acute bronchitis, specially of children.

Tonsillitis, laryngitis, pharyngitis, trachitis.

Emphysema.

Dry asthma.

6. **Sense Organs**
Eyes : Conjunctivitis, styes, chalazions.

Phlyctenular keratitis.
Iritis.

Ears : Otorrhoea.

Congestive deafness.

Furuncles of the meatus.

Menier's disease.

Nose : Rhinitis.

Sinusitis.

Anosmia, epistaxis.

7. Uro-genital Apparatus

Dysmenorrhoea.

Acute salpino-ovaritis.

Dyspareunia.

Pruritis of the vulva.

Fibroma, bartholinitis.

Furuncles of the vulva.

Renal lithiasis.

Cystitis.

Eczema of the scrotum, and of perineum.

8. Loco-motor System

Scapulo-humeral arthritis.

Dorsal arthrosis.

Gonarthrosis.

Arthrosis of small joints.

Spondylarthrosis.

Arthritis of the wrists.

Fibrous rheumatism.

9 Skin, Phanera

Chillblains. Acrocyanosis.

Pruritis *sine materia.*

Ecne. Ecne rosacea.

Eczema of the buttocks of children.

Alopecia. Acne.

Furuncles.

Flat warts on hands.

Varicose veins.

CHAPTER III
DYSENTRY-CO. OR B. DYSENTERIAE

(BACH NOSODE)
STOCK

The Shigellas belong to the large family of enterobacteriaciae. By their physiological and morphological characteristics, they are related to Escheria, Klebsiella; Proteus and Salmonella.

Shiga (1889) has given the description. At present 10 serological types are known.

The Shigellas are normally eliminated in the fecal matters of the persons infected, but there may also be healthy carriers in whose stools these may not be detected.

CLINICAL PATHOGENESIS

1. Generalities

Generally, but not obligatorily, subjects belong to the Phosphoric types, the blondes having black eye lashes, of pale colour, with red cheeks.

Nervous type, tuberculinics, with a *restless mind*, restless and apprehensive.

2. Neuro-endocrino-psychic System

(*a*) *Psychic* :

Anxiety from anticipation.

Fear without reason.

Fear of closed places (trains, planes, automobiles, buses etc.).

Afraid of going out, of meeting unknown persons.

Nervous stammering.

(377)

Tics of the face.

Restless, embarassed, depressed.

Incapable of struggle, to impose himself.

(b) *Nervous* :

Choreiform movements of muscles of the face or of the hands.

Sub-orbitary frontal headache or of the vertex.

Blinding headache with diarrhoea.

Supra or infra orbital neuralgia.

Tremblings of muscles of the face.

Irregular sleep, wake up at 2 to 3 p.m. with uneasiness in the epigastric region.

(c) *Endocrines* :

Hypertrophy of thyroid gland.

3. Digestive Apparatus

(a) *Mouth, tongue, pharynx* :

Lips are dry with fissures.

Bad taste in the mouth.

Tongue as if scorched and burning.

(b) *Stomach, intestines, abdomen* :

Desire for : Fats, sweetened foods, salty foods, milk.

Post prandial pain of the stomach, amel. by eating.

Distension of the abdomen, with uneasiness after meals.

Distension and abdominal flatulence.

Pain in the stomach between midnight and 1 a.m., better by vomiting of a large quantity of mucus.

Pyloric spasms of the babies :

Diarrhoea, frequent stools for 5 or 6 days.

Sensation diarrhoea.

Sensation of throbbing in the rectum, sensation of a plug in the rectum.

4. Cardio-hemo-vascular System

Palpitation with precordial uneasiness.

Extrasystole.

Tachycardia.

5. Respiratory Apparatus

(a) *Throat* : Frequent inflammation of the tonsils.

Inflammation of the pharynx.

Dryness of the throat.

(b) *Lungs, pleura* :

Thoracic pains by efforts.

Sensation of constriction on the lower ribs.

Pleural pains.

Loss of breath.

Catarrhs of the bronchi.

Cough with expectoration tinged with blood.

Spasmodic cough.

6. Sense Organs

(a) *Nose* : *Rhinorrhoea, spasmodic and vaso-motric* :

Acute catarrh of the nasal and ocular mucouses, occurring in some subjects during the flowering of the graminacae.

Root of the nose is painful.

(b) *Eyes* : Inflammation and irritation, conjunctivitis.

Inflammation of the borders of the eyelids.

Inflammation of the sebacious annexe of the lips of an eye.

Nicitation of the eyelids.

Floating bodies.

Yellow vision.

(c) *Ears* : Discharge from the ear.

Sudden swelling of the ears, bluish red colour, then desquamation.

7. **Genito-urinary System**

   (*a*) *Urinary* :

   Urgent desire for urination in train, aeroplane, trams.

   (*b*) *Genital* :

   Menstrual irregularity.

   Dysmenorrhoea.

   Throbbing sensation in the pelvis and perineum.

8. **Locomotor System**

   Articular pains of the joints.

   Backache.

   Pain in the knees.

   Inflammatory pains of the heels.

9. **Skin, Phanera**

   Integument, sensitive, painful when combing.

   Dryness of the integument, with abundant dandruffs.

   Cervico-scapular fibrocity.

   Facial, cervical, thoracic herpes.

   Vesicles between fingers.

   Dry dermatitis of the palms, with fissures, painful.

   Flat warts on hands.

   Urticarial eruptions.

10. **Modalities**

   Aggravation : In crowd, during journey.

             At night towards 2 to 3 a.m.

   Amelioration : While eating.

POSOLOGY

Dynamisations : According to the English authors : 12 c, 30 c, 200 c, 1 m, 10 m, 50 m, cm.

POSITIVE DIAGNOSIS

Nervous tension, apprehension.

Anxiety in anticipation.

Tics and choreiform movements.

Fear of a closed space.

Gastralgia and acute colitis.

Inflammation of nasal, ocular and pharyngeal mucous membrane.

Menstrual irregularities.

Articular pains.

Vesicular or dry dermatitis.

DIFFERENTIAL DIAGNOSIS

According to the English authors related remedies are : *Arsenicum album, Argentum nitricum, Kalmia latifolia.*

According to the present homoeopathy : *Levomepromazine* is related because of the psychic symptoms ; premonition of an event which is imminent but undefinable.

CLINICAL DIAGNOSIS

1. **Generalities**

   Acetonemia in children (Foubister).

2. **Neuro-endocrino-psychic System**

   Claustrophobia, timidity.

   Periodic headache.

   Choreiform movements.

3. **Digestive Apparatus**

   Aerogastria.

   Gastralgia ; gastric and duodenal ulcer.

   Spasms of the pylora in children.

4. **Cardio-vascular System**

   Thyroidian tachycardia.

5. **Respiratory Apparatus**

   Repeated bronchitis. Pharyngitis.

   Pleurodynia.

   Dry pleurisy.

   Chronic-bronchitis.

6. **Sense Organs**

   Eye : Blepharitis, conjunctivitis, styes.

   Ears : Otorrhoea.

   Nose : Hay fever.

7. **Uro-genital Apparatus** :

   Cystitis.

   Dysmenorrhoea.

   Menstrual irregularity.

8. **Locomotor System**

   Arthrosis of the jaws.

   Osteo-arthritis and periostitis of feet.

   Gonarthrosis.

   Osteoporosis.

9. **Skin**

   Herpes ; eczema between fingers ; psorisis.

   Dry eczema.

   Urtricaria.

CHAPTER IV

B. GAERTNER OR SALMONELLA ENTERIDITIS

(NOSODE OF BACH)

STOCK

Salmonella Enteriditis or Bacillus Gaertner belongs to the family of Enterobacteriacae and of the Salmonella group.

Salmonella Enteriditis is a Serotype of Salmonella, frequently found in animals which often causes food intoxication in men. Its antigenic formula is : 1, 9, 12 : gm and its biochemic characteristics are like those of most of the Salmonella. (The antigen H possesses only a phase designated gm. The antigen O is very near to that of S. typhi).

CLINICAL PATHOGENESIS

1. Generalities

The persons are lean, pale and hypersensitive.

Great deficiency of connective tissues.

Malnutrition.

Suits to punny, hypersensitive children.

They are often blonde subjects with red spots.

Blue eyes.

Hypothrepsia.

2. Neuro-endocrino-psychic System

(a) *Psychic* :

Intelligent persons, nervous, with *restlessness of hand and feet.*

They become restless when alone, or when crossing the street.

Excitable, irritable and depressed.

Chews his nails.

(383)

(*b*) *Nervous* :

Sleeps for a long time.

Wants light while sleeping.
Need for company. Cannot sleep alone.
Restless sleep, noctural fear.

3. Digestive Apparatus

(*a*) *Mouth, tongue, pharynx* :

Peri-labial herpes.
Dry eruption, desquamation of the lips.
Black teeth.
Salivation.
Fissured tongue.

(*b*) *Stomach, intestines, abdomen* :

Cannot digest fat foods.
Aversion to bread, butter, meat and fish.
Desire for oat soup, cheese, eggs, milk, pudding, sugar and sweets.

Vomits everything after taking sweets.
Stomach dilated with acidity.

Acetonemia in children : Headache and vomiting.

Constipation.
Foetid diarrhoea, every 15 days.
Stools with mucus, bloody.
Anal pruritis.

4. Respiratory Apparatus

Sensation of coldness in the chest.

Night cough.

5. Sense Organs

Nose : Catarrh, polyps.
Eyes : White sclerotic eyes. Styes.

6. Uro-genital Apparatus

(*a*) *Urinary* :

Burning of the urethra.
Presence of blood and mucus in the urine.

(*b*) *Genital* :

Female

Profuse, foetid leucorrhoea. Pruritus of the vulva.

Male : Hydrocele.

7. Locomotor System

Great pains of the hips and back.

Upper extremities.

Fibrosity of shoulders, rheumatism of shoulders, worse at night.
Rheumatism of hands.

Lower extremities.

Rheumatic pain of feet.
Depression of the vaults of the soles.

8. Skin, Phanera

Chapped hands in winter.
Chews the nails.
Pruriginous vesicles of the feet worse at night.
Round patches of urticaria.
Furuncles on arms and legs.
Circinatous sternal eruption.
Abundant sweats at night.

9. Modalities

Aggravation

Nervous, while crossing a street, at night, in winter.

Amelioration

While someone is near.

POSOLOGY

Dynamisations : 12 c, 30 c, 10 m, 50 m, c. m.

POSITIVE DIAGNOSIS

Deficiency of the mesenchymatous tissues.

Malnutrition.

Nervous, restless hands and feet.

Chews nails.
Nocturnal fear in children.

Cannot digest fat.

Pains of hips, back, upper and lower extremities.

Urticaria and vesicular eruptions, specially of hands and feet.

DIFFERENTIAL DIAGNOSIS

The English authors say that *Phosphorus, Silicea, Mercurius vivus* are related to it.

One should also think of *Tuberculinum* and *Luesinum*.

Among the modern homoeopathic remedies *Chloropromazine* and *Levomepromazine* (See Matiére médicale d'homoeopathie by O.A. Julian and Collab).

CLINICAL DIAGNOSIS

Pre-cancer state (Canceriques of Léon Vannier).

Hypothrepsy in children.

Nocturnal fear.

Fibrous rheumatism of Jacoud.

Furunculosis.

Onyxophagia.

Coeliac diseases.

Chronic gastro-enteritis.

Onyxurosis.

Chronic pancreatic diseases.

CHAPTER V

CLINICAL PATHOGENESIS OF MUTABILIS—B. FAECALIS, COCCAL-CO.

(NOSODES BACH-PATERSON)

(a) B. Mutabilis of Paterson

According to the bacteriological nomenclature corresponds to the Bacillus-Coli-Mutabile.

One should refer to Nelson Pharmacy of London. Neither its characteristics nor preparation of the stock is precisely described. According to J. Hui-Bon-Hoa, this nosode is so named because it undergoes a mutation immediately it is put to a culture and by a non lacto-lytic germ, it becomes a germ which attacks the lactose. It is a germ intermediary between Colibacilli and real non Lacto-lytic bacillus.

According to Foubister it is used in *Albuminuria*.

A second indication : *Morbid metastasis,* when a symptom, as for example, "an eruption on the skin alternates with asthmatic symptoms (J. Hui-Bon-Hoa). Its principal associated remedy is *Pulsatilla.*

(b) Bacillus Faecalis of Bach

According to the indications furnished by the Nelson Pharmacy it corresponds to Bacillus Feacalis Alcaligenes.

It is not a valuable remedy. Every time they are found in the stool, the clinical symptoms are those of *Sepia* (J. Hui-Bon-Hoa).

(c) Cocal-Co. of Paterson

Has no correspondence in the bacteriological nomenclature. It is indicated in septic states.

CHAPTER VI

BACILLUS NO. 7

OR

(a) B. ASIATICUS, (b) B. CLOACAE, (c) B. FREUNDI.
(NOSODES OF PATERSON)

STOCK

Face to face with the particular terminology of the English-men, we felt it necessary to ask for some informations from the Nelson Pharmacy of London.

Thus we know that some of the nosodes of Bach-Paterson have the common character that they do not ferment the lactose and so their identity corresponds to the international nomenclature. These are B. Morgan-Gaertner ; the B. No. 10 and the Cocal-Co. of Paterson.

Indications about the Bacillus No. 7, B. Asiaticus, B. Cloacae and B. Freundi are found only in the *Dictionaire française de medecine et Biologie* (Ed. Masson, 1970). Information regarding *Bacillus cloacae* or Aerobacteria Cloacae is as follows :

Gram negative bacilli of which the characters are related to *Aerobacter aerogenes*, isolated from water, from soil and very rarely from fecal matters of men and animals : probably non-pathogenous.

CLINICAL PATHOGENESIS

1. Generalities

Worn out subjects.

Great physical and mental weakness.

Prematurely old.

A subject who walks like an old man, swollen, slow, pale, voluted, walk slowly.

Face pale, heavy closed eyelids, swollen oedematous.

2. Neuro-endocrino-psychic System

(a) *Psychic* : Becomes fatigued at the idea of effort.

(b) *Nervous* : Muscular weakness.

Takes long time to fall asleep (about 2 hours).

Light sleep, wakes up at 2 to 3 a.m.

3. Digestive Apparatus

Gastro-intestinal flatulence.

Gastro-intestinal ptosis.

Aversion to fats.

Eructations, flatulence.

Pain in the region of liver.

Constipation. Hemorrhoids.

4. Cardio-hemo-vascular System

Hyposystole ; arterial hypotension.

Chilliness ; hyposthenic heart with slow pulse.

Excessive sweats.

Throbbing of the capillary vessels of the fingers.

5. Respiratory Apparatus

Inflammation of the tonsils.

Swollen tonsils ; bronchitis.

6. Sense Organs

(a) *Eyes* : Thrombosis of the central vein of the retina.

(b) *Ears* : Deafness of catarrhal origin.

7. Uro-genital Apparatus

(a) *Urinary* : Oliguria.

(b) *Genital* : Sexual weakness ; vulvar pains.

8. Locomotor System

Lumbar pains ; stiffness of the neck, "cracks like a nut".

Fibrosity of the neck and shoulders.

Fibrous rheumatism of the neck and back of abdominal muscles.

Dorsal pains, better by *rest and heat.* Worse in humid and cold *weather.*

Painful swelling of the articulations of legs.

Lancinating pains of the left hip.

Rigidness of legs and cramps at night.

Pain in knees.

Gout of the right toe.

Rheumatic pain of shoulders, elbows and wrists.

Swollen fingers.

Rheumatic pain of the thumb.

Stiffness of heels and the wrists.

9. **Skin, Phanera**

Fissures of the tips of the fingers.

Fissure of the palms.

Circinatous eruptions of palms, hot. desquamating.
Perionyxis.

10. **Modalities**

Aggravation : By cold, humidity ; at the beginning of movement.

Amelioration : Heat, rest.

Laterality : Right not specific.

POSOLOGY

Dynamisation : 6 c, 9 c, 12 c, 30 c, 200 c, 1 m, 10 m, 50m, cm.

POSITIVE DIAGNOSIS

General weakness.
Physical and intellectual weakness.

Gastro-intestinal flatulence.

Hypertension. Oliguria.

Polyarticular pains of the back, of extremities, of the type of "old rheumatism".

DIFFERENTIAL DIAGNOSIS

According to the English authors : *Kali carbonicum, Calcarea fluorica, Calcarea carbonica, Rhus tox., Causticum.*

New remedies : *Mandragora officianarum* may be mentioned.

CLINICAL DIAGNOSIS

1. **Generalities**

Tubercular condition.

Hypothyroidism.

Sexual weakness. Frigidity.

2. **Locomotor System**

Lumbago.

Gonarthrosis.

Painful flat-foot.

Rheumatoid arthritis of the knees and heels.

Rheumatoid arthritis of shoulders, elbows and wrists.

Rhizarthrosis.

CHAPTER VII

SYCOTIC-CO, SYCOCCUS-PATERSON, STREPTOCOCCUS-FAECALIS

(NOSODE OF PATERSON)

STOCK

Sycotic-Co. is a *coccus* which does not ferment lactose. It is morphologically similar to gonococcus. It is a gram negative diplococcus. These are the informations given by Paterson (Hui-Bon-Hoa).

Bacteriology describes *Streptococcus Faecalis* like an ovoid streptococcus, elongated, facultatively anaerobic, non-hemolytic, isolated from fecal matters of men and animal. Classified in the group D of the Mansefield and in the enterococcus group of Shermenn : it includes numerous types and sub-types of serology and presents two varieties : Str. faecalis, Var. liquifients and Str. faecalis, Var. zygmogenes.

CLINICAL PATHOGENESIS

1. Generalities

General irritation.
Irritation on the surface of the mucuses.

A pale subject having swollen face, yellow colour, anemic, premature gray hairs.

In women : Hairs on the face and on upper lips.

2. Neuro-endocrino-psychic System

(*a*) *Psychic* :

Mental irritability. *Punctilious.*
Angry.
Fear of obscurity, fear when alone.

(392)

Nervous, tense.

Sensitive to cold, chews nails, inconstant humours.

Tearful, timid, hypersensitive.

(*b*) *Nerves* :

Trembling of the facial muscles.

Blinking of the eyelids.

Sweats of the head at night.

Headache every fortnight, specially frontal, congestive, better by rest and heat ; aggravated by noise.

Leftsided facial neuralgia.

(*c*) *Sleep.* Restless, does not wish to remain alone ; nocturnal fright, dreams.

Abundant sweats of the head at night.

Takes long time to fall asleep.

Dreams of dead persons.

(*d*) *Endocrines.* Swollen face. Big neck with swollen thyroid.

Abundant sweat, specially of the head, hands and feet.

Slight oedema of the extremities. specially of the feet.

Loss of hairs.

Brittle nails.

Anxious, irritable, timid persons (fear of dogs).

3. **Digestive Apparatus**

(*a*) *Mouth, larynx, pharynx* :

Lips dry and fissured.

Tongue dry, cracked, painful, sticks to the palate.

Diminution of taste.

Ulceration and warts on the tongue.

Sialorrhoea.

Acid eructations, burning sensation in the stomach.

Vomiting at night, with amelioration.

Abdominal distension with pain in the iliac fossa. Constipation or morning diarrhoea.

Ano-rectal prolapsus.

Urgent desire for stools when waking up.

Soft, discoloured, brittle stools with bad smelling mucus.

(*b*) *Stomach, intestines, abdomen* :

Very capricious appetite.

Desire for butter, fat, cheese, milk, sweets, salt.

Aversion to eggs.

Nausea at the smell of cooking, after having taken eggs.

4. **Respiratory Apparatus**

(*a*) *Throat* :

Hypertrophy of tonsils, throat red, dry as if scalded.

Abundant mucus thrown in the morning.

Difficult deglutition, easily choked.

(*b*) *Lungs, pleura* :

Intercostal pains.

Fibrosity of the thoracic walls.

Pain in the region of the left shoulder blades, with rales on the upper base of the lungs.

Pleurodynia.

Sibilance and cough, 2-3 a.m. and when walking up.

Fits of spasmodic weakening cough.

Easy, viscous, expectoration.

Loss of breath in the morning.

Asthma and bronchitis aggravated during frost, by humid weather, better by sea-side.

5. Sense Organs

(*a*) *Nose* : Pains in the frontal and maxillar sinuses.

Acquous discharge from the nose ; coryza.

Dryness of the nose with crusts. Epistaxis.

Fissures of the nostrils.

Diminution of the sense of smell.

(*b*) *Eyes* :

Pain of the ocular globes.

Photohobia, hemiopia.
Vitral opacity.
Irritation of the conjunctivae.
Chalazion.

(*c*) *Ears* :

Pruritus of the auditive conduit.
Excess of cerumen.
Yellowish discharge.
Diminution of hearing.   Fissures behind ears.

6. Uro-genital Apparatus

(*a*) *Urinary* :

Irritating urine with strong smell.   Frequent proteinuria.
Tenesmus of the bladder, pollakuria.

(*b*) *Genital* :

Male : Balanitis, sexual weakness.

Female : *Pain of the left ovary* : Leucorrhoea, profuse, yellowish, foetid, corrosive ; pruritus vulvae.

Troubles of menstrual cycle, with prolonged delay. Algo-menorrhoea.

7. Locomotor System

Stiffness, fibrosity of the *neck, shoulders and back.*
Persisting intense pain of the lumbo-sacral region.
Pains of the hips, of the sacro-iliac region.

Aggravation of pain by prolonged sitting position, at night by the first movement.

Amelioration by heat and movement.

Nocturnal pains of the arms.

Pains in the wrists, hands and fingers.

Pricking and stiffness of the hands.

Painful swollen heels.

Pains of the soles.

8. Skin, Phanera

Oily, yellowish skin. Acne rosacea.

Fibrosic induration of the skin.

Vesicular eruption on the body and face.

Papillomatous formation on the right cheek (epithelioma).

Erythema.

Integument, sensitive, dry desquamating in spots.

Alopecia.

Brittle nails.

Fissuses on finger tips and heels.

Flat warts, on hands and feet.

Vesicular eruption, pruriginous, worse at night, worse by heat, by the detergents, by flour.

Erythematous dermatitis, fissured.

Pustulous eruptions on hands, circinatous eruptions on thighs, on the skin and on tibia.

Chilblains of feet, aggr. by heat.

Perionyxis.

Intertrigo of breasts.

9. Modalities

Aggravation : By cold, by humid weather, of pains in sitting position and by the first movement, at night.

Amelioration :

By sea-side, by heat, by prolonged movement.

Laterality :

Left, not predominant.

POSOLOGY

Dynamisation : 6 c, 9 c, 12 c, 30 c, 200 c, 1 m, 10 m, 50 m, c. m.

POSITIVE DIAGNOSIS

General irritation.

Pale yellow, swollen subjects.

Headache every 15 days.

Sleep with dreams, cannot remain alone.

Oedematous swelling of the extremities.

Fibrosity of the skin, and mucous membranes.

Fits of cough.

Maxillary and frontal sinuses painful. Irritation of the conjunctiva.

Frequent proteinuria.

Corrosive leucorrhoea, pruritius of the vulva, algomenorrhoea ; balanitis ; polyarticular stiffness.

Sweating of the heels and pains of the soles.

Vesicular dermatitis, papillomatous formations.

Fissures of the orifices and of the folds of the skin.

DIFFERENTIAL DIAGNOSIS

According to Paterson : *Pulsatilla, Thuya, Lycopodium, Sepia, Natrum muriaticum, Tuberculinum* or *Bacillinum, Kalibichromicum, Sulphur, Silicea, Calcarea carbonico* are related to it.

But in fact *Thuya* and *Medorrhinum* are to be kept in mind.

CLINICAL DIAGNOSIS

1. **Generalities**

   Tubercular condition ; cancer condition ; Anemia.

2. **Neuro-endocrino-psychic System**

   Nocturnal fears of children (Pavor nocturnus).

   Tics of the face.

   Students headache.

3. **Digestive Apparatus**

   Cortico-gastric distonia. Enteroptosis.

   Hepatosis. Acetonemia.

   Verminosis.

   Infantile exfoliative glossitis.

   Warts on the tongue.

   Hypertrophy of the tonsils.

4. **Respiratory Apparatus**

   Bronchial catarrh.

   Asthma. Fibrosity of the thoracic walls (Hui-Bon-Hoa).

   Hypertrophy of tonsils.
   Coryza of tuberculinics (Paterson).

5. **Sense Organs**

   (*a*) *Nose* : Adenoid vegetation. Anosmia.

   Coryza. Sinusitis.
   Polyposis. Nasal fissures.
   Epistaxis. Vaso-motric rhinorrhoea.

   (*b*) *Eyes* : Conjunctivitis.

   Chalazions, photophobia. Hemiopia.

   (*c*) *Ears* : Otorrhoea.

   Hypersecretion of cerumen.
   Pruriginous eczema, of the auditive conduit.

6. **Uro-gential Apparatus**

   Balanitis. Ovaritis.

   Cystitis. Urethritis.

   Proteinuria. Albuminuric nephritis. Nephrosis.

   Left salpingo-ovaritis. Sclero-cystic fibrous mastitis.

   Sclero-cystic ovaritis of the left side.

   Algomenorrhoea.

   Metritis of the neck (exo-endo cervicitis).

7. **Locomotor System**

   Chronic evolutive polyarthritis.

   Gonorrhial rheumatism.

   Fibrous rheumatism of Jacoud.

   Rheumatism of the thoracic muscles.

   Dorsal fibrosis (Hui-Bon Hoa).

   Arthritis of fingers of hands and of feet.

8. **Skin, Phanera**

   Acute aad chronic eczema.

   Zona. Hepes. Chicken pox.

   Intertigo of the folds of the breasts.

   Acne rosacea. Alopecia. Warts.

   Pre-cancerous keratosis.

   Scleroderma.

   Fissures of finger tips, of heels.

   Perionyxis.

CHAPTER VIII

BACILLE OF MORGAN GAERTNER
(PATERSON NOSODE)
CLINICAL PATHOGENESIS

1. Generalities

Subjects with fine brown hairs.

Pale face.

2. Neuro-endocrino psychic System

(a) *Psychism* :

Impatient, tense person, with *strong reaction* ; *irritable.*

Full of apprehensions, gets excited in company.

Chews nails.

Claustrophobia.

(b) *Nervous* :

Nocturnal fears cries out in sleep.

Neuritic pains of the arms.

Facial neuralgia, dominating left side.

Intercostal neuralgia.

3. Digestive Apparatus

(a) *Mouth, tongue, pharynx* :

Bad mouth, bitter taste.

Inflamed gums. Pyorrhoea.

Tongue burning, as if pricked by needles.

Thick saliva.

Fissures of the joints of lips.

(b) *Stomach, intestines, abdomen* :

Desire specially for sweets.

Desire for fat foods, eggs, viande, salted things.
Sometimes aversion to fat, eggs, viande.
Noisy *eructations with bad smell.*
Fullness of the epigastrium without eating.
Vomiting of food after meals, after-noon or at night.
Intestinal flatulence.
Flatulence of the left and right hypochondrial region.

Gall bladder, painful.

Intestinal lethargy, constipation.
Hard, dry stools with mucus.
Spontaneous explusion of muscus through rectum even when the patient is not constipated.

Rectal prolapsus.
Fissure and anal pruritius.
Painful hemorrhoids, bleeding, pruriginus.

4. **Cardio hemo-vascular System**

Thoracic pain, constriction in the chest, painful irradiation to the left hand.
Sensation of coldness in the chest.
Precordial uneasiness.
Nocturnal palpitation, wakes up the patient. Amelioration by eructations, by emission of gas, by movement.

5. **Respiratory Apparatus**

(*a*) *Throat* : Inflammatory congestion of tonsils.

Oedema of the uvula.

Sensation of burning in the base of the throat as if from acid.

(*b*) *Lungs, pleura* : Pleurodynia.

Short breath.

Tickling cough morning and evening, while walking up, while lying down.

6. Sense Organs

(*a*) *Nose* : Hypersecretion of nasal fossa and of maxillary sinus.

Crusty coryza with ulceration in the nose.

Nasal herpes.

Epistaxis.

(*b*) *Eyes* :

Chronic inflamation of eyelids. Blepharitis.
Styes, chalazions.
Ulcer of the cornea.
Vitral opacity.

(*c*) *Ears* : Furuncles in the auditive conduit.

Buzzing in the ears.

7. Uro-genital Apparatus

(*a*) *Urinary* : Vesical pain with frequent micturition.

Burning urines ; pollakuria.
Pain in the renal region.
Pyelo-vesical pain, congestion.

(*b*) *Genital* : *Irritation at the approch of menstruation.*

Painful menses.
Thick, brown, corrosive, bad smelling leucorrhoea.
Vulvar pruritus.
Warts on the breasts.

8. Loco-motor System

Cervical rigidity.
Rheumatic pain of the wrist.
Painful swelling of the thumbs.

Rheumatoid pains : Shoulders, arms, elbows, wrists, deltoid muscles (right).
Knees, numb and painful.
Excessive heat of the feet at night.

9. Skin, Phanera

Integument sensitive.

Loss of hairs in bunches.

Sudden oedema of the face.

Herpetiform eruption on the left side of the face.

Erythemato-squamous eruptious in round plaques on elbows, knees, integument, sacral region even on nails and heels.

Herpetiform eruption on soles.

Papulo-pustulous eruption on face, on brows, knees. Integuments, oozing, crusty, desquamating with fissures.

Giant urticaria on arms.

Warts on hands, big flat or lacerated.

10. Modalities

Aggravation : In company, after meals, before menses, by the heat of bed, at night.

Amelioration : By movement, by passing flatus, by eructation.

Laterality : Predominently right side.

POSOLOGY

Dynamisation : 6 c, 9 c, 12 c, 30 c, 2000 c, 1 m, 10 m, 50 m, cm.

POSITIVE DIAGNOSIS

Persons, pale, impatient, claustrophobic.

Flatulent dyspepsia, aerocolic.

Pain of the gall bladder.

Polyarticular rheumatic pains of upper extremities specially of the right side.

Vesiculous, vesiculo squamous, papulo-squamous, eruptions. Dysmenorrhoea.

Pyelo-vesical burning congestion.

14 F

DIFFERENTIAL DIAGNOSIS

Mme Paterson : *Lycopodium, Pulsatilla, Silicea, Kali bichromicum, Natrum muriaticum, Nux vomica, Sulphur, Sepia, Graphitis, Calcarea carbonica.*

CLINICAL DIAGNOSIS

1. **Neuro endocrino psychic System**

   Manic depressive psychoses.
   Jealousy. Claustrophobia.
   Nocturnal fears.
   Zona.

2. **Digestive Apparatus**

   Rhagades in corners of lips.
   Cortico-gastric dysthermia.
   Hepatocholitis ; cholecystitis.
   Ano-rectal prolapsus.
   Annal fissure.

3. **Cardio-hemo-vascular System**

   Angina pectoris ; myocarditis.

4. **Respiratory Apparatus**

   Asthma.

5. **Sense Organs**

   (a) *Nose* : Catarrhal rhinitis, sinusitis, nasal polypus.
   nasal herpes.

   (b) *Eyes* : Styes. Chalazions ; blepharitis.

   (c) *Ears* : Otitis, mastoiditis.

   Furuncle of the auditive conduit.

6. **Uro-genital Apparatus**

   (a) *Urinary* : Renal lithiasis ; pyelo-nephritis.
   Pyelitis ; crystitis.
   Enuresis.

(*b*) *Genital* : Pre-menstrual psychic syndrome.

Dysmenorrhoea.

Warts on the nipples.

7. Loco-motor System

Cervical arthrosis.

Progressive polyarthrosis.

Gonarthrosis.

8. Skin, Phanera

Alopecia areata.

Psoriasis, eczema, urticaria.

Warts on hands.

CHAPTER IX

BACILLUS NO. 10

(NOSODE OF PATERSON)

STOCK

It does not exist in its bacteriological nomenclature and its preparation is done by Nelson Pharmacy, without any other informations.

CLINICAL PATHOGENESIS

1. **Generalities**

    Subjects of *fluoride type*, blondes, or of brown and pale type.

2. **Neuro-endocrino-psychic System**

    Anxious, active, irritable, depressed.

    Frontal headache, specially above the left eye.

3. **Digestive Apparatus**

    Bad breath.
    Spongy gums.
    Anorexia ; aversion to breakfast.
    Desire for sugar, chocolate, fried fish.
    Cannot digest eggs and fats.
    Nausea and vomiting.
    Sometimes pains on the region of the gall bladder.
    Intestinal paresis.
    Anal pruritis.

4. **Respiratory Apparatus**

    Asthma.
    Cough worse in the morning ; expectoration difficult.

5. Uro-genital Apparatus

Urinary : Pollakuria.
Genital : Pruritis of the vulva.
Leucorrhoea, smelling like fish, greenish, corrosive.
Peri-vulvar irritation.

6. Loco-motor System

Pains in the two illiac fossae.
Painful thighs.
Painful coccyx.
Pain of the left knee.

7. Skin, Phanera

Greasy cyst of the neck.
Panniculitis of the thoracic walls.
Lipoma ; dartres.
Warts of the hands, numerous, flat or pointed.
Dermatitis of the folds of the flexions.
Sweats of the axillas.

POSOLOGY

Dynamisations : 6 c, 9 c, 12 c, 30 c, 200 c, 1 m, 10 m, 50 m, cm.

OSCILLOCOCCINUM

BIBLIOGRAPHY

Roy Joseph :

Towards the knowledge and cure of Cancer. (Vers la connaissance et la guerison du cancer.)—Edition du Raisin 1925.

Chavanon Paul :

Therapeutique O.R.L. (E.N.T.) homoeopathique. Imprimerie Saint-Denis, 1935.

Julian, O.A. :

Biotherapiques et Nosodes. Libraire Maloine, 1962, Paris. Mat. Med. der Nosoden, K.F. Haug Verlag. Heidelberg 1975, 2nd, ed.

Hui-Bon-Hoa, J.

Guerison d'un cas'd ulcére variqueux avec Oscillococcinum 200.
Annales Homeopathiques françaises, 1968 ; p. 90-938.

Wolter, H. :

Pathogenesie de Galinsoga. parviflora-Allg. Homoep. Zig. No. 3.

Schmidt, P.

Quelques indications cournates de remedes homeopathiques d' urgence. Annales Homoeopathiques, Fasc, No. 9, nov. 74, p 48-709.

HISTORY

In the year 1925 Joseph Roy is believed to have observed in some conditions of culture the existence of a germ animated by an oscillating movement. He named the nosode because of this fact.

These researches helped him to describe a biotherapic remedy which was called *Oscillococcinum* of which the clinical experiments in the infections of Influenza and E.N.T. were carried out in particular by Paul Chavanon. *Oscillococcinum 200* is actually a patent property of Boiron Laboratory, France.

STOCK

J. Boiron and J. Abecassis were kind enough to communicate to us the technique of preparation of that patent medicine which is as follows :

The stock of *Oscillococcinum* is an autolysate filtered from the liver and the heart of a duck.

It is characterised by :

1. Some criteria of preparation.
2. Some physical criteria.
3. Some chemical criteria.

Though the preparation is not utilised by injection.

4. Some trials of sterility are done.
5. Some experiments of innocuousness are done.

CRITERIA OF PREPARATION

It is processed in rigorous aseptic conditions in a place exposed to ultra-violet rays. All the glass utensils and materials used are sterilised beforehand.

In a bell jar with flat bottom of 1,000 ml is placed :
225 ml of solution of pancreatic peptone at 1%.
225 ml of serum glucosed at 10% tyndalised.

The duck is decapitated, the heart and the liver is taken out in a sterile way. In this jar are put 35 to 37 gr. of the liver and 14 to 15 gr. of the heart. Then the jar is put in the incubator at 37° for 40 days and thereafter the autolysate is filtered on fritted porous glass. It is that solution which is the stock of the remedy and is lyophylised in order to be preserved.

From that rehydrated stock, the 200th dilution (Korsakovian) is prepared which is utilised for the impregnation of the globules.

The experiments are done by the stock constituting the preparation of the M T. which alone may be put to analysis.

Physical Criteria

The stock is either in liquid form, yellow in colour more or less shaded, or in the form of a lyophilisate which is rehydrated during the control by adding a quantity of water equal to that which is taken out during the lyophilisation. Its physical properties are :

1. Index of refraction at 25° : $1,3430 + 0,0015$.
2. Density : $1,018 + 0,01$.
3. Determination of pH : pH equal to 3, 1% 0, 3.
4. Spectrophotometric absorption curve in UV.

The stock of *Oscillococcinum* diluted to 1/100 in isotonic solution of Sodium chloride at 9% presents a maximum of absorption situated between 260 and 275 nm.

The value of absorptions $E \dfrac{1/100}{1 \text{ cm}}$ is of 0·38% 0·05.

Chemical Criteria

1. ESTIMATION OF TOTAL NITROGEN

(a) *Principle* :

Estimation of total Nitrogen by the method of Kjeldahl.

(b) *Technique* :

For trial take 2 gr exactly weighed in a small glass tube. Introduce the tube in a distillation flask with long neck. Add 10 ml of concentrated Sulphuric acid and 0·05 gr of catalyser

(Potassium sulphate 100 parts+Copper sulphate 10 parts +Selenium 1 part). Heat it until the liquid becomes limpid.

Transfer the liquid thus obtained to a distillation flask along with the water for rinsing and dilute with distilled water.

Add some balls of glass or some grains of pumice stones in order to help ebullition.

The distillation flask is connected with a refrigeration system at the extremity of which there is an ampoule dipped into a beaker containing 25 ml O, 1N H_2SO_4 and the Taschiri indicator (Methyl red+Methylene blue) added to it.

Pass an alkaline medium in the distillation flask in the presence of Phenophthalene adding about 50 ml of Soda ash by means of a funnel with long stem and start rapidly the refrigeration.

Distil it for half an hour.

The Sodium displaces NH_3 of $NH_4/2\ SO_4$ formed during the mineralisation and NH_3 neutralises partially the Sulphuric acid.

Take out the beaker from the end of the refrigerator and rinse the ampoule. The excess of H_2SO_4 is titrated by n ml 0, 1N NaOH till a faint grey colour appears.

Percentage of total Nitrogen (expressed in Gramms for

$$100\ g) : \frac{0,1401\ (25-n)}{PE}$$

The total quantity of Nitrogen of the stock of *Oscilio-coccinum* should be within 0·297 wt% and 0,363 wt% (Poids ponderable).

2. ESTIMATION OF AMINATED NITROGEN

(a) *Principle* :

Estimation by formol titration.

(b) *Technique* :

Weigh exactly about 1 g. Oscillococcinum in an erlen

Meyer. Add 9 ml distilled water and 2 drops of Phenophthalene. Neutralise by 0,1 N Caustic soda in the presence of
a drop of Phenophthalene till there is a very pale pink colouration.

Add this formol to the preceding liquid, there is colouration.

Titrate then the acid liberated by 0·1 NaOH put in a flask
till there is a clear red colour in comparison to the standard :
10 ml of formol.

15 ml of distilled water.

2 drops of Phenophthalene.

Add 0, 1 N NaOH till there is a rosy colour add again 0,2
to 0,3 ml to obtain the clear red colouration.

Let n be the number of millilitres used :

$$\text{Amino nitrogen (expressed in g. for 100g)} = \frac{0.1401 \times n}{P}$$

The quantity of Aminated nitrogen should be between 0·207
wt% and 0·253 wt% (P/P).

3. PROPORTION OF AMINATED NITROGEN

The ratio : $\dfrac{\text{Aminated nitrogen}}{\text{Total nitrogen}}$ should be of 0·7+0·1.

4. ESTIMATION OF THE TYROSINE

(*a*) *Principle* :

(J. Loiseleur—Chemical estimation on proteins).

The phenolic group of Tyrosine is calorimetrically measured
by means of Follin's reagent. The final solution in which the
colouration is developed should be at a pH between 7, 1
and 7, 6.

(*b*) *Technique* :

Necessary reagents :

1. Follin's reagent is dissolved in a distillation flask of
1,500 c.c. capacity containing :

Tungstate of Sodium Na_2WO_4 $2H_2O$...100g.

Sodium Molybdate Na_2MoO_4 $2H_2O$...25g.

Water...   ...   .700 cc.

To this add :

Phospheric acid @ 85%   50 cc.

Concentrated hydrochloric acid   100 cc.

Now connect this flask to a reflux system with a condenser by means of a cork stopper and boil on slow heat for 10 hours. Then add 150 g of Lithium sulphate, 50 cc. of water and some drops of liquid Bromide. This mixture is boiled, after separating the refrigerator, for about 15 mts. to dispose of the excess of Bromide and cooled down to 1 litre. It is filtered.

The remaining reagent should not have a greenish colour, which will indicate the presence of the products of blue reduction. The reagent should be kept in dust-proof atmosphere because the organic products are apt to produce some little reductions.

2.   The buffer of alkaline Phosphate of J.J. Perez.

PO_4HK_2 0, 5 M.........50 cc.

NaOH   N   ....4 cc.

3.   Standard solution of Tyrosine @ 0,50%.

This solution is prepared by the dissolution of 0,5 g of Tyrosine, dried over P_2O_5 in 100 cc of N/2 SO_4H_2.

Method of operation :

Mix 1g of Stock for estimation with :

    10 cc of water.

    6 cc of Sodium chloride N/10.

    3 cc of Follin's reagent at 1/3.

    5 cc of Alkaline phosphate.

Leave the solution for 3 to 4 hours at the ambiant temperature and take calorimetric reading comparatively with reference to 1 gr of titrated Tyrosine solution treated in the same solution.

Percentage of Tyrosine in G% (P/P)$= \dfrac{0\cdot5 \times DE}{DT \times P}$

The percentage of Tyrosine should be between 0·45 and 0·55 g% (P/P=Poids ponderable).

5. CHROMATOGRAPHIC ANALYSIS OF AMINO ACIDS

(*a*) *Apparatus* :

The analysis is done on Jeolco auto-analyser 5AH.

Each experiment is compared with a standard solution of witness Amino acid.

Resins utilised for the separation are respectively Aminex A4 for the Amino acids and neutrals, and Aminex A5 for basic Amino acids.

The photometric measurements are done at 440 and 570 nm and at three sensitivities (the sensitivity of the apparatus used is inferior to 10^{-9} mole for an Amino acid).

(*b*) *Results* :

Particularly the following Amino acids are characterised : Lysine, Arginine, Glycine, Almine, Isoleucine, Leucine, Tyrosine, Phenylalanine.

The ratio : $\dfrac{\text{Alanine}}{\text{Glycine}}$ should be more than 1.

$\dfrac{\text{Lucine}}{\text{Isoleucine}}$ should be more than 1.

$\dfrac{\text{Phenylalanine}}{\text{Tyrosine}}$ should be more than 2.

The ratio of Argenine, though weak, is relatively constant 4, 5 mg+1 for 100 ml of autolysate.

As Boiron laboratory had not the necessary apparatus, this analysis was done by the Pharmaceutical Laboratory of Biochemistry combined Faculty of Medicine and Pharmacy, 8, Rokfeller Avenue, Lyon 8. M le Prof. Gras.

Sterlity Test

This test was done on three different mediums for 7 days as described in the French Pharmacopoea (8th ed., 1965, p. 1618).

- -Peptoned bouillon at 37°.
—Thyoglycolate bouillon at 37°.
—Glucosed Sabourand gelose at 24°.

The search was limited to a verification in male rats of (lot of 10 rats) or stock equal to $20 \pm 2g$ of innocuousness of the M.T. administered intra-peritonially in an arbitrarily selected very strong dose of 0, 3 ML/rat.

CLINICAL CORTICO VISCERAL PROTOCOL
OR CLINICAL PATHOGENESIS

There is no pathogenesis of this remedy according to the Hahnemannian method. We are, however, trying to give a clinical pathogenesis base on the works of P. Chavanon, our own clinical experience and the case reports of Hui-Bon-Hoa.

1. Generalities

Anxiety, paleness, chill.
Sensitiveness to hygrometric and meteorologic changes.
Tuberculous patients sensitive to cold.
Luetosic subjects with fixed ideas, obsessions.

2. Neuro-endocrino-psychic System

Agony, anxious without any motive.
Obstinate.
A busy body, maniac, cannot bear disorder, fear of dirt, fear of being polluted.

Has the need to wash his hands very often and is afraid of giving his hand to others for the fear of pollution, contagion.

Is afraid of storm.

3. Digestive Apparatus

Tongue white.

Swelling of the stomach.

Can digest neither milk nor eggs.

Putrid regurgitations.

Aquous or food vomiting.

Abdominal cramping pains followed by foetid diarrhoea.

Sometimes stubborn constipation.

Yellow conjunctiva.

Icterus or pains in the appendicular region.

2. Cardio-hemo-vascular System

Hypotonia.

Lipothymia.

Thermoregulation : Bruised sensation, chill, hyperthermia, headache with considerable throbbing.

3. Respiratory Apparatus

Oculo nasal catarrh.

Stuffed nose, nasal obstruction, sneezing.

Serous discharge from the nose, then muco-purulent.

Pain in the frontal and maxillary region.

Nasal voice, aphonia, dry painful cough.

Muco-purulent expectoration with humid cough.

Pains sometimes as if from needles in one or both the ears (In children, this symptom may not be found. Look at the tympanum which alone may be red at first, and swollen if there is purulent collection).

Diminution of auditive acuity.

Retro-auricular pain, spontaneous or felt on pressure.

6. Uro-genital Apparatus

Turbid urine, less abundant, deep colour.

Sometimes painful micturition.

7. Skin, Phanera

Varicose type of ulcers of the legs.

8. Modalities

Aggravation : By milk, by eggs.

Amelioration : By heat, by rest.

POSOLOGY

Dynamisation : There is only one dilution : 200 (K) (Korsakovian—single phial system). Classically 1 dose a day is used, or every 2 to 3 days.

At present we advise in acute affection repetition of dose every 2 to 3 hours (see Commentary).

POSITIVE DIAGNOSIS

Paleness, asthenia, hyperthermia.

Oculo-nasal catarrh.

Laryngo-tracheo-bronchial congestion.

Painful congestion of the tympanum.

Gastro-intestinal troubles of influenza.

Varicose ulcer.

DIFFERENTIAL DIAGNOSIS

In classical homoeotherapy it should be noted : *Eupat perf.*, *Mercurius bio-iodatus*, *Cinnabaris.* Among the biotherapics: *Pyrogenium* and *Luesinum.*

New Medicines

Luffa operculata : Fronto-occipital headache ; acute or chronic inflammation of the mucous membrane of the nasal fossa, lassitude and bodily fatigue.

Gaulphimia glauca : Hypersecretion of the nasal and ocular mucous ; sneezing, hypersensitivity to change of weather.

Galinsoga purviflora : Morning headache, makes mistakes when writing numbers and letters ; stuffed nose ; augmentation of diuresis ; articular pains, lassitude, feels as if bruised.

Ginco biloba : Pale face, drawn traits, numbness and chill. Laryngeal irritation with cough, frontal and left supra-orbita pain.

CLINICAL DIAGNOSIS

Influenza "at the beginning as preventive as well as during convalescence". (P. Schmidt)

Influenza, gastro-intestinal type.

Sinusitis, acute rhinitis.

Laryngo-tracheo-bronchitis.

Conjunctivitis of influenza.

Mastoiditis.

"At the beginning of a disease which does not develop". (Schmidt)

COMMENTARIES

This biotherapic is a faithful remedy at the beginning of influenza, at the beginning of rhinitis, at the beginning of otitis.

Given early it is very efficacious. Only in our time it requires repetition which Chavanon did not. To obtain good results in a case which begins and to cut short the manifestations of influenza of general type, or localised it is necessary to use one dose of *Oscillococcinum 200* at least every 2 to 3 hours.

Thirty years ago and even in our rural practice it was enough to use 1 dose in 24 to 48 hours.

At present if one wishes to obtain a rapid and sure result one should not hasitate to use it as indicated above.

Fifteen years ago Chavanon observed this fact and said that *Eupatorium perfoliatum* is to be associated with it.

Now the technique that we have described is more important.

Even the counter-indications have been somewhat changed.

Chavanon is formal : Do not use *Oscillococcinum* in a cancer subject. But at present, according to Hui-Bon-Hoa, it may be used in cancer subjects (ex-cancer subject).

In a case which he reports, he had a good clinical result in a patient who had varicose ulcer, only because the patient wrongly interpreted his prescription, "has taken *Oscillococcinum 200* daily, three times a day" for thirty days instead of three days as it was prescribed. So it is the posology which, according to us, was responsible for the therapeutic success.

It is for this reason one should take lesson from the facts, nothing but facts and should know to adapt to facts his method of prescription.

Thus we shall be always among those who, practice the art of cure enunciated by S. Hahnemann.

Finally here is the case report of Dr. Hui-Bon-Hoa published in the Annales Homoeopathiques françaises, 1968, p. 90-938.

"Mme S , 82 years, calls me for visit, on the 20th September, 1962. She has, since two years, a large varicose ulcer about the shape of the palm of the hand, of elliptic form, on the internal face of the left leg. The border is elevated, the base is greasy and sanious. The skin around is thickened, pigmented and grafted by an eczema, very pruriginous. The extremity is swollen, specially the foot. A.T. 18/10. No sugar in the urines.

Antecedants : Pulmonary congestion, cerebral congestion with the max. A.T. 24; fracture of the tibia 23 years ago, consolidated in a bad position, which has made the patient impotent (the patient is impotent beside obese) : eczema on hands and legs since three years ; rheumatic pains all over the body ; no tubercular or cancer antecedants.

Individual symptoms : Obesity, colour like coffee with milk +++aggr. in extreme temperature, closed room, before storm, fear of storm.

Anxiety for others in anticipation ; becomes anxious when her daughter goes out in a carriage.

A meddler and a maniac ; inspite of her impotence, she masturbates. "Fear of being polluted" even by her daughter who is a nurse. Terribly stubborn ; sensitive to music ; cannot digest milk and eggs.

Treatment : Carcinosinum 200 CH, a single dose.

2nd December, 1962 : Clear amelioration. The ulcer reduced. Eczema completely disappear. However the patient still does not sleep well.

Treatment : Hughe's treatment is tried.

...*Carduus marianus* M.T. 5 drops every four hours (also recommended by Dr. Windelband).

...*Calendula ointment* locally (Principle and Practice of Homoeopathy by Hughes, C. Ringer and Co., Calcutta).

...We added : Troformone (locally).

4th January, 1963 : Called for a visit. No amelioration. Patient fatigued. As it was the time when we were using *Oscillococcinum* systematically in the place of *Carcinosinum*, we prescribed :

Oscillococcinum 200, 3 doses, to be taken one hour before each of the three meals on the same day. We stopped the local treatment and recommended only cleanliness.

7th February 1963 : Complete cure of the ulcer. The patient was gay and smiling. She says that she is in good form and that she sleeps well.

Another detail that we should mention : Having wrongly interpreted our prescription the patient has taken *Oscillococcinum 200* daily three times a day till our visit, *i.e.* to say for 35 days.

In this particular case *Oscillococcinum 200K* of Dr. Jules Roy seems to have acted more vigourously than *Carcinosinum 200 CH*.

Finally in his work cited, P. Chavanon relates the following case :

In the month of March, 1928 I was called by telephone on a Saturday towards noon, to see a patient at St.-Germain-en-Laye. I had no time so I refused.

The sister of the patient, thought that the patient was transportable, decided to bring him to me urgently in a carriage at a time which was convenient for us.

At 15 hours the patient was at my house. He was very pale. He had 39·5° temperature. He was shivering though the temperature of my chamber was at 22°.

The distance could not be covered rapidly because the jerkings were very painful for the patient.

He was suffering from the left ear since 3 days, in course of which the fever rose gradually.

He had vainly tried *Belladonna 6, Capsicum 6* advised by Dr. Fortier-Bernoville on telephone.

I examined his ear. The right tympanum had become swollen to a bursting point having a very dark red colour (as if tumified and infiltrated by dark blood). The mastoid gland was sensitive.

It was our habit at that time about an otitis even at that stage, but I decided not to open it.

While I was explaining to the patient, he became suddenly very pale, and was so laid down. A robust boy of 20 years, suffering atrociously and any allopath would have opened his otitis widely.

I advised the sister to put the patient in the carriage (taxi), which was waiting at the door, take him down slowly up to the pharmacy in order to give him there a dose of *Oscillococcinum 200* (which I had not with me) and to continue afterwards the local treatment giving him the granules which I gave.

On Monday I was informed that gradually as the taxi advanced up to the door of Maillot, the patient was feeling well. Arriving at the door of Maillot the patient felt so much well that he preferred to take the tramway in order to arrive at Saint-Germain. He was feeling absolutely nothing and the temperature came down to 38·2°. He was only very weak and fatigued.

Then he continued the treatment. In the evening at 21 hours his temperature was only 37·5°. And the next day when she woke up he had 36·8°.

I advised to disinfect the nose carefully for some time, then there was no relapse.

OSTEO-ARTHRITIC-NOSODE

(O. A. N.)

BIBLIOGRAPHY

Srinivasan, S. :

A proving of O.A.N. (osteo-arthritic-nosode-hip). Read in ➤ the 18th All India Homoeopathic Conference at Madras, Rajaji Hall, on 10 Oct., 1970.

A proving of O.A.N.

The Homoeopathic Sandesh, V. xxv, No. 3, March, 1973, p. 115-118. (Fr. translation by M.H. Carette).

STOCK

Srinivasan says that the stock of O.A.N. was supplied to him by Dr. Foubister of London. I.B.L. Ainsworth from Nelson laboratory and also furnished the following information :

The two preparations of O.A.N. are done from the synovial liquid of articulations.

The O.A.N. originated from Dr. Foubister comes from the knee of a patient suffering from an osteo-articular affection, and the other stock from the hip of a similar case. Besides, we have the preparation R.A.N. (Rheumatoid-arthritic-nosode), which concerns the rheumatoid side in opposition to the osteo-arthritic inflammation.

Here is, therefore, a nosode which acts towards osteo-arthritic direction and the other one towards rhumato-arthritic direction.

The catalogue of Nosodes of Nelson mentions :

O.A.N. (hip—hanche)—6—200.

O.A.N. (Osteo-arthritic nosode, osteo-arthritic synovial tissue) 6—1 M.

R.A.N. (Rheumatoid arthritic nosode)—6—30.

HISTORY

Srinivasan S. of Madras (India) has made a pathogenesic experiment of O.A.N. and has communicated his attempt on the 10th October, 1970 at the 18th Indian Homoeopathic Congress of Madras. The experiment was done on 28 persons, of whom 3 young girls of 18 to 20 years old, 4 women (married), about 30 years old.

The remaining of the group was composed of men of 27 to 48 years, among whom 7 doctors of whom 4 received only placebo.

The proving started on the 2nd August, 1970, and the symptoms appeared about three days after the starting of the experiment.

Three young girls received 2 drops of the 13th dynamisation for 22 days and began again the proving from the 32nd day for 25 days.

Four women received O.A.N. by sub-cutaneous injections with the 14th dynamisation, and symptoms began to appear from the 4th day of the proving.

Six men received placebo by sub-cutaneous injections for 25 days, and two men received placebo by sub-cutaneous injections. No reaction was registered.

Finally, the last group composed of 8 men two of which, received placebo and the remaining (6 men) O.A.N. 13th dynamisation, one dose every day for 24 consecutive days.

The *Originality* of the present proving, by administering the medicine intravenously of the stock of medicine and the placebo, is notable.

EXPERIMENTAL CORTICO-VISCERAL PROTOCOL
PHARMACODYNAMICS OR PATHOGENESIS

1. Generalities

Extreme weakness with somnolence in the afternoon and profound sleep.

State of indifference.

Idleness, no desire to work, irritable, worse between 16 to 18 hours. Indecision, needs relaxing.

2. Neuro-endocrino-psychic System

Stage of stupor, *indifference* to others.

Has taste for nothing, nonchalance, *irritability*.

Irritability, *worse* towards evening.

Weakness, worse in the morning when waking up.

Great desire for sleep with deep sleep at night.

3. Sense Organs

Eyes : Styes of upper eyelid of the left eye.

4. Uro-genital Apparatus

Increase of sexual desire in men.

5. Loco-motor Apparatus

Swelling of the right wrist.

Pain in the right shoulder.

Muscular pain of the right hip.

Temporary redness and swelling of the right shoulder.

Redness and swelling of the right fore-arm and right wrist.

Pain aggravated by the first movement, ameliorated by continued movement.

Pain of the tendon Achillis.

6. Skin

Furuncle in the right aisle.

Furuncle above the umblicus on the right calf.

Furuncle on the scrotum.

Furuncle on the right arm, on the trapezium, of the right groin.

7. Biological Characteristics

S.V. accelerated from   16 to 20-33 in 7 persons.

12 to 17-19 in 5 persons.

Increase of leucocytes :   Eosinophiles to 45%   in 4 women and 5 men.

Polymorphes (?)

Polynucleairs (?) —33%

R.B.C. diminished by 5% in 11 persons.   Highly coloured urine and less abundant, worse at noon ; B.P. normal.

8. Modalities

(*a*) Aggravation by the first movement, at night.

(*b*) Better by prolonged movement.

(*c*) Laterality right.

POSOLOGY

Dynamisation to be had of Nelson 6—200.

This nosode is not sold in France.

POSITIVE DIAGNOSIS

Weakness with stage of indifference and irritability, aggravated in the evening.

Redness and swelling of the articulations, specially right side.

DIFFERENTIAL DIAGNOSIS

Anthracinum : See article.

Mandragora : Poly-articular, muscular pains, furuncle on the face, state of euphoria alternating with a depressive state.

CLINICAL DIAGNOSIS

Depressive neurotic states.

Cramps.

Muscular rheumatism.

Tendinitis.

Infectious arthritis.

Styes.

Furuncles.

CLINICAL OBSERVATIONS

S. Srinivasan presents in his first communication the following case reports :

A woman of 42, convalescent after an influenza was given the Nosode O.A. 24 for her extreme weakness, 4 doses on the first day. She took up her strength within 3 days.

—Catarrhal conjunctivitis, worse right side, instillation of Nosode O.A. 14 every second day. Cure during three days.

—4 cases of furuncles in children of 5 to 7 years. Cure in three days by 1 dose daily of the Nosode O.A. 14.

—2 patients : *compére loriot* on the upper eyelid of the right eye. Nosode O.A. 14, 4 times a day during two days. Cure.

—13 patients : Pain in the thighs, wrists, shoulders, worse right side. Nosode O.A. 14, 4 times a day during 3-4 days. All cured except one who continued the treatment for 7 days and was cured afterwards.

—Three cases of diarrhoea, frequent desire, mucus, rumbling in the abdomen, thirst, followed by weakness.

Nosode O.A. 14 every two hours. Cure.

—One case of arthritis of the right wrist, received O.A. 14 without success. Given other remedies : *Kali iod., Lyeop.*

OURLIANUM

BIBLIOGRAPHY

Julian, O.A. :

Biothérapiques et Nosodes. Edition Maloine Paris, 1962.
Materia Medica der Nosoden. 2e edition 1975, K.F. Haug-
Verlag, Heidelberg.

Pischel :

Kongressbericht über die 123 Jares Versammlung. Allg.
Homoeopath. Zeitung, No. 4, 1972. Observation du Dr.
Romer (Russelsheim).

Clarke, J. :

A Dictionary of Practical Materia Medica, London, 1955,
V. 3. *Appendix* : Parotidinum.

Romer, R. :

Meine Erfahrungen mit den Nosoden Parotidin (Ourlianum),
Pertussin and Histamine.

STOCK

Lysate from the saliva of a patient suffering from mumps,
diluted and dynamised according to Homoeopathic pharmacopraxis.

Actually no legal existence in France.

Nelson of London prepares *Parotidinum* (Mumps), Ourlianum in 30-200.

Reckeweg prepares injectable Parotis in combined dilution :
D 10, D 30, D 200 (Biologische Heilmittel. Heel-Baden-Baden).

There is no experimental pathogenesis according to the
Hahnemannian method.

It is necessary to mention here that the *Parotidinum* is prescribed in Mumps. It is an organotherapic and may eventually substitute Ourlianum.

CORTICO-VISCERAL CLINICAL PROTOCOL
OR CLINICAL PATHOGENESIS

Bilateral painful tumefaction of parotids.

Tumefaction very painful of a testicle, of the scrotum and hyperthermia.

Painful abdominal syndrome with hyperamylasemia, glycosuria (temporary), pancreatitis.

Meningitic syndrome with moderate hyper-albuminorachia.

Encephalitis or affection of the 3rd and 8th pairs followed sometimes by blindness and deafness.

POSOLOGY

Dynamisation : In neurologic sequalae : 30 CH, to be prescribed for a long time.

May be had of Nelson, London : *Parotidinum* (Mumps). Ourlianum 30-200 *should not be confused with Parotid* or *Parotidinum.*

CLINICAL DIAGNOSIS

Mumps in the terminal period.
Viral orchitis or orchitis during mumps.
Neurologic sequalae, deafness or blindness, post-mumps.
Pancreatitis.

COMMENTARY

During the 123rd meeting of D.Z.V. in 1971 meant entirely for the study of Nosodes according to the Materia Medica der Nosoden of Julian, Dr. Romer (Russelsheim) communicated on *Parotitis* (Ourlianum, Julian) in D 30, prescribed in orchitis during mumps and in a post-infectious syndrome in the case of mumps with very good clinical results.

PARATYPHOIDINUM B.

BIBLIOGRAPHY

Bernard, L :

Less états aigus en Médecine rural. Observations cliniques-Archives homoeopathiques de Normandie. No. 4, November 1956, p. 171.

Poisson, G. :

Observations de maladies guéries par le Nosode Paratyphoidinum-B. Archives homoeopathiques de Normandie, No. 19, Juillet, 1960, p. 131. Observations de maladies guéries par le Nosode Paratyphoidinum B. Les Annales Hom. Françaises. No. 1., October, 1959, p. 4.

Lamasson, F. :

Aspects bactériologiques et cliniques des différentes salmonellosis. Les Annales Hom. franç., No. 1⁻ ,Octobre, 1959, p. 16.

Poisson, G. :

Suite de réflexions sur l'emploi de Paratyphoidinum. Pathogénésis (clinical). L'Homoeopathie fr. No. 1, janvier 1956, p. 87.

Julian, O.A. :

Biothérapiques et Nosodes. Librairie Maloine, 1962.
Materia Medica der Nosoden. K.F. Haug Verlag, Heidelber 1975, 2nd ed.

Poisson, G. :

Indications actuelle de Paratyphoidinum B. Communication au Congrés de la Féd. Nat. des Soc. Méd. Hom. Fr. Reims. 1975.

STOCK

The Biotherapic *Paratyphoidinum-B* is prepared from the cultures from a mixture of different stocks of *Paratyphoidinum bacilli*. Because of its therapeutic value it may replace some of the Nosodes of Bach-Paterson (see the articles).

Para-B is a stock vaccin of which the base is Salmonella. Schottmuelleri prepared for making homoeopathic dynamisations.

It is composed of a suspension lysated, attenuated, corresponding to 10 milliards per millilitre of S. Schettmulleri (Marcy 222, 391 and 421). This lysate contains paratyphoid endotoxin of which the structure is analogous to that of *Eberthinum*.

TECHNIQUE OF PREPARATION

1. Stock Utilised

3 stocks of Salmonella Schottmuelleri, Marcy 222, 391, 421.

These stocks have the classical characters of the type.

They are controlled from the point of view of morphology, biochemic characters, and antigenes.

B. mobile, Gram—; colonies on gelose, round, opaque ; in turbid bouillon, abundant, in collerettes.

Lactose,—; glucose, arabinose, maltose, xylose, dulcite $+$ G ; H 2S ; Indol—; ant. O. IV ; ant. Hb.

They are conserved in lyophilised condition.

2. Culture Medium

(*a*) Maceration of chopped meat......................500 g.

Water...1,000 cc.

Leave in contact for 24 hours, then filter after having heated for 30 mts. at 100° and 30 mts. at 110°.

(*b*) Add :

Peptone.............. .... 12 g.

Sodium chloride...................5 g.

Powder gelose....................30 g.

Dissolve and put in incubator at 100° for 30 minutes.

(*c*) Adjust the pH at 7,2 by addition of soda.

(*d*) Put in autoclave at 110° for 20 minutes.

(*e*) Distribute in tubes in Roux boxes.

(*f*) Sterilise at 110° for 20 minutes.

3. Inoculation of the Cultures

The 3 lyophilised stocks are put in solutions, then inoculated on inclined tubes of the medium already described. After 24 hours of culture in the incubator at 37° the colonies are examined in order to be assured of the characteristic type of these cultures and of the purity of the stocks.

The culture of each tube is washed in a volume of 5 cm³ of solution of Sodium chloride at 9%, then taken up in vacuum pipettes for inoculation on Roux boxes containing 1,200 cm³ of the same medium.

The Roux boxes are in their turn put in the incubator at 37°. After 48 hours of stay in the incubator, the boxes are examined individually in order to be assured of the purity of the colonies.

Then to each of them is added 25 cm³ to 30 cm³ of distilled and sterile water. After the suspension of the microbian culture by manual balancing, the bacterian suspension thus obtained, is collected by aspiration in a sterile recipient.

The suspension is adjusted at 20 milliards of germs per cm³ by the addition of sterile distilled water.

The suspension thus obtained is heated at 56° for 45 minutes then placed immediately in refrigerator at +3, +5.

4. Lysis and the Obtaining of Endototoxins

The bacterial suspension is transferred in a resistant pyrex glass recipient.

It is then congealed at a temperature of 30° to 40° for 24 hours. Then the suspension is left to be decongealed and to remain at 20° during 24 hours. The process of congealation-decongealation is repeated for 3 times. *i.e.*, 4 operations in all.

Then centrifuged in sterile tubes at a speed of 6,000 tm for a time sufficient to obtain a complete sedimentation of lysated bacterias. The floating suspension of the endotoxin is then collected and submitted to a filtration on Seitz E.K.S. and preserved in refrigerator at + 30, ⋅ 50.

5. Detoxification

To the suspension of endotoxins is added an equal volume of sterile distilled water, and submitted to 3 heatings at 75° for 1 hour and at an interval of 24 hours.

The suspension thus obtained corresponds to an original concentration of 10 milliards of germs in a cm^3.

6. Distribution

Then it may be distributed aseptically in ampoules (sterile) *Controle* :

(*a*) *Neutrality* : The pH of the lysate should be between 7 and 7,2.

(*b*) *Sterility* : The inoculation on bouillon or gelose should not be followed by any culture.

(*c*) *Non-toxicity* : Sub-cutaneous injection of 1 ml of lysate should not cause any accident.

(*d*) *Activity* : Three tests are utilised :

1. Intra-cardiac inoculation on cobaye : It is followed by rapid death of the animal by respiratory trouble and after autopsy a hypertrophy of Peyer's plaques accompanied by a hyperplasic endothelitis and a splenomegaly with diffused lesions are seen.

2. Inoculation in the mesenteric ganglions : It gives the same characteristic lesions in weak doses.

Inoculation by splanchnic contact : This also causes similar lesions which show the neurotropism of the endotoxin for the vegetative system.

HISTORY

The first study was reported by L. Bernard in a communication to the Société Médicale Homoeopathique de Normandie and published in the Archives homoeopathiques de Normandie in 1956. Later on G. Poisson, member of the same society, took up the study and made different communications on the subject (see Bibliography). This Nosode has received a very valuable clinical study and has shown a therapeutic activity which should attract the attention of the practitioners.

There is no pathogenesic proving of this remedy according to the method of Hahnemann.

CLINICAL CORTICO-VISCERAL PROTOCOL OR CLINICAL PATHOGENESIS

1. Generalities

Chronic cancer state and chronic mesenchymatose (Sycosis). Recent or old history of a Salmonella affection.

Emaciation.

Intense headache, with or without vertigo, with or without epistaxis.

Insomnia.

Prolonged pyrexia : Without any apparent cause.

Intense fatigue : General sweat.

Chronic state of marasmus following an ancient salmonella infection (typhoid or paratyphoid).

2. Neuro-endocrino-psychic-System

(a) *Depressed condition :*

Cannot tolerate noise.

Passimist, sees the dark side of everything, future is dark, afraid of catastrophe.

Depressed, obsessed, *asthenic subject.*

Often they are fluoric.

(*b*) *Nervous* :

Continued headche, generalised, sometimes with vertigo ; frequent insomnia, accompanied by loss of appetite and nausea.

Meningitis.

Encephalo-myelitis.

Hemorrhage of meningitis.

Epilepsy.

Neuro-toxicosis of babies.

3. **Digestive Apparatus**

Stomatitis, pharyngitis.

Inflmmation of salivary glands.

Saburrale tongue, aphthe.

Fever, *vomitings*, *diarrhoea*, acute or sub-acute.

Denutrition—emaciation.

Chronic stage with headache, nausea, vertigo.

Morning or post-prandial diarrhoea.

Colic or burning of the intestines.

Acute or chronic cholecystitis.

Pancreatitis.

Abdominal pains.

Stubborn constipation.

Spleno and hepato-megaly.

Intestinal hemorrhage.

4. **Cardio-hemo-vascular System**

Dull sound of the heart, arythmia.

Pulse slow, sometimes irregular.

Phlebitis, at first slow, insiduous, specially of the lower limbs, of the left side. (Lamasson)

15 F

Thermoregulation : Prolonged pyrexias ; dehydration ; paleness.

5. Respiratory System

(a) *Throat* : Pharyngitis.

(b) *Lungs, pleura* : Cough without any expectoration. Diffused bronchial rales.

Pulmonary congestion and broncho-pneumonia appear and disappear rapidly.

Pneumonia and pleuro-pneumonia with slow resorption.

Abcess of the lungs.

6. Sense Organs

(a) *Nose* : Epistaxis.

(b) *Eyes* : Red conjunctivas.

(c) *Ears* : Acute otitis, sub-acute or chronic.

7. Uro-genital Apparatus

Pyelo-cystitis.

Cystitis ; chronic cystalgias.

8. Loco-motor System

Hydrarthrosis, localised on knees.
Purulent arthritis of the knees.
Vertebral osteo-arthritis with discopathia.
Erratic osteo-arthritis of the joints.

9. Skin, Phanera

Peri-buccal herpes.

POSOLOGY

Dynamisation : 4 CH, 5 CH, 7 CH, 9 CH.

For old case of paratyphoid etiology 15 CH and 30 CH may be used.

DIFFERENTIAL DIAGNOSIS

Is well related to *Eberthinum* but specially with *Colibacilium* and *Anti-colibocillary serum*.

New remedies : *Paronichia illecebrum*, *Acheranthes calea*, *Ipomia* and *Rajania subsamarata* (see. O.A. Julian and Collab. Matiére médicale homoeopathique, Librairie Lefrançois, 79006, Paris).

CLINICAL DIAGNOSIS

1. Generalities

Chronic mesenchymatous state, with evolution towards cancer.

Denutrition and emaciation with tendency towards general marasmas.

Chronic emaciation of patients having in the antecedants chronic etiology of Salmonella.

Pre-cancer-stage.

2. Neuro-psychic System

Depressive colibacillary psychoses.

Meningo-typhoid.

Neuro-toxicosis of babies.

Acute post-infectious encephalitis of children (measles, diphtheria, whooping cough).

3. Digestive Apparatus

Acute cholecystitis, sub-acute, chronic.

Angiocolitis with sub-febrile condition.

Enterocolitis.

Summer enteritis.

Intoxication by shell fish.

Hemorrhagic recto-colitis.

4. Cardio-vascular System

Bradycardia.

Phlebitis of the left lower limb.

5. **Pulmonary Apparatus**

Rhino-pharyngitis.
Dragging bronchitis.
Acute pneumopathies with slow absorption.

6. **Urinary Apparatus**

Pyelocystitis and cystitis, specially relapsing colibacillosis.
Cystalgias.

7. **Loco-motor System**

Arthrosis of the knee.
Purulent arthritis of the knee.
Vertebral and polyarticular osteo-arthritis.

8. **Infectious Diseases**

Dragging sub-acute pyrexias.

Typhoid and paratyphoid.

Angiohematic typhus.

Toxicosis of babies.

OBSERVATIONS

Here is a clinical case report of Dr. G. Poisson published in
lcs Archives Hom. de Normandie, No. 19, July 1960.

Case Report No. 1

The most spectacular case that I have seen came to consult
me on the 5th May, 1956. I will always see again and again
this young woman of 35 years, but she appeared to be of
60 years, emaciated, floating in her dress, having yellow waxy
colour, with weary and discouraged traits. Her hairs were not
done, stuck to the temples. Her eyes seemed feverish. Having
a weak and weary voice. She told me her history. Since more
than a year as a result of a car accident when she dashed
against a cyclist, she has a temperature rising from 37·9° to 38·4°
in the morning and 39° to 40° in the evening, headaches,
insomnia, intense weakness, extremely abundant night sweat

and vertigo. Gradually her general condition has become so
much weakened that she was forced to stop her activity of an
artisan in a little village where she worked.   She could no more
drive because she could no more remember what is to be done
to stop speeding.   Noises became progressively unbearable to
her, so much so that she had to stop the pendulum of the
clock ; her hands trembled, she lets falls the objects that she
carried ; she toppled down the glass articles.   She was not only
unable to open her shop, but was also incapable to give orders,
to receive salesmen, and to keep accounts.   She saw everything
in darkness and she always expected the worst.   Situation was
dramatic : Her weight came down from 68 kg. to 48 kg. then
39 kg.

Sometimes ago in the month of September 1955, she went
to a hospital where she underwent all sorts of examinations ;
X-ray of lungs which was normal, many negative hemocultures.
Wright's negative sero-diagnosis ; provac's negative intradermo-
reaction, cyto-bacterial examinations of urines which were
normal ; examination of stools was normal, X-ray of teeth
which was normal ; her eyes were normal.   Only the blood
counts showed the red globules as 2,740·000 and leucocytes
1,017·000. And the patient got out of the hospital without any
definite diagnosis.

But the personal history revealed rich informations : Numerous anginas and scarlatina in infancy, two jaundices one after
the other at the age of 11, a typhoid in 1946, a colibacillosis in
1950 and the last, in 1955, an extremely violent shock (let us
recall that she dashed against a cyclist one month ago), which
was the starting point of her present condition.

Then it was quite clear and logical : Cortico-thalamic stress
of emotional order which creats a cortico visceral reflex on the
intestines.   Colibacilli and Eberth bacilli came out of their den
which the ptosis offered to them, the diverticules and atonic
vesicle which explain the fluoric type of the patient, became
pathogenous.   Time helped to do the rest.   The women was

covered with many dresses and underwears, which took too much time to open which made the patient weary. Her skin is like that of seriously infected person ; her mucouses are pale, her arterial tension was 10 1/2-7. Her belly is distended and sensitive. I found neither big liver, nor big spleen. Her nails are full of white spots, the witnesses of great demineralisation.

And I prescribed : *Acetic acid 4, Metallum album 4, Silicea 4* and *Natrum mur. 7, Eberthenum 7.*

The 26th May, 1956 ; three weeks later her condition was unchanged. In the meantime I consulted with my friend Dr. Benard and I was advised to replace *Eberthinum* with *Paratyphoidinum*, because it was not a case of typhoid but the case of paratyphoid. The daily medicines were the same ; but I gave doses of *China* and *Colibacillinum 7, Para-B. 7* which I repeated several times.

Now let us hear the patient, in her letter, about the result :

"Without conviction I came to see you and brought with me the reports of all the examinations done. You encouraged me and gave me a treatment for 3 weeks. In your second treatment you gave me *Paratyphoidinum 7.* I took it. I was sceptic with a medicine of 250 frs (corresponds to 2.50 frs at present), while other medicines costing much higher failed to cure me. I took it on the following Sunday. On Monday I felt better. My temperature fell to 36·8° the first time in the course of a year ! I took the temperature many times believing that I had wrongly taken the temperature. I asked my husband also to take it thinking that the temperature was not rising because of a defect in the thermometer. The result was conclusive. From that time, my appetite came back and also the sleep. My convalescence was rapid. I could take up my work again. I was saved. You had found the exact remedy which suited me. I had taken several doses later on and I could assure you that it was absolutely radical. My case intrigued many persons and I assured you that I thought that it was my duty to explain the fact how I was treated ; what a remedy !

Your medicines had saved me. That my case may serve others to cure their diseases. I worked every day. I took my weight again and again. My present weight is 68 kg. However they used to tell me that I would not be able to work any more."

Such is the history of the cure told by Mme. B. herself.

On my part, I could have noted, gradually following the consultations the spectacular ameliorations. Two months after the taking of *Para. B.* I. found on my card an increase of weight by 13 kg.

The Red globules rose from 3,450000 to 4,320000. The rate of hemoglobin rose from 65 % to 80% ; the polyneutrals from 75,5 to 53,5 and Leucocytes from 23, 800 to 7,200.

Three years after, on the 3rd June, 1959, *i.e.*, to say after 15 days I saw the patient again. This was a woman well in flesh, with her full breast, well balanced body, high in colour, lively eyes, who smiled with her good teeth and she carry on her work soundly. She had again found the joy of living. She was toned up and dynamic. I gained much in this case because she gave me the idea of using *Para. B.* in psychasthenia and in depressive condition of *B. coil* infection.

That day she came to me for troubles of digestion of the type of *Nux vomica.* Periodically in September-October and in February-March she had troubles of digestion and she used to take *Para. B.* of which she had always a stock. Everything became normal.

I thought that this tendency to relapse is due to three cases :

1. I had never given her a prolonged ground treatment which would have swept off the sycotic colibacillary ground and the deep tubercular ground.

2. That the patient was of fluoric type with her ligamentary hyperlaxity, with her mal position of teeth, with her antecedants of scarlatina and repeated anginas—and that really

she had a hypotonic vesicle, some ptosis localised in her intestines and some diverticules of her intestinal walls which served almost unattackable refuge to *B. coli* and *Para B.*

3. Then there was in the small village where she lived an endemic paratyphoid of which the manifestations reached 2 acmes during spring and summer.

It was probable that there had been epidemics of paratyphoid in this country. Once the epidemic was stopped, there remained some carriers of the germs who may carry in them the germs in full virulence during weeks and months after the clinical cure of the patient, notedly on the surface of the gall bladder. These carriers of germs (who themselves may not give any sign of the disease) infected those who were around them. They infected by their evacuations the ground, the water sources and the vegetables. With their not well washed hand they infected the milk, the cooking utensils, the creams and pastries with, really speaking, the ready cultures of the germ.

It seemed that the last hypothesis was exact because since then I had seen another woman of the same village who obtained the same result as that of her fellow villager.

PERTUSSINUM

BIBLIOGRAPHY

Boericke, W. :

Pocket Manual of Homoeopathic Materia Medica. Boericke and Runyon, Ny., 1927.

Materia Medica and Repertorium. Trad. allemande. Verlag Grundlagen and Praxis. Margarette Harms, Leer. 1. Aufl., 1972.

Bernard, H. :

Nouveau Traité d'Homoeopathie. Coquemard, Angouléme, 1947.

Cartier François :

Thérapeutique des Voies Respiratories ; J.B. Baillérc et fils, Paris. 2e ed, 1920.

Clarke, J. :

A Dictionary of Practical Materia Medica. London, 1955, v. 3, Appendix, p. 1621—Coqueleuchinum.

Collet, T. J. M. :

Isopathie. Vigot fréres, Paris, 1902.

Fortier-Bernoville :

Nosodes. L'Homoeopathie Monerne, No. 2, 15, janvier, 1937.

Julian, O.A. :

Biothérapiques et Nosodes. Maloine, Paris, 1962.
Materia Medica der Nosoden. 2e ed 1975. Haug Verlag. Heidelberg.

Kollisch :

Homoeopathie. Maloine, 1955.

(443)

Romer, R. :

Meine Erfahrungen mit den Nosoden Parotidin, Pertussin und Histamin. Zeitschrift für klassische Homöopathie. Bd. 16, No. 4, 1972, p. 159.

Vannier, L. and Poirier, J. :

Précis de Matiére Médical Homoeopathique. Doin 1958, p. 159.

STOCK

The biotherapic *pertussinum* is prepared from the lysate obtained, without addition of antiseptic, from the expectoration of patient suffering from whooping cough not yet treated.

Composition : Lysate corresponding to 0,001 cm^3 of expectoration.

It is presented in ampoules of 1 mililitre for being used for homoeopathic dilutions.

1. Technique of Preparation

The collections are done according to the legal exigencies and in Petri boxes.

They are the object of different examinations :

(*a*) *Cytological examination* : Examination between lame and lamellas shows abundant mucus, some epithelial cells and some leucocytes.

(*b*) *Examination after May-grunwala-giemsa colouring* : Abundant microbian flora, some cells, some polynuclears, some lymphocytes.

(*c*) *Bucteriological examination* : It was not possible to detect the existence of any bacilli of Bordet Gengou in any of the collections.

2. Initial Dilution of the Expectorations

The expectorations are diluted in 100 times of their volume in distilled water.

3. Lysate of the Cells and Microbian Elements

The initial dilution of 1/100 is congealed at 20 ; then decongealed in the ordinary temperature four times one after the other.

4. Sterilisation and Distribution of the Initial Dilution

The lysate obtained before is sterilised by filtration on E.K.S. filter then distributed by fractions of 10 cm³ in sterile phials.

5. Stockage of the Initial Dilution

The fractions of 10 cm³ of the initial dilution are lyophilised so as to be suitable to be conserved without weakening. Each phial containing a quantity of product lyophilised corresponding to 0·10 cm³ of expectorations.

The lysate is characterised by the technique of preparation and by the control test.

6. Dilution

This content of each phial is taken up in 100 cm³ of sterile distilled water so as to bring the concentration of the final product to 0,001 by centimetre cube of expectoration.

7. Filtration and Distribution of the Final Dilution

The final dilution is filtered on E.K.S. filters then distributed aseptically in ampoule of 1 cm³.

CONTROL

(*a*) *Sterility* : Inoculation on bouillon or better on gelose should not follow any culture.

(*b*) *Non-toxicity* : By sub-cutaneous injection of 1 ml to rats weighing 20 g. does not cause any accident. A rabit should bear without any damage the injection of 5 ml of the product.

HISTORY

In his book "Isopathie" Collet T.J.M. relates first the treatment of whooping cough with an isotherapic.

Here is the case report :

In September 1879, when I was staying in Marolles-en-Hurepoix (Seine-et-Oise) there was an epidemic of whooping cough among the children of that country. The directress of the girls' school brought to me some of the children suffering from whooping cough. I took the secretions from the mouth of one of the girls and made from them the 6th dilution in alcohol. I advised to give 5 drops of this remedy in two table-spoonful of water to be given in the morning, two consecutive days every week for 4 to 5 weeks even when the children have no fits of cough, and this because of the tenacity of the disease and its easy relapse. The fits of cough diminished rapidly during the day although the fits were more frequent at night. But after eight days, in many of the children, there was great amelioration, although some of them had the cough from time to time. After 15 days all the children became almost normal. Nevertheless the use of the medicine was continued, 5 drops every week for two or three weeks more in order to be assured of the complete cure as the disease often reborns out of the ashes.

"In January 1894, remembering the good effects of the medicine among the students of the school, I advised the same remedy to a mother who consulted me for her child attacked by the same disease which was then raging in the country she lived, in Creuzot, near Saint-Thibault (Côte d'Or). I advised her to apply the same remedy and even sent her in a packet of powder of the ground globules of the 6th dilution of whooping cough of Marolles. I advised her to dissolve this packet in two tablespoonful of pure water and to give 10 drops of this solution in one half glass of the decoction of violet to be given in the morning before any food once a day, for one month or five weeks.

"From the very first day of the application of the remedy, the mother wrote to me that the young child was coughing much less. It had only two fits at night. After eight days it had only occasional fits of cough, with less of suffocation and had a good general condition. After 15 days the mother considered her child as cured, but continued according to my advise the remedy, once every eight days, for still 2 to 3 weeks, in order to avoid late relapses.

"Here are then some cures of whooping cough by the help of Isopathy, by a medicine taken from another subject ; but we have seen that in epidemic diseases it can be done specially when the isopathic remedy of the first subject has become well s uccessful."

Then J.H. Clarke published according to the informations supplied by Cartier a book "Whooping-cough cured with Coqueluchin", London, 1906.

He relates 14 cases of whooping-cough or whooping-cough like coughs treated successfully by *Pertussinum 30 C* repeated every 4 hours.

Clarke also relates a case of prevention with a favourable result.

Cartier confirms this case from one of his personal cases.

During the developed stage of whooping-cough *Pertussinum* seems to shorten the duration of the disease.

Then Duprat, Nebel in Switzerland, Pinart in Spain began to use this biotherapic.

Finally O.A. Julian has used in his practice the biotherapic *Pertussinum* in other affections of the respiratory tract and of the nervous system.

The biotherapic *Pertussin* has no pathogenesis according to the methodology of Hahnemann.

CLINICAL CORTICO-VISCERAL PROTOCOL
OR CLINICAL PATHOGENESIS

1. Generalities

Restlessness. Cries. Tears.
Anorexia. Asthenia. Anerzasia.
Predisposition to tuberculosis.
Jacquelin-Burnand Syndrome.

2. Neuro-psychic System

Convulsions. Hemorrhage from the meninges.
Paralysis. Neuro-motor deficit. Paresis.
Troubles of conscience.
Psycho-motor or sensorial troubles.

Somnolence and state of confusion, muscular jerkings (movements of the extension flexion of the wrists). Myelitis. Polyneuritis.

3. Digestive Apparatus

Ulceration of the tongue.
Vomiting.

4. Cardio-hemo-vascular System

Cyanosis, sweats, weakness.
Tachycardia or tachy-arythmia.
Thermoregulations : Slight hyperthermia around 38° to 40° with convulsions.

5. Respiratory Apparatus

Spasm of the glottis.
Dry cough, spasmodic of different intensity, comes suddenly.

Increasing jerking cough with cyanosis, with a phase of apnea followed by the taking of respiration.

Repeated fits which end in the rejection of mucosities and vomiting.

Laryngospasms.

Tracheo-bronchial adenopathy.

Dilatations of bronchi.

Dense, thick, mucus expectoration.

Dragging bronchitis.

Tracheo-bronchiac adenopathy.

6. **Sense Organs**

Nose : Epistaxis.

Eyes : Chemosis.

Ears : Oto-mastoiditis.

7. **Modalities**

Aggravation : By laughing, nervous shock, emotion, effort, rest.

POSOLOGY

Dynamisations : 4 CH, 5 CH, 7 CH, 9 CH, 15 CH, 30 CH.

In acute affections : 4 CH, 5 CH, 7 CH to be repeated frequently.

The high dynamisations 9 CH, 15 CH, once every 3 to 7 days.

In chronic anamnesic conditions : 15 CH or 30 CH, daily or every 7 to 10 days.

DIFFERENTIAL DIAGNOSIS

Aviaire : See article.

For whooping cough think of *Coccus cacti, Belladonna, Sulphur, Antim. tart., Kali carb., Kali bich., Pulsat. etc.*

CLINICAL DIAGNOSIS

Tuberculous state.

Syndrome of Jacquelin-Burnand (Atypical tuberculosis of sub-febrile form, general torpid toxemia, of slow evolution. broken down condition).

Whooping cough.

Spasmodic laryngitis.

Asthma (O.A. Julian).

Chronic bronchitis, bronchiectasis.

Spasmodic cough of persons suffering from bronchitis, or tuberculosis.

Convulsions (O.A. Julian).

Epilepsy (O.A. Julian).

Encephalopathy specially when there is whooping cough in the antecedants.

Mental backwardness (O.A. Julian).

Triosmia 21 (Mongolism).

COMMENTARIES

In practice *Pertussin* has become a very efficacious remedy. As regards whooping cough we may schematically mention the following treatment :

Give at 21 hours a dose of *Drosera 7 CH*, the 1st evening ; *Pertussin 7 CH*, the 2nd evening; *Cuprum 7 CH*, the 3rd evening ; *Hyocyamus 7 CH* the 4th evening and *Pertussinum 7 CH*, the 5th evening.

During the day symptomatologically should be given the following drainage :

Alternating every one hour : 8 drops of *Ipeca 4 CH, Drosera 4 CH, Coral. r. 3 CH* and then 7 drops of *Cuprum acet.4 DH*.

In the way one may get a cure in 8 to 10 days or maximum in 15 days. I affirm this from my long practice. Of course there are some particular clinical cases, or an epidemic genius. In that case one must try to find out one or two simillimum. But the schema of doses indicated above will differ very little. At the end of a whooping cough think of *Aviaire*.

However, if the whooping cough is not ameliorated within 3 to 4 days, give *Pertussinum 7 CH* one dose every day.

In asthma with fitful cough *Pertussinum* gives good service with *Cuprum* and *Astragallus* (See : Etudes Hahnemanniennes, cliniques et thérapeutiques, p. 21, by O.A. Julian, v., 2 Le françois, Paris 75006).

In the affections of children of neurologic order *Pertussin* may equally serve well in epilepsy, convulsions and tetanus, mental backwardness, specially when the pathological troubles are consecutive to whooping cough or if this disease is found in the antecedants.

In the Congress of German homoeopaths of "Deutschen Zentralvereins Homöopathischer Arzte" of 19 and 22 May, 1971 at Bad Durkheim, meant uniquely for the Nosodes,. in the presence of O.A. Julian, Dr. Romer of Russelhim reported some clinical cases regarding whooping cough of 2 adults and 3 children favourably treated by *Pertussin C30* globuli and with some homoeotherapics selected according to the law of simil-limum, such as *Kali bichromicum C30*, *Verbascum D4*, *Sulphur iod. C200* and *Mephitis C30*.

PNEUMOCOCCINUM

BIBLIOGRAPHY :

Seveaux, F. :

Recherches expérimentales d'Allergie Homoeopathique.
Cahiers de Biothérapie, No. 8, Décembre, 1965.

Julian, O.A. and Collab :

Matière médicale d'Homoeopathie, 1971. Librairie Le
François, Paris.

STOCK

The pneumococcus is a bacteria of Diplococcus type, of the
family of Micrococcaceae, Gram + .

The pneumococcus is a saprophyte host of the mucouses. It
is found in 50% of cases, in the saliva of healthy persons, in the
nasal mucous, mucous of pharynx and conjuctiva.

Sevaux did a study of clinical pathogenesis but there did
not exist any Hahnemannian pathogenesis.

CLINICAL CORTICO-VISCERAL PROTOCOL
OR CLINICAL PATHOGENESIS

1. Generalities

Constitution : Phosphofluoric constitution.

Temperament : Bilio-nervous, depressive, anxious.

Intoxication : Allergoso (psoro), mesenchymatosic (sycosic).

Cancer condition, tuberculinosis.

2. Neuro-endocrino-psychic System

(*a*) *Psychic* :

Depressive condition with anxiety.

Desire to remain at home, horror of going out.

Loss of the taste of life.

Loss of memory.

Impression that the patient is going to break down, that he can no more walk.

Great fear of becoming ill.

Great fear of death.

(*b*) *Nervous* :

Headache continuing for 3 to 4 days.

Right hemicrania or of the left side aggravated by walk which hurts the head.

Frequent headaches situated in the nape of the neck ; aggravated by nose.

The sensation of some liquid in the head when bending down.

Headache while coughing or while bending the head.

Vertigo.

Acute headache coming brutally, like pricking or cramping short lasting.

Pain as if caught in -a vice.

Pains aggravated by rest at night, ameliorated by movement.

3. Digestive Apparatus

Apthe in the mouth.

Somnolence at 3 p.m.

Bad digestion.

Frequent nausea after having eaten.

Gastralgia when hungry.

Better by taking some food.

Constipation with false urgency.

Cramps of the stomach with the sensation of burning.

Gas alternating with constipation and fetid stools.

Constipation.

Constipation during journey.

Bloating and pain of the left hypochondria calmed by passing wind.

4. **Cardio-hemo-vascular System**

Precordialgias, puncturing pains.

Emotive palpitations.

Frequent palpitation any time during the day.

Palpitation obliging the patient to stop while walking or getting up a staircase.

Electrocardiogram reveals right focal block.

Frequent redness of the face while entering a warm room.

5. **Respiratory Apparatus**

Pains on left frontal sinus.

Sub-orbitary frontal pains.

Cough after breakfast (No cough after 9 a.m.).

Dry cough in cold or in heat or trachitis.

Incessant cough without expectorations, specially at night with nausea.

Cough by heat while entering in metro.

Coughs specially while entering in a hot room and scrapes the throat.

Should bend down for coughing.

Much cough following frequent bronchitis during infancy.

Sensation of a feather in the throat.

6. **Sense Organs**

(*a*) *Eyes* : Fatigue at the neon lamp.

(*b*) *Ears* : Inflammatory otalgia, vertigo.

7. Uro-genital Apparatus

(*a*) *Urinary* : Urine escapes while coughing.

(*b*) *Genital* : Premenstrual aggravation.

Menstrual cycle short (22 to 24 days) stopping for 2 days.

Sensation of burning during coition when fatigued.

Late menses, less abundant, with heavy and swollen legs before menstruation.

Migraines and vertigo.

Sensation of heaviness in the uterus (crosses the legs).

No orgasm.

8. Loco-motor System

Cervicalgias.

Cervicalgias with frontal pains.

Cervicalgias with dorsal pains.

Dorsal pains.

Cannot stand erect because of pain in the back.

Pains in arms.

Restless legs, specially before the menses (*Zincum, Lachesis*).

Pains in the legs.

Legs heavy in the morning while waking up.

Trembling of the legs.

Cramps in feet.

9. Skin, Phanera

Moist hands.

Pruritus with disseminated eruption on the neck and on the forehead.

Small eruptions on the face.

10. Biological Characteristics

Right focal block revealed by cardiogram.

11. Modalities

Aggravation :

While entering in a hot room.

By inactivity.

By rest at night.

By prolonged sitting position, completely immobile.

By humidity.

Before menses.

Ameliorations :

By open air.

In the fields.

By a short sleep after meals.

By hot foot bath.

POSOLOGY

Dynamisations : From 5 CH to 30 CH, orally, drops or granules. Sevaux advises the mixture of dilutions, at first 5, 7, 9 CH, then 5, 7, 9, 15 CH and 5, 7, 9, 15, 30 CH (Dr. Julian also indicates the same technique).

POSITIVE DIAGNOSIS

1. Depressive condition, with pains of which the seats may be on any part of cervico-dorsal region.

2. Respiratory troubles, specially of the bronchi.

3. Palpitations with focal block, revealed by cardiogram.

4. Dysmenorrhoea with delayed menses and premenstrual syndrome.

DIFFERENTIAL DIAGNOSIS

Medorrhinum : See article.

Thuya : Hydrogenoid condition, fixed idea, varicosity of the wings of the nose.

Natrum sulphuricum : Hydrogenoid condition, melancholy, worse during change of season, consequence of a traumatism.

Flatulence, diarrhoea, periodical cutaneous troubles.

New remedies :

Acidum hippuricum : Multiple arthralgias, right sided headache. Hepatic nausea, bloating of the abdomen.

Aranea diadema : By its hydrogenoid constitution is related to *Thuya* and *Natrum sulphuricum*.

CLINICAL DIAGNOSIS

1. **Neuro-psychic System**

   Anxious and depressive condition.

   Hypochondriasis.

   Hemicrania.

   Neuralgia of the skull.

2. **Digestive Apparatus**

   Cortico-gastric disthermia.

   Insufficient liver.

   Aerogastria and aerocholia.

   Constipation.

3. **Cardio-hemo-vascular System**

   Cardiac neurosis.

   Basedow's heart.

   Tachy-arythmia.

4. **Respiratory Apparatus**

   Sinusitis ; trachitis ; dragging bronchitis.

   Emphysema.

5. **Uro-genital Apparatus**

   Sinusitis.

   Trachitis.

6. **Uro-genital Apparatus**
   Weakness of the bladder.
   Oligomenorrhoea.
   Frigidity.
   Menstrual migraine.
7. **Loco-motor System**
   Cervicoarthrosis.
   Dorso-lumbar arthrosis.

PROTEUS

BIBLIOGRAPHY

Sevaux :

Experimental research of homoeopathic allergy. Cahier de Biothérapique, No. 8, December, 1965.

Hui-Bon-Hoa :

Intestinal nosodes. Proteus. Annales homoeopathiques françaises, 6e année, No. 9, p. 691-695, 1964.

Julian, O.A. :

Biothérapiques et Nosodes : Bacille Proteus. (Nosodes intestinaux de Bach et Paterson), p. 245-247, Ed. Maloine, 1962.

Hui-Bon-Hoa :

Les Nosodes intestinaux. Ed. Coquemard, Angouléme, 1966, Bulletin du C.H.F., 1967, p. 69.

Poisson Georges :

A propos de plusieurs observations d'infection urinaire á Proteus. Annales homopathiques françaises, p. 21-672, No. 8, October, 1958.

Schmidt Roger :

Proteus—A Bach-Nosode. Journ. of the Americ. Inst. of Homoeop., In : Rev. de Presse, Anglaise par le Dr. J. Hui-Bon-Hoa. Annales Homoeop. Fr. 1966, No. 2., p. 162.

STOCK

Proteus belongs to the great family of Enterobacteriacae. Described in 1885 by Hauser, its bacteriological study has been done very recently by Prevost, Moller and others.

(459)

This is a gram negative bacilli, polymorphous, very mobile, without capsule, without spore.

The biochemic characteristics are :

(*a*) Possession (except for *Providencia*) of a urease which hydrolyses the urea in Ferguson medium with alkalinisation by the liberation of carbonate of ammonia.

(*b*) Presence of a typtrophanedesaminase.

(*c*) Great proteolytic activity.

There are four varieties, *viz* :

Proteus vulgaris, Mirabilis, Rettgeri, Morganii.

The groupe *Providencia* is now added to them.

Proteus are Gram negative rods, flourishing on ordinary mediums attacking the glucides, with formation of acids and sometimes some gas. Very mobile, provided with peritricic flagella ; they never attack lactose.

They ferment the glucose and transform the phenylamine in acid phehyl-puruvic.

The pathogenous power takes the directions to intestines in the form of gastro-enteritis, diarrhoeas. Even their origin is due to genito-urinary infection and may be responsible for mastoiditis, otitis, meningitis, peritonitis, overinfection of wounds and ulcers.

In nosodotherapy, it is John Paterson of Glasgow, after the work of Bach, Wheeler and Dishington, who described the clinical indications and the prescription of homoeopathic dynamisations.

In France, we owe to F. Sevaux, a study of clinical pathogenesis (see above) in Cahiers de Biothérapie, No. 8, December, 1965.

In 1968 appeared a study of G. Poisson on bacteriological study as well as on their clinical indications.

CLINICAL CORTICO-VISCERAL PROTOCOL
OR CLINICAL PATHOGENESIS

1. Generalities

Proteus, the bacteria frequently found in the intestines is a biotherapic of which the sphere of action concerns essentially to the phenomena of the allergy of the digestive system such as it was described by Monod.

Constitution :

It suits to three constitutions : *Carbonic, Fluoric, Phosphoric.*

Temperament :

A digestive, with brown hair, lean, pale.

A spasmodic parathyroidian.

Intoxication :

An allergosic (psoric).

It is necessary to note that this remedy is rarely indicated when there is no nervous symptoms as says Hui-Bon-Hon.

It is a subject at first irritable then despressed, tense, aggresive specially after nervous overwork.

2. Neuro-endocrino-psychic System

(*a*) *Psychic* : Sensation of great nervous tension, of great overwork.

"Tempest under the skull".

"Explosion of anger when contradicted".

Throws away the objects near at hand, kicks.

The child rolls on the ground.

Slight agony while ill.

Thinks of suicide though he has not the wish for it.

Tense, irritable, depressed, and is capable of murder when he is angry.

Dislikes company.

Rigid attitude, often with fixed ideas.

(b) *Nervous system* :

Vertigo.

Vertigo increasing with the rising of the sun.

Insomnia worse in village.

Frontal headache with the sensation of heaviness.

Headache aggravated before the menses, for a week.

Headache begins in the morning.

Headache with diarrhoea and pasty tongue.

Convulsions, epilepsy, meningism during fever.

Pain of the neck when rising up in the morning.

3. **Digestive Apparatus**

(a) *Mouth, tongue, pharynx* :

Fissures of the joints of the lips, not easily avails to the treatment.

Salty taste in the mouth.

Sensitiveness of the gums.

Ulcer in the mouth.

(b) *Stomach* :

Acidity, pyrosis.

Painful hunger, not ameliorated by food.

Nausea and migraine after meals.

Frequent hiccough for a few seconds, coming at least once in a day after meals.

Aerophagia, the patient puts his fingers in his throat to vomit up air.

Vomiting by the least excess.

Gastric pains, no fixed time, sometimes at night.

According to the English authors, Proteus is to be prescribed specially in the cases of duodenal ulcers, which manifests itself brutally by hematemesis or perforation.

(c) *Intestines* :

Emotive diarrhoea.

Diarrhoea with headache and pasty tongue.

Alternating diarrhoea and constipation.

Constipation with false urgency.

Yellow, soft stools after breakfast.

Hematemesis, melena.

Presence of oxyuris in the stools.

Anal pruritus.

Aversion to butter, pork, viande, eggs, specially hard eggs, green haricots, salades, onion, cucumber, chocolate which he cannot digest.

Desire for fat, sugar, salt, butter and eggs.

4. Cardio-hemo-vascular System

Sensation of heaviness in the precordial region.

Pain aggravated by effort.

Palpitation in elongated position.

Palpitation by the least emotion.

Frequent right sided focal block.

Spasms of vessels, *sensation as if the fingers are dead.*

Intermittent claudication.

Bleeding hemorrhoids, with intense itching.

Venous congestion of legs.

5. Respiratory Apparatus

(a) *Throat* : Sensation of thick mucus flowing from the cavum. Nasal obstruction, aggravated in closed rooms.

Subacute pharyngitis with difficulty to speak.

Cough and expectoration.

(*b*) *Lungs, pleura* :

Bad tenacious cough, weakening with expectoration.

Thoracic constriction, with the sensation of oppression and suffocation.

6. Sense Organs

(*a*) *Nose* : *Nasal obstruction* worse in a closed room.

Impression that thick mucus is dropping from the back of the nose.

(*b*) *Eyes* : *Burning pains in the eyes.*

Pains ameliorated by pressure.
Coloured phosphenes with vertigo.
Eyes, red, fatigued in light.
Intermittent weakness of the sight.
Meibomian cysts.

(*c*) *Ears* : Sharp or burning pains of the type of otitis but without fever.

7. Uro-genital Apparatus

(*a*) *Urinary* :

In men and in women :
Turbide and fetid urine.
Whitish filaments in the urine.
Cystitis after having taken food.
Violent burning in the urethra.
Pain in the renal region.

(*b*) *Genital* :

In women : Menses with clots.

Abundant white discharge, worse during ovulation.
Brownish bloody discharge before the menses.
Thready clots at the end of menses.
Regular menses with clots for seven days.
Pruritus of the vulva.

Vaginitis.

Furuncles of the ano-vulvar region.

8. Loco-motor System

(a) *Upper limbs* :

Hands as if dead at night.

Hands *burning at night.*

Hands *numb* in the morning.

Retraction of palms and of the little finger.

Cannot close the hand.

Deforming rheumatism of the hands.

(b) *Lower limbs* :

Intermittent claudications.

Pains in the calves : Pains obliging the patient to walk with a stick.   Cramps in the feet.

Feet numb, as if frozen, aggravated by cold weather.

Sciatic pain.

Contused condition of the feet.

Hammering of the toes.

(c) *Pains of the neck better by pressure.*

9. Skin, Phanera

Sweats under the arms, hands moist.

Very abundant sweats under the arms falling in big drops with moist hands.

Oozing dermatitis on the back of the hands.

Pruriginous vesicles of the external face of the wrists, fingers.

Herpetic eruptions.

Eruptions, papulo-pustulous, erythematous, dry, desquamous of the chin and of the upper lip.

Severe pruritus.

Doubled nails.

Fall of hairs.

Thoracic panniculitis.

10. Modalities

Aggravation :

In the morning, when waking up, by effort, while getting up a staircase.

By drinking wine.

In stormy weather, by heat, by exposition to sun.

In the winter, by cold.

While lying down.

At night.

Amelioration :

In moderate temperature, while lying stretched, in mountains by pure whisky (a mixture aggravates).

One hour after rising up, after eating.

POSOLOGY

Dynamisations : From 5 CH to 30 CH.

By mouth : Globules. Rectal suppositories.

The 5 CH is used daily.

The high dilutions from 7 CH to the 30 CH in aspaced doses for desenibilising but according to clinical necessity may be prescribed daily. To be had of Nelson, London : Proteus (Bach) 12 c, 30 c, 200 c, 1m, 50 m, cm.

POSITIVE DIAGNOSIS

The predominance of the troubles of the digestive system or troubles coinciding with the ingestion of foods that may cause allergic troubles.

The brutality of the nervous symptoms with the important sensation of intra-cranial tension.

The urinary troubles of the type of acute or subacute cystalgia. Morphopsychic rigidity with fixed ideas.

DIFFERENTIAL DIAGNOSIS

Psorinum : Cortico-somatic inhibition, chilliness, sadness, periodical migraines, need for eating at night, morning diarrhoea, weakness of the back and of the articulations, bad smelling, eruptions, appearing in winter and disappearing in the summer

Sulphur : Allergic condition (Psoric). Skin, burning with eruptions, itching. Impatient, quarrelling, asthenic.

Tuberculinum : Unstable, emotive, aggravated by physical effort, or by intellectual effort ; emaciation, sweats, morning diarrhoea. Aggravation by humid cold and during change of weather.

Colibacillinum : (See article).

Paratyphoidinum B : (See article).

CLINICAL DIAGNOSIS

1. Generalities

Cortico-somatic inhibition.
Morbid-metastasis.
Long and dragging convalescence.
Early senescence.
Neuro-arthritic diathesis of Charcot.

2. Neuro-endocrino-pyschic System

Beard's disease (neurasthenia).
Myelasthenia.
Melancholy state.
Migraines.
Neuralgias.
Hysteria.
Convulsions.
Epileptoid syndromes.
During fever, reaction of meninges.
Meniere's disease.

Characterial troubles with aggressiveness. (See Pathogensis of D.N.A., R.N.A. by O.A. Julian in Recherches théoriques pratiques en Homoeopathie, t. 2, p. 83, 1973. Le François, 75006 Paris).

3. Digestive Apparatus

Digestive migraines.

Cortico-tuberosity.

Aerophagia with troubles of pseudo-angina.

Aphthe and ulcers of the mouth.

Cortico-gastric dysrythmia.

Cholecystitis.

Spasmodic colopathies.

Hemorrhoids and anal pruritis.

Oxyurosis.

4. Cardio-hemo-vascular System

Angor pectoris.
Coronarian heart.
Obliterating arteritis.
Nocturnal acroparesthesia.
Raynaud's syndrome.
Phlebitis and sequalae of phlebitis.

5. Respiratory Apparatus
Pharyngitis.
Purulent bronchitis.

6. Sense Organs

(a) *Eyes* : Cyste, meibomian of the eyelids.
(b) *Nose* : Chronic hypertrophic rhinitis.
(c) *Ears* : Otalgia, otitis, mastoiditis.

7. Uro-genital Apparatus

(a) *Urinary* : Cystitis. Pyelitis. Pyelonephritis.

(*b*) *Genital* :

Female : Ano-vulvular furuncle.

Vaginitis. Vulvitis.

Leucorrhoea. Salpingitis.

Metritis of col uteri.

Male : Balanitis.

8. **Loco-motor System**

Carpo-pedal spasm (hand of accoucheur).

Functional or professional spasms (writer's cramp, cramp of pianists, of dancers...).

Torsion neurosis of Ziehn-Oppenheim.

Ischemic retraction of the muscles (Volkmann's disease).

9. **Skin, Phanera**

Herpes. Hyperhydrosis. Ephydrosis. Pelade.

CLINICAL CASES

Here are two case reports of Dr. G. Poisson (Annales homoeop. Fr. No. 8, October, 1969, p. 21, 677).

Report 1

The first case concerns Mme P...Suzanne, came to consult for the first time on 12th April, 1962, having 51 years of age.

Interrogation revealed to us that she had passed twenty years of her life in India, in Malaysia and in Indochina. She had suffered from itch and prickly heat. She was copiously vaccinated.

She had malaria for which she had taken large quantity of quinine; she became progressively very heavy, her weight increased from 61 to 74 kg ; three months ago she had her last menstruation. She is now before us, on the threshold of menopause, psoric, but above all decidedly sycotic. The built is like that of a carbonic and she administers with much practical mind her business of tobacco and a restaurant.

She is big and fat; she is chilly; she is constipated. Her traits are rough, with prominent nasogenian furrows; the skin is shining, the nails are soft; she sweats easily, and she exhales a complex smell of tobacco, fried foods and soup beats. Her weariness appears on her face and on her gait ; she is soon out of breath and complains of heavy legs.

She came to consult us specially for an intense fatigue, of pain in her lumbar region, which caused sleeplessness since some months, and painful micturitions which are frequent. Some uriographis were done and some V.U.I. have been done which revealed a chronic right sided pyelitis.

Classical antiseptics, sulfanimides and antibiotics gave no relief, but on the contrary made her more weak. Numerous washing of the bladder with silver nitrate and cyto-bacteriological examinations of urines revealed always and hopelessly Proteus.

By examinations were found :
——White tongue.
——Cramp rings in the iris.
——Arterial tension 17-10.
——Intense costo-lumbar pain by pressure (right side).

——A pain along the trajectory of the urethra of the right side and specially to the point of juxta umbilical and prevesical. (Points—Acupunctural).

——A pain by pressure on the 12th point of the meridian of conception (point of *Thuya*).

——A pain on the point of *Ignatia* (above the Mc. Burney).

——A pain of the 30th point of the stomach (point of *Kali c.*).

——A pain on the 8th point of the silver (specially of the left side) and on the RP 6.

——There are warts and interdigital mycosis.

You see that each of the above indicates sycotic remedies.

And you have recognised the important remedies of sycosis: *Graphitis, Kali carb., Thuya., Nat. sulph.* without omitting *Solidago* and *Ignatia*.

They should be given one after the other in the course of different consultations. But specially, on 12th April, 1962 the patient received an Isopathic (urinary) in 30th CH, 5 drops once a day.

On 8th May, 1962, there was no amelioration on the urinary sphere and there were always some Proteus in the urines. The idea came to me then to give her 5 doses *Proteus 12 CH* (which the patient had from Nelson, London), one dose every 10 days. The three first doses gave her an important jerking, but she had confidence and sustained it well.

30th June, 1962 : The patient was feeling much better but the *Proteus* is still there. I prescribed her four doses of *Proteus* 18 CH, one dose a week.

2nd August, 1962 : The patient does not suffer any more. She sleeps well, she has lost weight progressively ; the A.T. is 16-8. But she is still feeling fatigued.

I gave her *Proteus 30 CH*, three granules a day, helped by well indicated *Mercurius solubilis*.

And on 8th October, 1962, we had the satisfaction to see that all the urinary symptoms have disappeared and with them the lumbar pains, the fatigue ...and the *Proteus*.

Later on, 27th October, 1964, Mme P...had a short relapse (the result of a long overwork in her profession) which was rapidly stopped by the daily dose of *Proteus 30 CH*. Finally in the month of December, 1966, Mme P...underwent a surgical operation for galucoma and bilateral cataract and had a second realpse. It was the result of the long immobile condition in clinic ; no antibiotic gave her relief and in February, 1967 she was cured again within 48 hours with the treatment by *Proteus*, 2 granules 4 times during 24 hours.

Proteus 30 CH is nevertheless continued during some days in order to consolidate the results, two doses in 24 hours, then once a day. Parallelly I applied on her a double cervical and lumbar manipulation, which freed her instantaneously from her headache which appeared during her confinement in the clinic. There was also lumbo-vertebral pains.

Thus *Proteus* in 12 CH then 18 CH, 30 CH, cured three times our patient, like a real antibiotic. There was no doubt a cause at the basis of her diseases which required operation which she refused before she came to consult me.

Case Report 2

The second case is that of a young woman living at Caux, Marie-Claire M...

Typically carbonic and *Pulsatilla.*

I have treated her in the year 1960 and 1961, at the age of 20 years, when she was a young girl.

The girl was working (still work) in a factory of electric piles and manipulated the whole day graphites. She was constipated as you may easily think of it, and the girl came to consult me because of her abundant menstruations with a phase of amenorrhoea for 2 to 3 months, painful, stopping at night, heaviness and cyanosis of lower limbs and hands.

Pulsatilla in 5 CH then in 12 CH, then 30 CH, twice daily helped by *Calcarea carb.* and *Graphitis* in 5 CH, 9 CH, and in 30 CH have shortened the delay to 18 days.

The duration of the abundance augmentated; she had to use linen several times a day.

But the menses remained very painful and alone an Isotherapic of menstrual blood in 30 CH, prepared from the first menstrual flow, was given 5 drops in 24 hours, for weeks and months almost cured her. She was so much so cured that she married in 1962.

Two years afterwards, in July 1964, at the age of 24 Marie-Claire had a nephritic colic of the right side. She was hospitalised and a right nephrotomy for the ablation of a big stone was necessary.

The consequences of the operations were not simple : a pyelo-nephiritis developed with B. coli, then Proteus, resistant to all antibiotics. And after 4 months in November 1964, I saw her coming in my chamber with great lumbar pains, pollakuria, burning during micturition and Proteus in the urine.

Proteus was given in the 30 CH, which relieved the patient in 24 hours.

But on 23rd March, although there was no pullakuria, neither any dysuria, Proteus were regular in the urines. It was then that I decided to give *Proteus 50m*, three globules every two days.

On 17 April, the patient wrote to me that she was no more suffering at all and that this time Proteus disappeared from the urines.

Thus, again Proteus (of Nelson), highly diluted became vitorious.

In these two observations, let us note in passing, that it were the cases of two carbonics (therefore subject to spasms), of two Graphities, the one physiopathological, the other experimental, both constipated ; and one need not underline the part played by constipation in the production of these urinary manifestations because of Proteus.

PSORINUM OR PSORICUM

BIBLIOGRAPHY

Hering C. :

Quelques remarques au sujet de Psorin. Archiv für Homöopathische Heilkunst. V. XIII, Cahier 3, Leipzig, 1833, S 32 et S 163.

Stapf E. and Hering C. :

Psorin (Psorinum). Archiv für Homöopatische Heilkunst, V. XIII, Cashier 3, Leipzig, 1833.

Kent James Taylor :

Kents Arzneimittelbilder. Trad. du Dr. Edwards Heits. Karl Fl. Haug-Verlag, Ulm/Donau, 1958.

Tyler M.L. :

Psorinum. Traduction française par le Dr. Perichon—Bastaire—Annales hom. Fr. 14e année No. 9, 1972 et, p. 65-741, 15e année No. 1, janv. 1973.

Kent J.F. :

Psorinum Tr. par le Dr. Perichon-Bastaire-Annale hom. française, november 1972, 14e année, No. 11.

Hui Bon Hoa J. :

Psorinum. Annales homéop. fr. 1968, p. 46-894.

Lefort :

Psorinum. Aspect de l'Homoeopathie. Ed. Franise, Paris, 1963.

Boiron J. :

Matiére Médicalc de Psorinum. Rapport du Congrès de Tours de la F. N. des S.H. Fr. 1955. Ed. Pernet.

Michaud J. :

Psorinum. Cours C.H.F., Janvier 1971.

Granier M :

Homéolexique, t. 2, p. 524-525, 1874.

Andrade :

Observation sur 1 cas de Psorinum. L'Hom Moderne, 1930, No. 20, p. 645.

Clarke J. :

A Dictionary of Practical Materia Medica, London, 1955, v. 3, p. 891.

Sevaux :

Contribution a l'ètude des hautes dilutions homoeopathiques—Psorinum 7 CH. Observations. L'Hom. fr., 1961, No. 1, p. 27.

Belot :

Une observation de Psorinum. L'Homeop. fr., 1961, No. 1, p. 45.

Caulier :

Quelques observations de Psorinum. L'Homoeop fr., 1961, No. 4, p. 211.

Grisselich :

Le médecine homéopathique. Librairie J. B. Baillére et fils, 1891, Paris.

Julian O.A. :

Materia Medica der Nosoden. 2ę ed. K. Haug-Verlag, Heildelberg, 1975.

Biothèrapiques et Nosodes. Librairie Maloine, Paris 1962.

Illing :

Kongressbericht über die 123 Jaresversammlung par le Dr. Pischel. Allg. Hom. Zeitung Heft 4, 1972.

Hering C. :

The Guiding Symptoms of our Materia Medica, Phila., 1889, Gregg Press, 1967, v. 8, p. 538-566.

Allen T. F. :

The Encyclopedia of Pure Materia Medica. v. 8, p. 164-177, Ny., 1887. Réédité par, Gregg Press, 1964.

Allen H. C.:
The Materia Medica of the Nosodee. Boericks et Tafel., Phil., 1910, p. 344-409.

Attomyr :
Allg. Homoop. Zeitung. ö. 4., S. 14.

Gross-Lilienthal :
Archiv. f. Homöop. Heilkunst, B. 15, Heft 3, S. 117.

Hartmann :
Psoricum. Allg. Homöop Zeitung Bd. 1.

Tyler M. L. :
Homoeopathic Drug Pictures. The Hom. Pubg. Co. Ltd. 152, Landor Road, London SW 9, Ed. 1952, p. 671-678.

HISTORY

Psorin or Psoricum or Psorinum, as the facts proves is the second Biotherapic-Isopathy (after Lachesis) whose author was C. Hering, active and moving homoeopath, "author of that extravagant doctrine" Isopathy (Griesselich). In 1831 he communicated the idea that the serpent poison or rabic virus was a remedy again hydrophobia, the virus of the small-pox and that of the itch may be remedies against each of these diseases."

And Hering assures that he had the occasion to communicate this experience concerning the serpent poison and its medicinal effect from 18th June, 1830, which was published in the Archiv, lo Band, 2 Heft, S. 24, 1831.

In the year 1833 appeared in the Archiv für die Homöopatische Heilkunst, t. 13, cahier 2, 1833, p. 163-167 the pathogenesis of Psorin (Psoricum) with an introductory chapter of Stapf where the latter wrote : "The very important symptoms mentioned above are those of one of the most active and equally the most useful medicines of which the communication for the Archiv is due to M. le "Hofrath" Hahnemann. These symptoms are due to two persons for their observations and for their good name M. S.. r de L et M.O.R...de P. who experimented on themselves by taking repeated doses of Psorin 30 C in some granules noting down the symptoms faithfully and conscientiously.

Stapf indicates that it is, thanks to Hering and his communications as well as those of Attomyr, Gross...that we possess with Psorin a very efficacious remedy in many severe diseases.

Some remarks are to made :

1. Psorinum is no more a simple biotherapic ex-isotherapic leading towards etiotherapic ; it is a homoeopathic remedy having been the object of an experiment according to the methodology of the proving of Hahnemann.

2. It is Hahnemann and not Hering who wrote to Stapf for publishing the pathogenesis of Psorinum.

3. One can prove that it was Hahnemann who wrote the homoeopathic pathogenesis of Psorin to Stapf because this remedy was the object of homoeopathic proving. It is no more a nosode-isotherapic-biotherapic, but a homoeotherapic. However, he has published it neither in his Materia Medica Pura, nor in his Chronic Diseases.

4. We should also mention that the experimental technique regarding Psorin followed done by the two provers, *men*, is not described.

5. While writing the present pathogenesis, we have specially taken into consideration the original text and have incorporated the results of Kent's and Tyler's descriptions etc...

6. If one reads attentively the pathogenesis of Psorin in the original text one finds a series of symptoms developed in a woman. But it is nowhere mentioned that a woman took part in the proving of this medicine.

STOCK

As we have seen in our historic study, it was C. Hering, who in 1832, has stated as follows :

During the experiments on the serpent poison, I have given out the idea that the hydrophobic virus should be a powerful pathological agent. I presented the same hypothesis regarding the virus of variola. I expected no less as regards the psoric virus, and I invited my colleagues to make provings.

I waited for a long time to publish my own observations and that because of the regard I had for Hahnemann, of whom the opinion I wished to know and because I knew that his desire was that nothing should be published on this subject until it was well ripe. It was I who had to give it a name because it was I who first proposed, and prepared and applied the new remedy. I thought the most suitable name should be *Psorinum.*

He has also indicated the method of collection : "It should be taken from a robust and healthy individual having the viril age, whose family is known, and also the diseases that existed in the family. That one should select a family in which existed only the chronic benign diseases. In order to collect Psorin one should look for *an well developed itch,* having vesicles of the dimension of pin heads, of an yellowish colour and accompanied with itching specially in the evening. These vesicles multiply themselves at night".

"It is necessary that it should not be complicated with other diseases".

Hering indicates further on : "I had in Surinam numerous occasions to observe how great is the diversity of the cutaneous eruptions which we designate by the name of Psora".

In a study regarding the stock of Psorinum J. Boiron indicates : (Boiron J. : Mat. méd de Psorinum. Rapport du Conrés de Tovrs de la Fed. N. Des S.H. Fr., 1965) :—

"It is very difficult to affirm that the first "Psorines" were produced surely from the pustules of real itch. This affection was so much widespread at that time that it was probably at the basis of the great majority of "Itching psoras". But even if one admits that the patient who was the object for the collection was really "galeux". there still remains a certain indetermination about the collection itself".

In fact, and this is a very important fact, the collection was not done from the surface of a furrow, of which no mention has ever been made, but from a vesicle, where, consequently, is not found any sarcopte, even in a person suffering from real itch.

What is then the psorine which has served as the basis of the pathogenesis of Psorinum ?

It should be only a purulent serosity, *without specificity* originating from an eruption or from the scratching of the unhealthy infected skin.

Our present knowledge about itch gives us to think that it is nothing of the kind. Buiart, in his Traité de parasitologie tells us that the existence in the itch, caused by sarcoptes, of not only the furrows dug by the acarus (female) entering under the skin digging galleries where they lay egs, but also cause the eruptions of some vesicles and pustules, at a distance by the parasite.

According to Delafond and Bourguignon. *The Papulo Pruriginous Eruptions* are due to the saliva of the parasite. In order to prove this fact he reduced in bouillon about a hundred sarcoptes and inoculated them under the skins of man and dog. The inoculation was followed, on the point of inoculation and in other distant points, by an eruption with great itching at night, which persisted for 15 days to two months.

On their side, Mandoul and Brumpt note under the furrows of itch the existence of samll vesicles like the heads of pins called "Pearly vesicles of Bazin", which are due to a flow of lymph caused by the venomous saliva of the parasite".

Therefore there exists a *poison*, a toxin secreted by the sarcopte and consequently the itch appears to us only as a local reaction because of the presence of sarcopte, accompanied by the lesions caused by scratching, but also a more general eruption caused by that toxin. Consequently, the presence of vesicles may be related to the sarcoptic affection and the content of the vesicles and pustules should be, well, a product which is specific, of the real itch.

. This fact upsets the barrier which separated the humoral theory of psora from its "Sarcoptic" theory. The sarcoptes may cause a general intoxination and may cause a *humoral modification* of the whole organism.

The itch infection will give rise to Psora.

STOCK

At present the Biotherapic Psorinum is prepared starting from the lysated stock obtained without addition of antiseptics, from the serosity of the furrows of itch taken from a patient, not yet treated.

COLLECTION OF THE SEROSITIES

The collections are done under the conditions required by the paragraph 1 of the letter of 26th January, 1956 (ref. Ph 3 B/S et V/J 166) established by the Service Central de la Pharmacie (3e Bureau—Serums and Vaccins).

TECHNIQUE OF PREPARATION

1. Reception of the Collections

Thsee collections are kept in sealed capillary tubes. They are the object of different controls.

(*a*) **Cytological examination** : The examination between lame and lamellas shows sufficient number of weakened polynuclears, some numerous cells. some rare hematies and a great number of mobile or immobile germs. No sarcopts.

(*b*) **Examination after colouring according to the method of Gram** : Shows a very polymorphous microbian flora, however, with the predominence of Gram positive germs. Presence of polynuclears and cells completely lysated.

2. Initial Dilution of Serosities

The serosities are diluted in 100 times of their volume, of distilled water.

3. Lysate of the Cells and of Microbian Elements

The initial dilution 1/100 is congealed at 20° and decongealed at the ordinary temperature four times.

4. Sterilisation and Distribution of the Initial Dilution

The lysate obtained before is sterilised by filtration on *EKS* filters, then distributed in fractions of 10 ml in sterile philas.

5. Stockage of the Initial Dilution

The fractions of 10 cm³ of the initial dilution are lyophilised so as to be suitable for conservation without weakening. Each phial contains a quantity of lyophilised product corresponding to 0, 1 mililitre of serosity. That lysate is characterised by its technique of preparation and by the control tests.

6. Dilution

The content of each phial is taken in 100 ml of sterile distilled water so as to bring to a concentration of the final product to 0,001 mililitre of treponemic serosity.

7. Filtration and Distribution of the Final Dilution

The final dilution is filtered on *EKS* filter then distributed aseptically in ampoules of 1 ml.

Afterwards they undergo the following control ;

(*a*) *Sterility* : Inoculation on bouillon or on gelose should not be followed by any culture.

(*b*) *Non-toxicity* : By sub-cutaneous injection of 1 ml to some 20g rats will not cause any reaction. The rabbit should sustain without any bad effect the injection of 5 ml of the product.

EXPERIMENTAL CORTICO-VISCERAL PHARMACODYNAMIC PROTOCOL OR PATHOGENESIS

1. Generalities

Typology : A certain type with prominent outlines, male or female characterises Psorinum. It may not be specific for "Psora" a role attributed by Hahnemann to *Sulphur*.

But this Nosode-Biotherapic (with reserves that we have exposed in the history) may be characterised as *cold Sulphur*, and we may stay with Kent :

"If anyone has the repulsive look and smells bad, he has the need for Psorinum".

He is a person having a very prominent mask of cortico-visceral reactional inhibition, an abnormal sensibility to cold, a marked inhibition of his physiological functions, and having a foetid, repulsive cutaneous elimination.

Hypotonic, sad, desperate, *lean or emaciated*, worn out skin, having *dirty look*. He is afraid of air current and water. He is a gentleman who does not dare to take up his hat. He is the Candida of Voltaire who has become cold, pessimist, desperate. Lefort has found a small poem of Maurice Donnay which gives the portrait of Psorinum :

"He was ugly and lean,
Having sucked milk thin,
Of a pessimist wet nurse.
And one was a nurse sad.
When he died of an eczema
He wished to be creamed.
And on his grave a symbolist
Wrote the words "he was sad.""

Everything irritates him, he becomes *quarrelsome, startles at the least noise*, prefers solitude, and is afraid of the future, because he is afraid in advance that everything that he undertakes, must be a failure.

This anxiousness, this cold interior, gives him the impression of external coldness and even in a hot weather, he is *chilly*, covered with several underwears of wool, shivering by the least wind.

Bizzare and fixed ideas, he has loss of memory, takes time to recognize a spot where he finds himself. Loss of power for work, great weakness, desperate of his disease which he thinks will never be cured. General weakness, chilliness, itching, *bad smell of his body, fetidness of eruptions*, profuse sweats, dry, dirty, rough skin, loss of reaction, and morbid metastasis characterise Psorinum type.

For H. C. Allen Psorinum should be prescribed according to the totality of symptoms and not as a specific for psoric diathesis.

Psorinum according to Clarke is not a remedy reserved for adults. It can equally be prescribed to children. It is the "whinning baby", having no sleep, very dirty

We may summarise the Psorinum type in the following triad :

(*a*) Coritico-visceral inhibition which leads to a state of netabolic energy.

(*b*) Periodicity and alternation of morbid purturbations.

(*c*) Neuro-metabolic regulation by autodrainage or rather by cleansing through the skin.

2. Neuro-endocrino-psychic System

(*a*) *Psychic* :

Sad, quarrelsome, pessimist subject. Anxious, desperate of everything and for nothing. Unreasonable fright, fear of everything, feels himself inferior physically and socially and even in his affections.

Misanthrope with a clear *inferiority complex* (Sulphur— Superiority complex) : *Failing memory*. Cannot remember what he has just said.

Nominal, temporary aphasia : Defect of comprehension and of using words.

Very much forgetful.

Early senescence : Appearance of an old man, neglected, hobbling about to break down.

If the patient is a young adult, he has the look of a present day "Hippy" badly adapted to the society.

Religious melancholy.

(a) Dreams of business, of thieves, of voyages, of dangers :

Restless sleep, non-reposing. Somnolence during the day, and takes long time to fall asleep.

Gay, well disposed, has pleasure and satisfaction for work, then *morose*, full of cares, and sad.

Sad with the ideas of suicide and expansiveness.

Restless, explosive, always thinks that he will die, then suddenly very gay, sad immediately afterwards, many times during the day.

In hopeless, thinks of failure ; these ideas follow him, begun at night out of a dream.

In children, fear at night, with cries and the need of a light for sleeping.

(b) Nervous :

Migraines of frontal and occipital type often concomitant with hunger pains better by eating.

Should wake up at night for eating.

Indicative symptom ; feels himself clearly better the day before the attack of migraine.

Periodical migraines ; aggravated by the least air current and ameliorated by hotly covering his head, and by eating.

Migraine comes soon after the suppression of an eruption, or menstruation.

Migraine better by an epistaxis.

Frontal pain with the sensation that the skull has not enough place to contain the brain, soon after waking up ; after ablution and breakfast, feels himself better.

Very heavy and boring sensation in the left temple.

Sensation as if the whole head on fire.

Violent pain in the head as if beaten by a stick.

Pain in the temples after an intellectual effort.

Vertigo : Everything turns around him.

Sensation of numbness of the half of the left forehead.

Pain in the occipital region, as if constricted.

Sensation of as if bound by a rope specially behind the head, with the sensation of being compressed.

Tremblings of hands and feet.

Tenacious neuralgia.

Enuresis in full moon.

(c) Endocrines :

Typhoid : Great chilliness ; the necessity of covering himself hotly in all seasons. Sensitiveness to the open air.

Dysthyroidia regarding the skin : dirty, greasy, lusterless, rough hands, may be caused by scratching, fissures.

Seborrhoea of the integument.

Thin hairs.

Anxiety with premonitions, restless and tremblings of the hands.

3. Digestive Apparatus

(a) Mouth, tongue, pharynx :

Dry lips, *swelling of the upper lips.* Lips, burning and swelling of ganglions under the chin.

Teeth are yellow, and shaking with red, bleeding gums with bad smelling pus.

Tootache and the tip of tongue is burning.

Foetid, repulsive breath.

Fad, sweetish taste.

Acid eructations, having the taste and smell of rotten eggs.

Voracious appetite : Wakes up at night to eat ; sensation of great hunger the day before the attack of a headache.

Dislikes viande of pork and desires for beer.

Painful pricking in the splenic and hepatic region.

Disheartening taste in the mouth aggravated after eating, and smoking.

Taste of oil in the mouth during the whole afternoon.

Bad taste in the mouth, forcing him to drink for being relieved of the bad taste.

Sticky saliva, having a nauseating taste ; feels as if the teeth are stuck together.

Dryness of the mouth and of the lips.

The right half of the upper lip seems swollen.

Morning nausea : Fetid eructations, vomitings at first of the foods then sticky liquid, acid.

At table, sudden heat all over the body with heavy sweats of the face, thirst, dryness and burning in the mouth : headache.

(b) *Stomach, intestine, abdomen* :

Yawning at noon and in the evening.

Distension of the abdomen, passing of flatus having the smell of rotten eggs.

Constipation because of rectal atony, forcing the patient to make some efforts to pass stools which are normal.

Diarrhoea with urgency ; putrid stools like that of routten eggs, of dark colour, comes out in a gush.

Involuntary stools occasionally at night.

Hematemesis ; rectorrhagia.

Diarrhoea, vomiting, dehydration in children of the first age ; stools with the smell of rotten eggs as well as of the acquous eructations, which are brown, gushing out, bloody ; general weakness.

Abdominal colic from the morning, when in bed ; sensation of fatigue and pressure in the epigastrium better by passing stools.

4. Cardio-hemo-vascular System

Hyposthenia of the myocardia ; pricking pains in the region of the heart ; palpitations.

Hypotension :

Worn out patient, dyspnoea after a short walk ; aggravated by open air and difficulty of respiration when standing.

Need for lying stretched, at rest, which ameliorated ; aggravated while in a sitting position or while standing. Face pale, yellow, waxy or cyanosed, sounds of the heart weak, dull, vitrious look, pulse, rapid, irregular.

If he wants anything for life, he has the impression that his heart is going to be torn.

Thermoregulation : Intermittent fever, after catching cold with sticky and peachy sweats, bad smelling ; intense heat, humid.

5. Respiratory Apparatus

(*a*) *Throat* :

Pain in the throat, difficult to swallow and sensation of swelling in the interior.

Painful vesicle on the tip of the uvula.

Tickling in the throat causing cough.

Dull pricking sensation in the left tonsil.

Bilateral adenopathy of the neck, painful, radiating towards the head.

Aggravation by taking hot drinks ; better by drinking cold water.

Nasal voice.

Repeated anginas.

Big tonsils, painful, and radiation of the pain towards the ears.

Sticky mucus coming from the back of the throat and expectoration with the taste of rotten eggs.

(*b*) *Lungs, pleurae :*

Pricking pressure on the left false ribs.

Cough with greenish yellow expectoration.

Dry cough with pains as if from a wound behind the sternum.

Cough with the sensation of weakness in the chest.

Expectoration of mucus and acid secretions after prolonged cough.

Dry cough with nausea and tickling in the throat the whole day.

Difficult respiration specially in the evening.

While respirating, a pricking pain from the back to the chest.

After a deep respiration, pricking on the right side of the chest with the sensation of oppression and weakness.

Respiration, short in the open air, better when lying down or during a travel.

Oppression in the chest with intense dorsal pain.

The loss of breath is the worst with pain in the chest, when in a sitting position because of which he could not write for six weeks. Better in lying position.

Loss of breath even when walking in the open air, which forces him to return home and to lie down. There is no trouble when doing light manual labours.

Sensation of constriction in the chest.

Terrible pain in the chest, as if a weight of 100 kgs. is crushing him. Loss of respiration while trying to bend forward which is intolerable.

Pain in the chest as if the lungs are going to be torn out.

Alternating asthma and eczema without complete disappearance of the one or of the other.

6. Sense Organs

(a) *Nose* :

Sneezing without cold, with perforating pain in the right nostril.

Chronic congestion of the nasal mucous.

Nose stuffed, discharge of bad smelling retro-nasal liquid. Loss of smell.

Strong cold, for several hours, relapsing.

Hypertrophy of the nasal mucous with permanent dropping from the nose.

(b) *Eyes* :

Dazzling when walking in the street.

Pressure in the right eye, worse while lying.

Ocular fatigue towards the end of the day, likes one hour's prolonged reading in the light.

Around the eyes, deep, wide, bluish circles.

Sensation of sand in the eyes.

Bloody secretion from the conjunctives.

Eyelids stick in the morning, redness of the borders of the lids which stick together.

Cannot bear strong light ; photophobia.

Border of the eyelids are red, as if styes are going to be formed, as if something is moving before the eyes.

Darting in the right eye.

Pruritus of the right eyelid.

If the look is fixed for a long time, lachrymation.

In the corner of the eyelids formation of vesicles resembling styes.

Impression that the objects seen in a room are trembling.

Relapsing pterygium.

(c) *Ears* :

Pains and ringings in the ears.

Lightning like sensation in the ears when he swallows the salvia.

Pricking pains of the auditive conduits ; momentarily better by scratching the ear, then aggravated ; frequently repeated pain, when at rest specially in the evening.

Alternating ringing of the right and the left ears with buzzing in the ear, causing lowering down of the power of hearing.

Pain in the ears as if from a wound, painful, with the sensation of heat, radiating towards the skull, worse in evening, as if someone is drawing the hairs.

Pruritus and pains (pricking) of both the ears.

Inflammation of the pavillion of the ear with discharge of the auditory conduits of a bad smelling pus.

Pain as if from an abscess in the left ear and at the same time a button like eruption on the pavillion of the right ear which breaks into four parts.

Chronic otorrhoea with the discharge of pus, yellow brownish fetid for years specially in children.

7. Uro-genital Apparatus

(a) *Urinary* :

Dysuria, painful with post-micturition terminal drops.

Involuntary loss of some drops of urine after micturition.

Pricking pains in the urethra.

Burning of the urethral orifice at the beginning of micturition.

Enuresis, aggravated during the full moon.

(*b*) *Genital* :

Masculine : Purulent, painful vesicle on the scrotum. Loss of spermatic liquid before micturition.

Marked repulsion of all sexual contact.

Total impotency. (In a robust man it durated for four weeks).

The genital organs are soft and lax.

Feminine : Menstruation late by eight days, less abundant.

Frigidity with apathy, depression, sensitive breasts, nipples are red, irritated, pruiginous and *hypermenorrhoea.*

8. Loco-motor System

Drawing pain of the neck, radiating towards the shoulders, while waking up in the morning.

Pain of the neck, intense, only in a room, disappears in the open air, and begins again when he enters into the room.

Constant drawing in and between the shoulder blades, irradiating to the ribs like a rheumatic pain.

Dorsal pain, as if the third vertebra is crushed.

Pain of the back as if beaten.

Pain of the lumbar region radiating towards the knee.

Weakness of the kidneys with the sensation of heaviness and weight.

While waking, pains in the bones of the tibias.

In the evening, during rest, cramping pain in the left scapulohumeral region.

Rigidness of the bones of the hands and while waking up rigidness of the hips.

Tearing pains of the left knee and left shoulder.

Pain in one leg which cannot support the weight of the other, should constantly change position in the bed.

Gouty pain of the whole left foot.

Tendency of the left foot to turn inward while walking.

Drawing pain of the left elbow.

Itching of the left arm, left elbow, right biceps and carpa of the right hand.

Weakness of all the articulations as if they are going to crumble down.

The pains are aggravated during rest as well as the itchings.

Hurts easily the heels.

9. Skin, Phanera

Dirty skin, oozing oily giving out an unhealthy smell, some times nauseating, of rotten flesh, and filling the room for a long time.

Face pale, seborrhic, dry hairs, sticking together, difficult to dress and comb.

General pruritus, need for scratching until the skin becomes red and dermic lesions are formed, with crusts.

Pruritus aggravated by the heat of the bed.

Multiform eruptions on the skin : Vesicles, papules, pustules, being infected by scratching, oozing, bad smelling, pruriginous and of chronic appearance.

Seasonal eruptions specially in the winter season :

Specially behind the ears, in the auditory conduit ; around nails of hands and feet, in folds of the joints.

Striated and breaking nails.

Eczema of the integument : With brittle hairs, aggravated at night, by hot humid compress, ameliorated in open air.

Formation of subcutaneous nodules on the face, on the neck, and on the legs, persisting for a long time.

Ulcerations on legs, in joints, of herpetic type and prurigi-nous.

Sweats of the palms and of the face.

Cannot bear sun.

10. Modalities

Aggravation :

By cold ; in open air ; by walking ; by washing ; by pressure ; by coffee ; the suppression of a discharge or an eruption.

Amelioration :

In the morning, while waking up.   By the heat.

By lying with lowering the head.

By eating ; by bleeding from the nose.

By drainage through respiratory system or through skin : expectoration, sweats, eruption.

Laterality :

Right, but not characteristic.

POSOLOGY

Dynamisation :

Specially the 30 CH which, according to us seems to be the most active.   Although the pathogenesis of Psorin has excited the imagination of homoeopaths, the fact is that Psorin has a very feeble pharmacodynamic reaction.   It acts slowly, whence there is necessity for prolonged use.

POSITIVE DIAGNOSIS

1.   Subject, sad, apathetic, with a clear inferiority complex.

2.   Anergy, cortico-visceral, loss of memory, intensely chilly, canine hunger, great weakness.

Perpetually old, the skin has a dirty look, yellowish, which emits a smell painful to the entourage, sweats and eruptions, fetid, generalised itching.

4. Clear general amelioration the day before a toxinic crisis (migraine, asthma, eczema...). Worse by cold except the itching which is aggravated by heat.

5. Alternation of morbidity and endocrenal hypo-function (thyroid, testicles, ovaries).

DIFFERENTIAL DIAGNOSIS

For classical Homoeopathy, the following medicines are to be differentiated : *Sulphur, Thuya, Tuberculinum* (when Psorin does not act prescribe *Tuberculinum*—Kent), *Hepar sulphur, Silicea, Petroleum, Graphitis, Arsenicum, Lycopodium, Causticum.*

For modern homoeotherapy the following medicines may be indicated :

Cortisone

Unstable mind, alternating euphoria and melancholy ; from excitation to depression ; dryness of the mucous of the rhino-phorynx with cough, dry eyes, the eyelids stick together ; dorsal and sacro-illiac pain as if the back is going to break down ; discoloured skin, vesiculous eruptions, dryness and fissures of the skin, of the face, of hands with disquamation on the roots of the nails ; sexual asthenia.

Histaminum hydrochloricum

Disthyrodian subjects, irritable, with vertigo and sensation of heat, burning in the head, of the face, looseness of the teeth, pruritis and burning gastric pains, burning in the anus, of vagina, of nose, throat, ears of the precordial and thoracic regions ; red pruriginous papules.

Penicillinum

Asthenia, frilosity, subfebril state ; intellectual obnubilation. Headache, right orbitary neuralgia, teeth painful,- precordialgia, repeated rhino-pharyngitis, exudative dermatitis, asthmatiform dyspnoea with dry cough.

Proteus

Tense, irritable, depressed, frontal headache, vertigo ; sensitive gums, painful hunger, easily vomits. diarrhoea, aversion to pork, sensation of weight on the chest, specially on the precordial region, cough, expectoration of mucous, burning pains of the eyes, in the ears, while urinating. Eruption, papulopustulous, herpetic, falling of hairs.

Sarothamnus Scoparius

Sensorio motor asthenia, sensation of coldness except on the head, *precordialgia*, sensation of boiling in the head ; constant hunger inspite of nausea, takes long time to fall asleep ; eczematous eruptions, and loss of hairs by bunches.

Tellurium

Amnesia ; frontal headache, cutano-mucous dryness, burning vesiculous eruptions, itching, sweats of feet, very bad smelling ; foetid suppuration of the ear ; cervico-dorsal and right lumbosciatic neuralgia.

CLINICAL DIAGNOSIS

1. **Generalities**

   Allergosic state, Tuberculinosic, Cancerosic.
   Allergic conditions.
   Hyporesistivity to infections.
   Early senescence.
   Meteoropathy.
   Hyposthenic energy.
   Morbid metastasis.
   Demineralised children.

2. **Neuro-endocrino psychic System**

   Depressive condition ; melancholia.
   Anxiety, neurosis with hypothyroidism.
   Migraines. Neuralgias.
   Enuresis of children and of olds.
   Barré and Lieou syndrome.

3. Digestive Apparatus

Alveolo-dental pyorrhoea (Fauchard's disease).
Agueusia.
Dysthermia, cortico-gastric.
Digestive migraine.
Athrepsia ; cholera infantile.
Muco-membranous enterocolitis.

4. Cardio-hemo-vascular System

Rheumatic myocardia.
Card othyreosis.
Hypotension.

5. Respiratory Apparatus

Asthma. Emphysema.
Bronchiectasis.
Winter bronchitis.

6. Sense Organs

Spasmodic rhinitis.
Purulent rhinitis.
Adenoid vegetations.
Blepharitis— Conjunctivitis—Eczema of the eyelids.
Chalazions—photophobia.
Chronic suppurated otitis.

7. Uro-genital Apparatus

Urinary : Cystitis.   Urethritis.
Enuresis of children and of olds.
Genital—masculine :
Impotency.
Prostatitis ; prostatic adenoma.
Genital—feminine :
Frigidity.
Hypomenorrhoea and spaniomenorrhoea.
Metritis.

8. Loco-motor System

Rheumatisms : Cervicalgias ; dorsalgias ; lumboarthrosis ; coxarthrosis.

Repeated dislocation of the elbows and ankles.

9. Skin, Phanera

Polymorphous erythema.

Prurigo and prurigo scrophulous.

Calvitias (baldness, diffused). Ringworm.

Hyperhydrosis of the palms.

Herpes. Impetigo.

Versicolor pityriasis.

Marginal eczema of hebra.

Pre-mycosic erythema.

Chronic eczema of integument.

CLINIC OF PSORINUM

The somewhat dry but interesting reading of this Biotherapic, becomes an attractive description and a remarkable living portrait with the study that E.F. Lefort presents in his book 'Aspects de l'Homoeopathie (Ed. Farnese, Paris, 1963, 135—151).

Here are some long extracts :

"This parent sad and miserable of Sulphur" who is Psorinum has a very less attractive look.

"His attitude, his gait, express his weakness; it is difficult for him to be in a verticle position and he walks vaulted, as if carrying with difficulty the weight of his diseases.

"Without energy ; he sweats because of his weakness and he is eternally cold, because since sometimes he has lost all his bodily heat.

"He fights unceasingly against himself, in order that the chilliness does not take upper hand and he protects himself by multiple dresses so as not to lose the least of the heat that the miserly nature has dispensed for him.

"We know well this patient. He has two waist coats, two shirts, two sweaters, a flanel band, a skin of cat on his back, a breast plate on his chest. It becomes hopeless to tell him to take off all the dresses in our chamber and to tell him to put them again on. When there is burning heat in the month of August he may be persuaded to take off two or three waist coats, but he says that he cannot do without them.

"How much we will prefer *Silicea*, which is also chilly but sparely dressed, affirming that does not serve anything, because hotly covered or not he will always have cold.

"The unfortunate *Psorinum* will keep a voluminous grade-robe. The most timid tentative to escape from it, will result in a new ennui. The least that may arrive to him in this case is a coryza, a dry coryza but violent, for which he immediately adds a foulard or an extra knitted vest.

"He never takes the risk of cutting his hairs. If he has a haircut he will have immediately a cold.

"This mass of dress, that muffled up look, when seen from a distance does not give us the idea that he is a person who is sure of himself, who is sure of his health.

"When seen from near, our idea becomes confirmed.

"To the suffering, timid, recoiled, trembling, and emaciated look is added a less attractive face. The pale colour, shining, dirty face with greasy skin of the forehead, small ridges, acne, fissures at the joints of the lips, dry lips, deep red, the upper lip swollen, thin hairs which are dry, blepharitis for which he can hardly open his eyes. These are all for his face.

"The rest is not better. The hands are restless because of slight tremblings, are covered with small warts. They are never clean, and they are not in fact so because Psorinum never washes them. Basically he is not so dirty but his phobia of coldness is such that he is afraid of water and of soap and use only parcimoniously.

"His whole skin is marked by this dirtiness, which is sometimes covered with dust, sometimes greasy, with squamous eruptions or oozing eruptions in the folds of the flexions, with intolerable itching.

"It is here we touch some more miserable points about *Psorinum*.

"Shivering throughout the day, one may think that he will find his well-being in the heat of the bed, which is refused to him during the day. He is always weary and if it happens for example, that he has taken a walk in the open air, he returns home, completely extenuated and desires to lie down. But no.

"Because immediately he is under covers and begins to be heated, his itching starts, and the unfortunate passes white nights scratching the skin and he is taken possession ridiculously and enervatingly, by the alternative of making him hot in order to be exasperated by the itching or to uncover himself in order to escape from itching and to catch cold which will cause to appear his asthmatic fits.

"One thing however will make him to rise up, oh ! with what a precaution, the hunger which makes the wolf to get out of the wood. Because he has the desire for eating at night, like *Anacardium*, he feels better by eating. The more foreseeing relations of Psorinum, will keep a box full of eatables (not pork by any means) in his bedroom so that he may get up and eat and lie down again and perhaps will find rest.

"Those among them who will be able to do so, will not taste from the hands of Morpheus, forgetfulness, calm and rest.

"They sleep in a curious fashion, sometimes the head pushed into the pillow (no doubt for getting more heat), sometimes on the back with stretched limbs because he cannot bear the touch, not even of the bed cover inspite of cold.

"The dreams of Psorinum, because, to be sure he dreams, are full of anxieties as those during his sleeplessness. They are

17 F

full of dangers, of thieves, and very often he finds himself closed in a certain place, like the heroes of *"Huis Clos"* of Sartre.

"He wakes up in sweats, fasigued by the horrors of his dreams, suffering from a headache, as if beaten by hammer, and thus many times during the night.

"During the day he feels his fatigue of the night. He wishes always to sleep. He is already less solid in his legs, so much so that they give way suddenly and for nothing, which causes some torsions. He looks for the occasions for sitting down and then he breaks down which he should not.

"If Psorinum has a child, because alas he may have one, the latter (quite the opposite of that of *Lycopodium*, because it cries during the day but does not disturb its parents at night) is quiet during the day but begins to howl from the evening throughout the night up to the morning. This adds more to the insomnia of its father.

"Here is then the aspect of Psorinum. An unfortunate being who walks, worn out, fatigued, vaulted, with the diseased look not good to look at, and little appetising to approach. Because to be complete, he gives out a bad smell. His eruptions, his scratches, increases that fetid odour which is known as the smell of a carion. He has, the unfortunate man, let us say for his defence, all the reasons to exhale around him that mustiness which are less desirable. He is covered with eruptions, he sweats constantly, all these are macerated in his linens that he never takes off and he never washes himself.

"One thinks irresistibly about Psorinum when one sees the portrait of the descendants of Charles Quint. Philippe II (who died with the whole body covered with crusts and wounds), pale, prognate, with the expression of dark mysticism, so faithfully carved by Titien and by his favourite painter Marc Antoine. Philippe III still more pale who came down from Phillippe II, and followed by Phillippe IV are portraited by

Valzsquez, as pale, adenoidians, globulous eyes, pale face, without expression, broken down by the weight of his heredity which went on aggravating from father to son as one can see in the museum of Prado, the hallucinating image of a race and of a dynasty, which gives one to think of the lasts of Valois, going side by side with the decadence of their country.

"The other example is more noble and brings to the most seducive summits. It is the question of one of the most delicate writers, the most productive, and the most complete of the century of a novelist whose reputation only went on growing. He is Marcel Proust.

"It requires a long study about his case, and one may speak about it for hours, and can write about it pages after pages without being able to draw any conclusion.

"As regards this man who was throughout his life ill, others will ask what influence had his pathological conditions on his works. We cannot occupy ourselves here with this fact.

"Only know that Marcel Proust, after having been a normal child, had suddenly at the age of seven, an attack of asthma and from that day, he was, till he died at the age of 50 years, an unfortunate being, subject to miseries which did not give him the least possible breathing time.

"He was extremely sensitive to cold. Finally it became legendary. He is described as a youngman and going out in full dress, so much stuffed with padding under his breast that some tampoons came out of his false collar. He never took off his pelisse, even in summer, and I do not know who, meeting them in a dinner described Mme de Nailles and him as "similar to two laplanders, swollen with furs". What teaches, let us say, is that the dear countess whom we believe to be a *Lachesis*, because of her loquacity, was really a *Psorina*.

"Those who have mixed with them, have always noted the atmosphere of their room where nothing was ever opened, and this claustration was made thicker by the smell of medicines :

"The room was full of yellow volutes of fumigations impregnated by their acrid smell. Through this cloud one could see Mar el, pale, slightly swollen, his eyes shining in the mist, dressed in a night gown, and in several vests superposed.

"That swelling of traits which are not like those we have described about Psorinum whose lips are swollen, is explained by the cardio-renal insufficiency which accompany asthma and if he seemed on the other hand slightly big, it was because he was fully covered, within which was his lean body.

"A being sufficiently big, almost fat, the shoulders high, noted Boylesve, cramped under a overcoat. He keeps on his overcoat because he is a patient who is afraid of bad temperature. But his face is extraordinary, with the skin like that of a plucked pheasant, almost blue, with large eyes like an Egyptian dancing girl, hollow, supported by two thick amber lines which are becoming larger, abundant hairs, straight, black, not well cut or not cut since two months ; a neglected mustaches, black ; his false collar is worn out which, without exaggeration, has not been changed since eight days. I looked for his hands, but they are imprisoned in white gloves remarkably dirty, but on the contrary I noted a fine wrist, white and fat. The figure seemed to have been moulded, then made thicker incompletely and haphazardly......"

"One also finds in him the fear of taking cold and of coryza which are going to follow each other and Proust, was always afraid of cutting his hairs like that of Psorinum.

"His insomnia is well known which forces him to take 1·50 g. of *Vernol* every day.

"Edmond Jaloux also noticed his tuffed hairs, black, always very long which formed around his face a thick cover. "There was even in his physique" he writes, "in the atmosphere which was floating around him something so singular that one experiences a sort of stupor at his sight. He did not participate with the current humanity, he seemed to come out always from a dream, and also as if from another period, perhaps of an other world, but which ?"

"And now we are going to study his psychology. At a first consideration he seems quite different from that of *Psorinum*.

"Psorinum is sad. Proust is also sad. He is sad because of his health, of the asthma which is in the way of all his activities and he is tormented in his life. If he had not the disease, he could have been a man of humour, his books are not lacking in them and when he is in his good days, he becomes gay in society and witty.

"Psorinum desires to be alone, avoids society, does not like to be consoled. But Proust mixed with people assiduously, he is pleased in salons, looked for friends and when he is sad he wished to be surrounded with his friends and to be consoled. He had for his fellow-men delicate attentions, and spoke with them with affectionate words, even he addressed them with tender epithets. He is nearer to *Pulsatilla* than to *Psorinum*. At least we believe so.

"Because after deep examination of his behaviour in his existence we see him gradually detatched from his Pulsatillian attachments.

"It is there that one should note that there is the necessity for a homoeopath to be a psychologist, and a very subtle psychologist. We should be never hasty to make a judgement, we should not be content with a nearabout, and we should not believe in appearances only. Sometimes in fact, a single word, gives us light about the mentality of an individual, but also sometimes it helps us to make a false judgment. We must go beyond things

"Examining him more closely, we must never forget that Marcel Proust is before all a man of letters.

"A man of letters in the most complete sense of the word. His whole life is going to be guided, transformed, fashioned by this fact. He has dreamt from his very infancy to write big books, it is his aim, the only aim which has absorbed him entirely.

"We should therefore consider stating from the above fact that he cannot be judged in a common way.

"His sensitivity is at first acute because of his disease, by his physical weakness it has become more sharp.

"Having on the one hand decided to write a big book and on the other hand knowing that his days are counted, he was afraid that he will not be able to manage to do it well. He is anxious in a permanent way, restless, anxious, as a Psorinum is uncertain and is tormented like him.

"The very little credit, that was given to his first writing *Les Plaisirs et le Jours*, the successive refusals of the publishers for his first novel "Du cöté de chez Swan" published on his account by Grasset, were at that time sufficient food for his hopelessness.

He amassed the materials.

Having said this, it appears clearly that his taste for the world, his assiduity in the soirées, his readiness to mix in the society and meet famous men were in reality in the basis of the preparation of his great work to which he projected himself. Every visit transformed into a sitting for work. He questioned passionately, noted with precision André Maurois, with incredulity, bringing back his interlocutor who wanted to avoid him, and each specialist was consulted. Reynaldo Hahn on music, Jean-Louis Vaudoyer on painting, the Daudet family on flowers ...to women he asked to enlighten him about them...

He amassed the materials.

This lasted for years. Two years in course of which he was taking and heaping up numerous notes which are going to serve him to paint the picture of a world, of the whole of a period, a period which was menaced to be lost and thanks to him it was rediscovered.

"Then he put himself to work, and then only really he was alone, alone in the solitude of a writer who began to grow dark, corrects pages after pages, completes them, polishes indefatigably his style, alone in the solitude of the artist.

"He entered in literature, says Maurois like other entering into religion.

"He escaped from it only to glean a documentation which must be very clear to him, which must be as minute as possible, leaving nothing to chance, leaving nothing to imprecision. He did so in a very unexpected way, generally during night, when he did not sleep and also the exigency of an ill person. He must have the information immediately. He used to send a messenger at night at the house of his friend, himself being very much suffering or very much occupied, when it is difficult for him to go personally. Thus one night someone rang at the house of a friend...it was his *valet de chambre* who asked in a most natural voice : "Monsieur sends me to ask Monsieur and Madame what happened to the heart of Shelley".

"That retired life was followed and completed by his imperious need of silence. He had such horror of noise that he matted his room with cork, and if he ever went on a journey (he hardly displaced himself), he used to reserve rooms in a hotel : one which he occupied, and the two other on each side of his living room would remain empty, in order to isolate himself. He moreover asked the hotel keeper that no one should walk above his head, because he could not have rented the whole house.

"The single trait may be interpreted as a need for solitude. The silence is by no means the companion which is obligatory and necessary for a retreated existence.

"One cannot, while speaking of Proust, avoid to enter into his tendency towards his abnormal sexual behaviour. There

again, one finds at the first examination, that his sexual behaviour is different from that of Psorinum. The latter, we know,
is first of all indifferent as regards love and secondly he becomes
soon impotent. But he is not sexually inverted. The discretion
of Marcel Proust in this regard obliges to look for the obscure
motives of that anomaly. If he has spoken in his books about
the inverted persons, he has spoken it tactfully and with care
in order to enter upon this subject as far as it concerned him.
He was not like Guide who displayed himself so much in his
works and whom he advised, "You may write anything, but
never write I".

"Then we may suppose that his little attraction for the
sexual act, turned him away from women, then in a second
time, because he is not impotent, he tried to find out something
in his own sex.

"There is again an other trait which at the first sight presented him as different from Psorinum, but a deep study helps us
to bring him near Psorinum. We have not pretended in this
sketch which is forcibly evasive and very limited that Proust
was a Psorinum totally, but we have found some symptoms so
that this famous example helps us to retain the picture of Psorinum in our memory". (E.F. Lafort)

The reading of this romantic description will help us to
retain better the picture of Psorinum in our mind.

CLINICAL OBSERVATIONS

Finally, we think that some clinical cases will make concrete
the prescription of Psorinum.

Here are at first two case reports of J. Michaud which he
related in his lecture of the 8th January, 1971 in C.H.F.

Case 1

M.B....aged 45 years, consults for an asthenia lasting
since two years. This is the only symptom told by the patient.
At the first sight, it is the question of habitual asthenia by
overalimentation of the patient, who took 4 meals a day,

14 tarts of bread with butter, without counting pork, beer and coffee. The tandem *Nux vomica Antimonium crudum* would be evidently the prescription, if after questioning the patient we would not have discovered :

1. A cough with continual expectoration in the morning, since years.

2. Attacks of pleurisy during adolescence.

3. Some numerous eliminatory reactions on different dates : darts and impetigo in the infancy, furuncles twice, nephritic colic very recently.

The prescription of Psorinum because of the antecedants is confirmed by some informations got from the patient, who said that he is extremely chilly and that she is forced to rise up at night to eat.

Case 2

Mme L., 51 years, is asthmatic since the age of 15, and takes cortisone without interruption ; his attacks are almost suppressed but is replaced by a dysponea almost permanent. She is a patient of bad moral, sad, discouraged, anxious, subject to frequent diseases of the liver. Her menopause took place at the age of 49 without any other history. One would think of *Nux vomica, Sepia,* but a more minute interrogation revealed that there were several eliminatory reactions through the skin in the form of furuncle and zona and that the patient had itch. This last fact decided me upon the prescription of Psorinum which became successful where some remedies like *Poumonhistamine* and *Kali carb.* proved insufficient.

Case 3

Dr. Illing (Kassel, Germany) reported, during the 123rd Congress of the D.Z.H.A. of 19-22 May, 1971 and of which the summary appeared in Allg. Homöop. Zeitung ; Heft 4, 1972, p. 171. Here is the case : A patient 52 years, tall (190 cm), lean, complains of an essential hypotonia, R.R. 80 equal to

90/60 and is subject to some relapsing infections. Many medicines were prescribed but gave no effect ; subjectively he complains of chilliness, the face is of dark colour, dirty, voice melancholic, thinks of his future although everything goes on well. *Psor in 30DH* was prescribed to him and one year after T.A. 110-120/80 (R.R.) and no infection.

Case 4

Baudemprez : Study of Psorinum. A personal case. Revue Belge d'Homoeopathie, No. 1, 1964, p. 341.

M.B...18 years, student, comes to consult me by the end of August 1961, for a large eczema, oozing, of the peri-anal region.

The affection is three years' old, was obstinately rebellious to all treatments : local topics, anti-histaminic, cortisone and even radiotherapy. Some Homoeopathic treatments brought some amelioration.

Locally, the cutano-mucous zone presents an appearance of induration, and bleeding, of bright red colour ; it oozes intermittently, the itching is intense, worse by the heat of the bed ; the affection clearly aggravated in the winter, by cold wind and by dry cold wind (this is spontaneously told by the patient) ; sometimes there was intense darting in the place of itching so much so that the sitting position becomes almost intolerable. The patient is a tall young man, weak and cyphotic. Hereditary and personal history are of no importance. However he had a mononeucleosis in his childhood ; he eats well but has pyrosis and flatulence after fats and eggs ; he liked salted food, the thirst is of no particular importance. He is relatively chilly, not much, although his eczema is worse in dry weather. He has a sad mood, seems to have already resigned to the success of our treatment.

The First Prescription

Lycopodium—Result : Its total failure. I gave too much importance to flatulence, acidity, sullenness, the expressions of hepatism. On the other hand as the patient was not excessively chilly I did not prescribe him *Psorinum*.

During the second consultation, I studied again carefully the case trying to valorise :

1. Horribly sensitive and pruriginous dermatosis, aggravated during the night, by the heat of the bed, worse in the winter and by north wind.

2. The general symptom of insufficient reaction in a young subject who does not react to any medicine. *Prescription* : *Psorinum* 6, 12, 30, 200 on the 18th October, 1961.

I see again my patient on the 19th December, 1961. The amelioration is spectacular ; there is still a slight induration on the surface of the old eczema, more oozing. Slight itching at night. Prescription : Placebo.

The 20th March, 1962, the patient came smiling and says that he is entirely cured and in fact the examination is quite negative.

Very recently I took news of this young man from one of his near relatives and I know that he is prefectly well.

Case 5

Case of Dr. H. Bernard—in l'Homoeopathie Moderne, No. 20 of 15th October, 1936, p.648-649.

M.F...65 years.

Came to consult for a chronic bronchitis which begins at the beginning of the cold season and which durates throughout the winter. He says that it was due to a gas, towards the end of 1915. (There was no Yperite at that time). He was for that pensioned at 10%.

"A man of medium stature, rather big, gray hairs, clear eyes, with an air of apprehension. Face slightly swollen, the look is dirty and shining. He exhaled when one approaches him a smell of "uncleanliness". He is an easy-going peasant. His wife who accompanies him is perfectly clean.

"Very much chilly, heavily covered, is afraid of the least air current ; asked me to keep on his hat.

"His bronchitis particularly aggravated, he says, during the new moon. If he has cold at that time, he sneezes ; at first the discharge from his nose is thin, then it becomes greenish ; his cough becomes frequent, more loose and he expectorated some purulent expectorations which smells bad. By auscultation nothing particular was found ; big rales of bronchitis, tendency to emphysema. Sometimes cough causes nausea.

"No digestive troubles except some morning diarrhoeas, starting at 6 A.M. when he wakes up : yellow stools, glairy, of bad smell. The least cold on the belly gives him colics ; he wears a flannel band. Good appetite, always hungry. At night he has "some langour" in the stomach, which is ameliorated by munching a lump of sugar ; this happens towards 2 A.M.

"No urinary troubles ; slight costo-lumbar pain.

"Nothing in the heart.

"Some migraines with the changing of the moon", generally unilateral sometime on one side sometime on the other. Cold in the head aggravates.

"Cutaneous lesions from scratching on the legs and on ankles which aggravate in the evening and by washing.

Treatment :

One dose of *Psorinum 200* to be taken after 10 days. Drainage with *Ipeca 6*, two granules while going to bed : *Chelidonium 3x, Berberis 3x, Hepar sulphur 30* three days a week.

"Although I have well noted the modality of the treatment, the patient imagined that he should begin the treatment only after 10 days. He took *Psorinum 200* when waking up in the morning at first.

"From the next morning, intense diarrhoea. The patient, thinking to have cold on the belly lied down within being

anxious. The diarrhoea persisted two days, glairy and weakening ; the cough increased and the expectorations were of unexpected abundance and foetidity. The absence of fever made
the patient patient and he did not wish to take any medicine,
believing on the power of the little globules.

"Three days afterwards everything calmed down progressively. To-day he is not coughing any more. Advised him not to
take any medicine for 10 days.

"At the end of these ten days the cure was maintained.

"The patient has passed an excellent winter ; only one
bronchitis which lasted six days without leaving any trace ;
maintenance treatment.

"I mention that this patient was a farmer and therefore gives
much importance to the phases of the moon. The aggravation
mentioned during the new moon which gave me to think of
Silicea is really an aggravation during storm, humid and cold
weather which was at that time very frequent. We found the
periodicity of *Psorinum* in the lunar aggravation of the
margines.

"One may also think of *Hepar sulphur* which I gave as a
functional remedy, but the special hunger was present here.

COMMENTARIES

We have presented here the polychrest *Psorinum*, biotherapic
and homoeotherapic in a manner as complete and as clear as
possible.

However, we are inclined on the basis of our experience, to
make a certain reserve, because in fact, its action is slow,
irregular and capricious.

In order to be certain about its action, there is every ground
to prescribe practically uniquely in the 30 CH.

From the fact that *Psorinum* would be rarely prescribed
alone one may think that it is an *adjuvant* which acts deeply,
in the "depth of the tissues" as says Leriche.

The use of 30th CH exclusively will allow us to get some therapeutic results which are, if not as spectacular as those of *Luesinum* or *Medorrhinum*, not negligible.

Psorinum has therefore been used in high dilution 30 CH, since the publication of Materia Medica der Nosoden in Germany, by the German homoeopaths with some good results.

Psorinum has therefore clearly an *etiological* indication, in dragging morbid processes, in the form of alternating noso-graphic forms and where a heterogenous intoxination cause some attacks having acute form of morbid expressions, or alter-nating morbidity.

But *Psorinum* is also used *among other homoeopathics* in what is known under the name of *Psora* of Hahnemann.

The *Psora* of Hahnemann really speaking, according to the conception of the founder of Homoeopathy is now strongly shaken if not completely ruined.

This is the reason why some homoeopathic doctors, specially the Germans, do not desire any more to make any mention of *Psora* and rejected this *Psora* among the things forgotten in the history.

We must not believe that this attitude is recent.

Thus in Homoeolexique published by Michel Granier of Nimes edited and published by Adrien Delahaye, place de l'Ecole de medicine, Paris, 1874, we find the following article on *Psora*.

("*Psora* : ψωρα, gale). A new word introduced in the medical science by Hahnemann, in order to express a fact well recognised in almost every period of history, which has become only as an important subject of special and explicit considerations, since the time of this author. This fact is the presence in the constitution of living beings in general and particularly in some amongst them, of an element or a morbid cause not yet well defined, resulting out of an abnormal condition of the cutaneous function : humorous, gaseous, virulent and miasmatic nature, rather perhaps simply dynamic ; an element supposed by the ancients flowing in the economy of the human body, and who attributed to it some incomplete dangerous phenomena, particularly the morbid metastasis or the changing of places of the diseases. For Samuel Hahnemann this element is nothing but a contagium or psoric miasm, with which the economy would remain infected in subjects having had the itch at some periods of their own lives, or even in those having this element, influencing all the tendencies of their nature, from their forefathers who were infected by this disease. To-day this element is extended to different chronic cutaneous affections, under the different names given to darts, so numerous or so varied in their forms impress on the skin a somewhat abnormal contamination ; to eruptions and vegetations no less diverse and numerous, in the forms of pustules, papules, vesicles, bullas, phlyctenas, crusts, tumors, cancroids, strumouses, fibroids etc .. of ulcers of different natures, some simple efflorescences, liver spots, ephelides, or reveals itself in the form of more abundant or rare secretions by sensitiveness to cold, to heat which may vary upto the most complete indolence, up to intolerable pain, to unbearable itching or by simple emanations of smell also of different natures, in a word by a somewhat chronic impairment, of the normal condition of the skin. From this very legitimate extension of the element of chronic diseases and of its transmission by heredity, results the psoric heredity of all the present generations and generations to come and consequently the subjection of all, in only a different measures, to chronic diseases as well as to hereditary diseases. The psora resulting out of an abnormal condition of cutaneous reaction is, generally, in subjects who are infected by it and particularly in the system that it affects, an obstruction added to the original insufficiency of the economy for the complete function of the vital force." (Dr. Gastier)

Let us suppose a philosopher doing research about the truth in medicine. He has examined all the systems and all the theories. He comes to the doctrine of our school. He reads with religious attention the works of Hahnemann. He is at first struck by the logic of the Master. Hahnemann demolished the old systems to build on them his new one. He purifies the fields of medicine from all vain hypothesis. He declares once for all the essentiality of all diseases. He proclaims the most beautiful dogma of the therapeutics ; the individualisation of morbid cases. And the researcher bow down in admiration before the genuis of Hahnemann. But then the Master formulates his idea about the genesis of chronic diseases. These diseases and the results of three occult powers : the *psora* the *syphilis* and the *sycosis*. The *psora* above all is the fruit that the first man gathered from the tree of science of illness, and the juice of this fruit endangers in a fatal way almost all the chronic diseases. The remedies that will cure these diseases are called by a name, have their root in the field of old errors ; they are called antipsorics. Such psoric disease is cured by such remedy, this remedy is placed for this reason in the ranks of antipsorics will cure such a disease : that disease is placed for that reason in the rank of psoric diseases. One error always calls for another error. The viscious circle is formed. He who has formed this circle is glad to be enclosed within it. What do you think that the philosopher would think ? Alas ! The hypothesis is always living. Hahnemann has not therefore broken down the heads of the ancient hydra. The genesis of diseases is not therefore any more a mystery ? The individualisation is not therefore dogma ? A Gaubius said that it is better to stop walking than to a advance in the darkness, and Gaubius while speaking thus, has lost himself in the darkness of humorism, and gave himself up while sleeping to the acrimonious chemical and mechanical current of humours. There is the nature of man. Hahnemann with his torch of genius, dissipates the darkness of the old systems and wanders later on in the fallacious darkness of hypothesis. He has therefore, himself gathered the fruit of the fatal tree, and vivified the legend of human destinies that the most pure genius will commit at least one error and a very great mistake. Hahnemann has committed his mistake (See. Systéme).

We see that at least Granier (and others of his French contemporaries) is not tender about the idea of Psora of Hahnemann.

The contemporanian French homoeopaths do not reject as strongly the Psora.

After the first World War, between 1920-1940, the Psora is in major part identified with the *Tuberculinism* (L. Vannier, Fortier-Bernoville, Rouy, H. Bernard and R. Zissu).

As regards the therapeutic indication of *Psorinum*, Jacques Michaud in his lecture of C.H.F. of the 8th January, 1971, indicates the directive lines of the prescription :

—Either as a remedy of diathesis ;

—Or only as a homoeotherapic remedy ;

—Or like a reactional remedy ;

—Or for ameliorating a patient who cannot be cured of a dragging disease ;

—and finally, as complementary of *Tuberculinum.*

Place of Psorinum is between *Sulphur* and *Thuya,* complimenting *Tuberculinum.*

In the strict application of analogical reasoning, *Psorinum* therefore finds its place in the simple analogical progress.

If we pass, with Hahnemann, over this level in order to arrive at the idea of morbid processes of chronic diseases the prescription of Psorinum will take another dimension. It is this idea of processes which escapes the author homoeopaths of the second half of the nineteenth century and our contemporaries.

If we put ourselves in the field of the real, we will keep as a historical souvenir the etio-pathologic concepts of psora formulated by Hahnemann.

First of all it is necessary to free it from the mystery and the dust.

In the place of the word Psora, we have suggested the word *Allergoso.*

The *Allergoso* represents according to us (O.A. Julian) a structural state, morphological, dynamic, contradictional setting of the organism containing a molecular code, genotypic and peristastic (the idea of physico-chemical ground as well as the socio-familial ground on which the individual develops).

The genotypic code is polymorphous, toxinic, infections, traumatic.

This polyetiology leaves in the cell memory some informations from which results a contradictional cortico-visceral conditioning.

Since then Allergoso represents a structural stage of equilibrium which becomes unstable, of excitation and cervico-visceral inhibition, differenciated quantitatively and qualitatively on the cellular, tissular and organic levels.

Clinical expression shows some incongruous and contradictory nosographic forms.

This is even the meaning of morbid metatasis and alternance of morbidity.

The clinic describes a subject presenting alternate excitation and cortico-visceral inhibition with restlessness, anxiety, depression or hyperacitivity.

This is the mute phase of the nosographic state which explodes according to the focalisation : angina-pectoris, cerebral ictus, intermittent claudication, acute attack of gout, hyperuricemia, eczema etc...

Thus this moving contradictional course may end in this long historical process of manifestations, to a degenerative somatic process of sclerosis by inhibition of the exchanges or to cell anarchy by disordered excitation, following a physiological rupture.

On the biological plane this Allergoso is characterised by :

(*a*) The perturbation of tests of hepatic flocculation.

(*b*) The anomalies of proteinogram and by the reticulo-endothelian memoranda.

(*c*) The falling of histamino-pexic power of the serum according to Parrot and Laborde.

(*d*) By a cancerometry of perturbed Arthur Vernes.

This biological complex objectively characterises Allergose.

The significance of perturbations of proteinogram, of the reticulo-endothelial memo, in the tests of hepatic flocculation is well known.

Let us say only some words regarding two other tests :

(*a*) Concerning the histaminopexic power of the serum Parrot and Laborde have verified that the normal human serum captivates in virto the histamin.

The mixture of human serum (submitted 24 hours in the dialises) with a known dose of histamin (solution of chlorohydrate of histamin by million) is placed in contact of a soft muscle of ileun of a cobaye standardised beforehand.

If the serum fixes the histamin, the contraction of the muscle will be less important than that caused by the same dose of histamin without serum.

The serum of a normal subject causes histimin to lose about 15 to 30% of its activity, therefore histamino-pexic power : 15 to 30%.

The serum of an allergic subject does not generally modify the histaminopexic power.

On the contrary our clinico biologic study on one thousand clinical observations has helped us to determine that in the allergose there is constantly a sinking down or a very great fall of the histamino-pexic power. (O.A. Julian)

This biological statement is confirmed by the clinico-biological experiment of numerous other biotherapists who have the knowledge of our work.

(*b*) The Cancerometry of Arthur Verne is a blood test done with photometre of Vernes.

It consists in the measurement of cuprum acetate of glucoproteins of the blood of which the rate rises in cancer subjects as well as the dose of the dissimulated body reducers. (C.E.A.) by the test of Vernes Orcinol.

In case of an Allergose with some evident clinical manifestations there will always be registered a serious unwedging of the test of Vernes.

Having thus defined Allergose (ex Psora) and described its clinical and biological aspect we can now envisage its therapy.

The Biotherapy of Allergose (ex-Psora) indicates with S. Hahnemann the homoeopathic *Sulphur* is to be prescribed in high dynamisation and for a long time.

It will be helped by the biotherapic *Psorinum* of which we have just read the pathogenesis. With Boeninghausen we mention after *Sulphur* the following Homoeopsorics : *Ammon carb., Baryta carb., Calc. carb., Graphitis, Iodium, Lycopodium, Magnesium, Magnesia muriaticum, Natrum carbonicum, Acid nitric, Petroleum, Phosphorus, Silicea, Sepia, Zincum and also Carbo. animalis, Causticum, Kali carbonicum, Natrum muriaticum.*

The works of O.A. Julian indicate moreover the following homoeotherapics : *Agave tequilana, Argenium metallicum, Berberis aquafolla, Beryllium metallicum, Bunias orient., Cobaltum nitric., Cortisone, Corticotrophine, Tellurium, Thalamus.*

This new study of ancient Psora of S. Hahnemann actualised in the form of Allergoso of O.A. Julian, finds a kind of second youth and merits to attract the attention of all biotherapic clinicians.

But let us finish tne monograph by underlining that *Psorinum* is a remedy which is applied, by virtue of analogical reasoning to all *analogous morbid condition* and not only to Psora : Allergose.

PUTRESCINUM

HISTORY

This product has been preconised by Paul Chavanon in 1955, when the Nosode *Pyrogenium* was not among the authorised products.

STOCK

Pharmacopraxy is of Hahnemannian system of a derivative of ornithine, the Putrescine or tetramethylenediamine.

This product exists as "product under seal" in the commerce and its fabrication is assured by a homoeopathic laboratory of France.

CLINICAL PATHOGENESIS

There is no Hahnemannian proving of this product.

CLINICAL INDICATIONS

Those of Pyrogenium (see monograph) and my personal clinical impression is that Putrescinum seems to be sometimes more active than *Pyrogenium*.

POSOLOGY

Dynamisation : 7 CH.

PYROGENIUM

BIBLIOGRAPHY

Allen H.C. :

The Materia Medica of Nosodes, p. 400-427, Boericke and Tafel, Phil., 1910.

Boericke W. :

Pocket Manual of Homoeopathic Materia Medica. Boericke and Runyon, Boericke and Tafel, Phil., 9th ed. 1927.

Homoeopatische Mittel und ihre Wirkungen. Tr. in German by M. Harms, 1972. Verlag Grundlagen und Praxis, M. Harms, Leer.

Julian O.A. :

Biothérapiques et Nosodes. Maloine, 1962, Paris.

Maroger F. :

Pyrogenium. L'Homoeopathie Moderne, 15 déc., 1936, p. 20.

Chavanon :

Thérapeutique O.R.L. Homoeopathique. Imprimérie St-Dénis. Nirot, 1935.

Poursain : Quelques cas cliniques de *Pyrogenium* ; L'Homeopathie Française, oct., 1931.

Boocock ; *Pyrogenium*. Homeop. Recorder, 1892, T 7, 196.

Aguilar E. : *Pyrogenium*. Homoeopathic Recorder, 15 Sept., 1924, in l'Homoeopathie française, Oct., 1931.

Loos-Julia. *Pyrogenium*. Journal of the Amer., Institute of Hom. 1909.

Flury R. :

Pyrogenium. Klassische Homöop. 1972, 16, H. 4. p. 167-71.

(520)

Junod F. :
Revue de presse : Flury : *Pyrogenium*. Annales Homeop. Fr.
No. 9, Nov. 1973.

Borliachor : *Pyrogenium*, dans la Matiére Médicale de Nash.
l'Hom. Fr. 1948, No. 8, Oct., p. 379.

Foubister : Pratique de *Pyrogenium*, B.H.J. 1971, No. 2, in
Revue de presse Homeopathique de Langue Anglaise, par
R. Sèror (Oloron), Cahiers de Biothérapie, No. 33, mars
1972.

Ferrion : Quleques observations sur *Pyrogenium* chez les
cardio-renaux et hépato-renaux. L'Hom. Fr. 1949, No. 4.,
p. 174.

Bardoular : Indications de *Pyrogenium* en Homeotherapie
vétérinaire. L'Hom. Fr., 1956, No. 8, p. 484.

Dufilha : *Pyrogenium* et Penicilline. L'Homeop. Fr., 1952,
No. 5, p. 275.

Tyler M.L. : Homeopathic Drug Pictures. The Homeopathic
Pubg. Co. Ltd., 152 Landor Rd., London S.W. 9.

Julian O.A. : Materia Medica der Nosoden. K. Haug
Verlag, Heidelberg 1975, 2e ed.

Flury R :
Pyrogenium. Zeitschrift fur Klassische. Homöopathic Bd. 16
Heft. 4, 1972.

STOCK

The biotherapic Pyrogenium is prepared from a stock
obtained by the mixture of autolysates of the flesh of beef,
pork, human placenta, being the object of visa No. 2222, SV,
1669, of the Merieux Institute.

COMPOSITION

Lysate diluted, corresponding to 0,001 ml of an autolysate
prepared from :

Beaf	⎫
Pork	⎬ à à
Human placenta	⎭

No preserving or stabilising agents.

It is delivered by the Institute Merieux in ampouls of 1 ml for preparation of homoeopathic dilutions.

TECHNIQUE OF PREPARATION

1. Collection of Beef, Pork and of Human Placenta

The beef and pork are collected cleanly in the slaughter house, immediately after slaughtering the animals. When they arrive at the laboratory, they are dressed carefully.

The placentas are fresh and collected during night. They are, after their arrival in the laboratory, washed in physiological serum, then put to the hanger in order to eliminate the blood.

2. Preparation of the Pulpe and Autolysate

The viandes and the placentas are transferred to the chopper, and the pulp thus collected is placed in the glass vases, ambiant temperature (18'—20') for three weeks.

3. Separation of the Liquid of Autolysate

The content of the vases is centrifuged in mugs of 1 litre, 30 mts. at 3,300 t/m. The floating liquid is filtered through paper and then centrifuged. Thus one collects about 5 cm³ of liquid of autolysate per kilogram of pulp.

4. Final Lysate by Congealation-decongealation

The liquid thus obtained is congealed at 20° then decongealed 4 times consequtively, then centrifuged once again.

5. Distribution and Stockage of the net Lysate

The lysate undergoes a sterilising filtration on EKS filter, and is distributed aseptically by fraction of 1 cm³ in sterile ampouls of 5 cc, then lyophilised. These ampoules form the stock of the base defined by the technique of preparation and its tests of control.

6. The Obtaining of the Diluted Lysate

The content of a lyophilised ampoule (1 cm³ of net lysate) is. diluted in 1,000 cm³ of sterile distilled water. The solution. undergoes sterilising filtration on EKS filtre, then distributed. aspetically in sterile ampoules of 1 cm³.

TECHNIQUE OF CONTROLS BEARING ON THE STOCKED LYSATE IN LOPHILISED FORM

1. Total Nitrogen

Determined by the Kjedahl method, the rate should be between 7 and 9g for 1000 cm³.

2. Electrophoresis

The electrophoresis should correspond to the values given below. The fraction of proteins rendered insoluble by denaturalisation and fraction of soluble proteins which are distributed in the following manner :

—Protein 1 : mobility—1.90×10^{-5} representing 73% of the soluble proteins.

—Protein 2 : mobility—4.15×10^{-5} representing 4,5% of soluble proteins.

—Protein 3 : mobility—5×10^{5} representing 14,4% of soluble proteins.

—Protein 4 : mobility—5.75×10^{-5} representing 8,10% of soluble proteins.

The protein 1 is a protein of mobility comparable to that of gamma globulines, and should represent 73% ± 3% of soluble proteins.

3. A Chromatographic Examination is done.

HISTORY

Drysdale a homoeopathic doctor had first the idea of using. Pyrogenium as a therapeutic agent. This doctor was interested in the works of chemists who towards 1860 studied the products. resulting out of the decomposition of meat.

He tried at first a product prepared by *Panum* which did not give him satisfaction, so he fixed his choice on the preparation of *Paterson* (1879) of which, here is the original description of preparation :

"Half a pound of meat of beef is put to be macerated in water for 14 days in the month of July 1879. It is filtered through a linen. 12 ounces of this clear solution is measured precipitaled with 12 ounces of 98° strong ethylic alcohol and it is left at rest the whole night. The precipitate thus obtained is almost the half of the vase used for precipitation.

"The floating alcohol is decanted and the precipitate is collected on the linen, washed by ebullition of 5 mm with 12 ounces of alcohol.

"It is washed again with boiling alcohol then the precipitate is swept off from tue linen and conserved 36 hours under sulphur vacuum, time during which it becomes dry and become blackish. Its weight is 15 grains.

"This product is then transformed in the first decimal dilution in a mixture of water and glycerine".

This preparation is as seen, very complicated. It is roughly an acquous extract of putrified meat, purified by precipitation in partially denatured alcohol because of the fact of the use of boiling solvent. The washing in hot alcohol has again this regrettable effect of dissolving an important part of the ptomaine base, which has been researched by Drysdale.

Other authors have preconised some slightly different operatory method.

We will cite only the process of Dr. Dias Da Cruz cited by J. Favre (Propagateur de l'Homoeopathie, 1910, p. 136) :

"A vase, containing 500 g of water and 200 g of meat free from fat and chopped in small pieces, is exposed to dry air for 20 days. Thus a reddish liquid is obtained, which is thick and fetid. This liquid is filtered and evaporated in *bain-marie* until it becomes dry. It is macerated in alcohol for 2 hours. The dry residue then forms a compact mass of deep colour. This residue is left to become dry. Then it is mixed with 30 g of distilled water and filtered after two hours. The liquid, having a clear amber colour that is thus, obtained, is the acquous extract of *Pyrogenium*. To this a double volume of glycerine is added and this preparation is considered the mother tincture to be run for making, the different dilutions".

The pathogenesis of *Pyrogenium* was, already said, laid down by Drysdale, completed by Wyborn (1899), and published in a complete form in the monograph of Kent (Allegemeine Homöopathische Zeitung, 1905) as well as in the Materia Medica of Nosodes of Allen (1910).

Besides common *Pyrogenium* many other preparations were experimented between the two world wars, particularly *Pyrogenium "H"*, prepared from the base of human flesh and *Pyrogenium "P"* of which the basis is placenta.

Drysdale obtained favourable results in some infectious febrile conditions. Another author Sherbino used it in high dynamisation, while Clarke was inspired by Flury, for his pathogenesis.

Swan utilised a product prepared from a septic abcess and named it *Sepsinum* or *Septiseminum*, but it created a confusion calling it also *Pyrogenium*.

P. Chavanon also gave attention on *Pyrogenium* and prepared a stock by putting "in a recipient, a bit of all the organs brain, marrow, meninges, bone, tendons. kidneys, ganglions, intestines, pancreas, spleen, lungs etc. I have left it to be putrified for 14 months in on alternated series of three months aerobia and three months anaerobia. Then I have selected experimentally the optima dilution of the product obtained, and given them to different pharmacists who imbibed labelled globules in it and labelled *Pyrogenium P.C.*—stock, October, 1934.

Its action is so powerful that I prescribed to patients once in 24 or 48 hours according to the resisting power of the person" (P. Chavanon). (Therapeutique O.R.L. Homoeopathique, p. 107, Imprimérie St-Denys, 1935)."

It is important to note that the only stock at present legal in France is that which we have discribed under "Stock".

Then it is necessary to note that there is no experimental pathogenesis according to the method of Hahnemann and the description which follows is a "clinical pathogenesis" (M.L. Tyler, Homeop. Drug Picture, p. 690).

CLINICAL PHARMACODYNAMIC CORTICO-VISCERAL PROTOCOL OR CLINICAL PATHOGENESIS

1. Generalities

The clinical picture regarding *Pyrogenium* goes from localised small infection to the great septicemia.

The key symptoms :

Not obligatorily present together, but to characterise the physiognomy of this remedy are :

—*Dissociation of the pulse (rapid) and of the temperature (tendency to hypothermia).*

—*Putrid breath*, discharges and dejections.

—*Restlessness.*

There may be an infected condition, general and local or localised.

General :

It is a patient more or less prostrated, anxious but above all having some clear symptoms of restlessness, cannot remain quiet on bed. He cannot find any place of rest which may ameliorate his condition.

To the motor restlessness is added a psychic restlessness, with incessant talking, or a mild delirium.

Pale face, eyes surrounded with blue circles, checks sometimes burning, nostrils flapping.

Local :

Formation of suppurating collection with lymphangitis of the corresponding territory.

2. Neuro-endocrino-psychic System

Prostration followed by restlessness : *At night the bed feels too hard*, which forces him to move constantly in order to ameliorate the painful parts of the body.

The patient thinks that his personality is changed when turning his body from one side to another.

He makes mistake regarding the localisation of the different parts of his body. Cannot realise if he dreaming or if he is awake. *Loquacious* patient, speaks too much with a rapid ideation changing disordered.

Cannot sleep because his mind is full of obsessing ideas.

Head congestive with pulsations and throbbing.

Throbbing in the temples better by pressure.

Pressive headache : Pain in the ocular globes and of the occipital region, aggravated by cough.

Arterial beatings in the ears.

3. Digestive Apparatus

Horrible breath, repulsing, foetid, putrid.

Dry mouth, the teeth are covered with fuliginosities, the tongue coated, cracked, sometimes varnished red, sometimes covered with thick yellow coating.

Great thirst for cold water but which the patient immediately vomits up when it becomes hot in the stomach.

On the contrary, the patient can retain hot water which calms down the nauseating condition.

Repeated vomiting, of a brown liquid like coffee in fecaloid with intestinal paresia.

Foetid diarrhoea, brown or black stools wilh involuntary emission of a gas and of fecal matter or *constipation* from intestinal atony with dry, black stools with the small of carrion.

Vesico-rectal tenesmus.

Distended abdomen, bloated, sensitive and painful.

4. Cardio-hemo-vascular System

Sensation as if the heart has become fatigued.

Feels himself completely drained with palpitations and beating in the ears.

Is concious of his heart.

Rapid pulse, small, filiform, dissociated in relation to the temperature.

Tedency to collapse.

Thermoregulation :

Irregular fever, having the difference of 2° to 3° between Hypothermy and Hyperthermy in the space of a few hours.

Hyperthermy and hypothermy alternate with a purse always very accelerated not in relation to the degree of heat.

Chill specially of the painful region followed by heat and pains in the extremities.

Periodic chill at 19 hours.

He is afraid of air, cold and is better temporarily by heat.

Putrid and nauseating sweets.

5. Respiratory Apparatus

Rapid jerking respiration, fanning of the nasal wings, fetid breath.

Taste of pus while coughing.

Cough with abundant expectoration of *putrid* mucus.

Cough aggravated in *hot room* and by *movement*.

Pains on the sides of the chest, aggravated by movement. Ameliorated by lying down on the painful side.

6. Sense Organs

Nose :
Secretions having putrid smell. (furuncles of nose—Chavanon).

Eyes :
Chalazions of the eyelids, infected.

Ears :
Furuncles of the auditive conduit. (Chavanon)

7. Uro-genital Apparatus

(a) Urinary :
Urine less abundant, of dark colour, with albumins and cylindres.

Vesical tenesmus.
Urine of putrid smell.

(b) Genital :
Localised mastitis, abscess of the breast. (Chavanon)

Foetid lochia, of brown colour, with chill, fever and abundant sweat.

Foetid menstruation with fever.
Uterine hemorrhage with black putrid blood.

8. Loco-motor System

Bruised pains all over the body.
Stiffness with numbness of the extremities of the limbs.
Sensation as if the bones are broken.
Constant need for moving, the bed feels hard.
Sensation of coldness on the painful parts.

9. Skin, Phanera

Skin, cold livid, covered with abundant sweat, cold, viscous and fetid.

Varicose ulcers, persisting, foetid, late to cicatrise, specially in old men.

10. Modalities

Aggravation : By movement, by touch.
By cold, specially in humid cold.

Amelioration : By the heat, by cold bath, by hot drink.
By movement, by stretching, by changing position.

POSOLOGY

Dynamisation : 4 CH, 5 CH, 7 CH, 9 CH.

The most useful dynamisations appear to be the 5 CH and 7ʃCH, may be prescribed together.

POSITIVE DIAGNOSIS

Oscillating fever ; pulse very rapid (dissociated with the temperature).

Restlessness and painful sensation.

Foetidity, putridity of the breath, of excretions and evacuations.

DIFFERENTIAL DIAGNOSIS

Classical homoeotherapy : One should think of *Baptisia*, Arsenicum, Crotalus, *Bothrops*, *Hepar sulphur*, Mercurius sol, Arnica, *Carbolic acid*, *Anthracinum* (see article), *Lachesis*, Staphylococcin, Streptococcin, *Echinacea*, *Rhus tox*.

Modern Homoeotherapy

Achyranthes-calea : Muscular stiffness, dryness and burning of the mucouses and of the skin ; fever rising between 38° and 40°, congestive headache, throbbing, aggravated by light.

Acidum butyricum : Anxiety, foetid smell in the mouth, bleeding gums, bad smelling stools, foetid leucorrhoea, osteo-muscular pains of the arms, of feet.

Rajania-subsamarata : High fever, prostration, muco-purulent diarrhoea. Metrorrhagia of black putrid blood, circumscribed inflammation of skin with tumefaction and ulceration.

Paronichia-illecebrum : Feeling of a double personality, hyperthermia, involuntary passing of stools and urines, foetid nauseating breath, abundant sweats with the smell of curd.

CLINICAL DIAGNOSIS

1. Generalities

Septicemia. Pyohemia.

Ptomain poisoning.

Infectious influenza with gastro-intestinal complications.

Toxicosis.

Tuberculosis with cavity (adjuvant treatment).

Mastoiditis.

2. Nervous System

Meningitis ; encephalitis (Adjuvant treatment).

3. Digestive Apparatus

Typhoid.

Infectious enteritis.

Cholera infantile.

Toxicosis of babies.

Septic appendicitis.

Anal fistula.

Sub-phrenic abscess.

Abscess of the liver.

Acute cholecystitis.

4. Uro-genital Apparatus

Acute albuminuric nephritis.

Puerperal fever.

Uterine hemorrhage (after failure of Ipeca).

Perinephritic abscess.

Abscess of the breast.

5. Respiratory Apparatus

Phlegmon of the throat.

Purulent pleurisy.

Abscess and gangrene of the lungs.

6. Skin

Eschars of decubitus.

Phlegmon. Abscess.

Furuncles. Anthrax.

Panaris.

COMMENTARIES

Pyrogenium is a good helping Biotherapic in certain acute or subacute affections, the nosographic conditions of which we have mentioned in the paragraph on clinical diagnosis.

It is well related to the homoeotherapics *Hepar sulphur, Biothrops, Lachesis* and others, also to the biotherapic *Anthracinum.*

In infectious states, if the antibiotics are avoided, it may be given with *Echinecea* 3 DH, *Argentum met.* 7 CH, *Ferrum phos.* 7 CH prescribed in ampoules, injectable sub-cutaneously, 1.M or 1 V. It may prove a very efficacious treatment.

We should also think of the new remedies *Acid butyric, Achryanthes calea, Rajania subsamarata, Paroñichia illecebrum,* and of the biotherapic *Anthracinum.*

Paul Chavanon was the great pioneer who has cleared as a specialist of O.R.L., thanks to Homoeotherapy and to Nosodotherapy, a vast field of pathology of infections.

It is for this reason that in his magnificient work (Therapeutique O.R.L. homoeopathique, 1935), he has indicated the coupled therapeutic of *Hepar sulphur* and *Pyrogenium* to be prescribed in :

1. Suppurations of bone cavities with spontaneous drainage (ex : maxillary sinus).

2. The suppuration of bone cavities not well drained (example : mastoid) where he does not advise *Hepar sulphur.*

3. Suppuration in the soft tissues where the collection in question is very often spontaneously drained (abcess of the tonsils).

4. Suppuration in the soft tissues where the collection may be suddenly dangerous (Ludwig's angina, furuncles of the lip (upper or of the nose).

Finally, Chavanon writes that "in the very grave conditions. immediately when one can obtain pus, should make from it some dilutions, 30 or 200.

It is the most powerful remedy of all.

Here is the question of preparing an Isotherapic in 5 CH or 7 CH, according as it is prescribed by the present legislation.

Thus, thanks to some fearless homoeopaths, the great chapter of infectious diseases was courageously approached.

To be sure, in the time of antibiotherapy which has incontestable success but aleatory because the couple Microbe-antibiotic if manifested by some antagonistic immunological conflicts of which the microbe is not always dead, our position of a different biotherapy taking into account of the ground, of the microbe and of the pathological conflict, has its full value.

It gains some ground there where for sometime it seemed to have fallen back.

Homoeotherapics or biotherapics judiciously associated are and will remain as an excellent therapeutic arm.

Before terminating, let us cite some clinical cases of Pyrogenium.

Case 1 (Dr. Chavanon) :

The wife of one of my friends had an abscess of the breast, after lactation for a few days. I was asked about my opinion on that question because the colleague who treats her became hopeless seeing the thing aggravated, inspite of the vaccins and incision.

From my bag I gave her *Pyrogenium* P.C., immediately and then *Hepar sulphur* P.C. after 12 hours.

Twently four hours after *Hepar.* therefore in 36 hours, the orifices that were suppurating warped, the swelling of the breast diminished and the new places which were becoming hard became normal.

"The surgeon was shocked, asked me what is to be done for one of his relatives who has a phlebitis after delivery. Give her the same *Pyrogenium* every morning after waking up ; but do not give her *Hepar sulphur*, it would cause disaster. Watch over the temperature.

"At the end of 48 hours, the temperature became normal and the patient got up after 3 days, completely cured at the deep stupefaction of the colleague.

"The latter then came to me, and said : Please excuse me ; I thought that your remedies were only water, and that you were quacks. I believe Pierre Mauriac. "Pierre mauriac", I replied to him, criticises a method (no doubt in the name of his scientific spirit) which he does not know and thus he columnises honest men who work hard in order to make the progress of medicine and to cure better and more rapidly." (P. Chavanon)

Here is now a short case report of Dr. Ferriot published in l'Homoeopathic franscaise, 1949, No. 4, p. 174.

Case 2 :

Mme P .... 68.

Mal compensated mitral insufficiency, passive congestion of the bases, big liver, obesity very marked.

Temperature 38°4. Tachy-arythmic pulse of about 130.

Disturbance in the form of gastric embarassment with abdominal pains have begun about 5 days ago.

By examination, great pain on the Mac-Burney's point, presence of a breast plate and muscular defense leave no doubt for the diagnosis.

The age, the condition of the heart, obesity, the starting of the disease, inclined me to avoid if possible the operation.

Treatment : Hydric diet, *Pyrogenium 30 K*, two granules morning and evening.

In 48 hours the temperature is about 37° with amelioration of all the symptoms.

In eight days, everything was cured. (Dr. Ferrie)

Case 3 :

Extract of the article : "Mes premiéres guérisons (My first cures) by Nicole Fredon Montessuit in" Annales Homoeopathiques Franscaises No. 9, November, 1974, p. 50—710.

About 6 weeks after his influenza, my husband has remained immobile for a longtime in a tempest of snow, insufficiently covered, before going to take a course of ski.

The next day at noon, he feels himself very bad, shivers, shudders, is very pale, inspite of all the covers piled over him he could not be heated.

The temperature is at 40°1. Ausculation revealed clear congestion of the left base.

I became somewhat mad—Homoeopathy ? ......Allopathy ? What to do ?

I thought about *Aconite* : face to face with the sudden explosion of the disease, caused by exposition to cold air.

But my husband has no thirst—Then I felt the pulse.

It beats at 80. To be sure, I felt the pulse twice. It is absolutely slow : dissociation of the pulse and temperature and it is *Pyrogenium*.

After having asked the advise of Dr. Schmidt, I gave XM dilution.

The fever being 40° 1 how there can be homoeopathic aggravation ? One hour after the temperature is but the same my husband is feeling better.

The night was much better for him as well as for me, because I felt him always burning. But in the morning, the miracle ! The temperature 37-40°. Pulse 84. He feels himself perfectly well no more coughs, asks for eating. The congestion completely disappeared in 3 days and there was no need of any other therapeutic !

SCARLATINUM

BIBLIOGRAPHY

Julian O.A. :

Biothérapiques et Nosodes. Maloine, 1962.
Materia Medica de Nosoden. 2e ed., 1975. K.F. Haug
Verlag, Heidelberg.

Pischel :

Kongressbericht uber die 123 Jahresversammlung der
D.Z.V.H.A. Allg. Homöop. Zeitg. No. 4, 1972.

Cartier F. :

Traité complet de Thérapeutique Homoeopathique, t. 4,
p. 128, Baillére, Paris. 1929.

Clarke J.H. :

A Dictionary of Pratical Materia Medica. London, 1955,
t. 4. Appendix, p. 1634.

P. Valerry-Radot, J. Hamburger and F. Lhermitte :

Pathologie Medicale. Flammarion Medicine, 1971, Paris.

STOCK

Lysate from the squams of a patient suffering from Scarlatina diluted and dynamised according to Homoeopathic pharmacopraxy.

This nosode is not at present sold in France.
Nelson, London delivers in 12 CM.

Reckeweg prepares it in injectable ampoules (D 15), D 20,
D 30, D 200 (and a separate dynamisation D 10).

The D.H.U. (Germany) prepares *Scarlatinum* in D 12 or
D 30 in dilution. Clarke prescribed *Scarlatinum* 30, on the
contrary stauffer (Germany) prefers the prescription of *Streptococcinum* 30.

There is no experimental pathogenesis according to the method of Hahnemann.

CLINICAL CORTICO-VISCERAL PROTOCOL OR CLINICAL PATHOGENESIS

Erythematous angina, painful with dysphagia, hyperthermia at 39°-40°.

Weakness, headache, vomiting, sometimes abdominal pains, asthenia.

Tumefaction of tonsils ; pharynx, red.

Cervical adenopathy. Tachycardia.

Diffused erythema on which are seen small plaques ; granite look of the skin.

Enanthema with the tongue of raspberry colour.

Nephritis with azotemia, hematuria or proteinuria.

Arthralgias. Rheumatism of fingers and hands.

POSOLOGY

Dynamisation : 12 and CM (Nelson) D 10 in injectable ampoules (Reckeweg).

DIFFERENTIAL DIAGNOSIS

See monograph on *Streptococcinum*.

Think of *Belladonna, Mercurius cyanatum, Arum triphylum, Echinacea angustifolia, Ailanthus gland.*

CLINICAL DIAGNOSIS

Delayed Sequalae of Scarlatina

According to Reckeweg.

Cardiac neurosis.

Coronary troubles ; angina pectoris.

Thrombopenic purpura (Morbus Werlhoff).

Chronic polyarthritis.

General asthenia from myocardia.

Psoriasis in swollen persons.

Ligamentary laxity.

Albuminuric nephritis with oedemas.

CLININAL OBSERVATION

Zinke, during the congress of D.Z.V.H.H., 1972, reports the clinical observation regarding an angina with hyperthermia as follows :

Profound asthenia, infectious look.

Grave hyperthemia of tonsils swollen, pillars; the uvula dark red, the submaxillary glands swollen, painful.

In the antecedents ; suffered from Scarlatina treated by *Penicilline*.

Since that time the general condition is bad and every year : Angina+Penicilline.

Prescription : Scarlatinum D 12, twice 2 globules the first day.

Immediate amelioration which the patient had not had till then.

Repeated once D 12 and 14 days after one dose of D 30. Cure.

SERUM OF ANTI-COLIBACILLARY

BIBLIOGRAPHY

M. Fortier-Bernoville :

Quelques réflexions sur la colibacillose. Bull. de la Soc. d'Homoeopathie de France, 1930, p. 246-251.

M. Martiny :

Quelques suggestions thérapeutiques sur le traitement de la Colibacillose. Bull. de la S.H.F., 1930, p. 251-254.

Kollitsch :

Traitement des colibacilluries. L'Homoeopathie Moderne, No. 16, Oct. 1934, p. 396.

Fortier-Bernoville :

Arsenal thérapeutique et plan général de traitement de la Colibacillose. L'Homoeopathie Moderne No. 16. Oct., 1934.

Julian O.A. :

Biothérapiques et Nosodes. Maloine, 1962.

Wurmser L :

Biotherapiques anticolibacillaries. Bulletin du C.H.F., 1961, p. 27-31.

Julian O.A. :

Materia Medica der Nosoden. K. Haug, Verlag, Heidelberg, 1975, 2e ed.

STOCK

The biotherapic anti-colibacillary serum is a purified form of the stock serum anti-colibacillary, of caprine origin.

COMPOSITION

1 ml. concentrated purified serum corresponds to 5 ml. of a crude serum originating from goats immunised by subcutaneous injections of *Escherichia coli*, free of any preserving or stabilising agents.

1. Technique of Preparation

(*a*) *Stocks used* : 3 stocks comprising of Escherichia-coli Marcy, 423, 430 and 431 each, having the classical characteristics of its type, are used.

Escherechia-coli are colonies of normal, shining, opaque, mobile, gram—, rod-shaped bacilli thriving on lactose, glucose, arabinose, xylose, maltose, mannite rhamnose G citrate— ; 1+ M+ ; VP— ; H2S— ; Gelatine O ; and milk coagulated.

These are checked with a morphological, biochemical and antigenic point of view and are conserved in lyophilised condition.

(*b*) *Preparation of the microbian suspension* : The stocks are cultivated on gelose then diluted in physiological water so as to obtain a microbian concentration of 10 millilards of germs per millilitre. This suspension is heated one hour at 70° and formulated at 2%. Thus the antigene is obtained for the immunisation of goats.

2. Immunisation and Bleeding of the Goat

The injections are given sub-cutaneously in the following sequence :

7 injections of 1 ml at 5 days interval.
5 injections of 2 ml at 5 days interval.

8 days after the 12th injection, drawing of 250 to 300 ml. blood.

On the very day of the bleeding an injection of 2 ml of antigen ; 6 days after another injection of 3 ml of antigen ; 8 days thereafter drawing of 250 to 300 ml. blood. Recharging and bleeding follow in the above order.

3. Collection of the Crude Serum

The blood is collected in mugs of sterile centrifuger and centrifuged 24 hours after the bleeding. The serum is sterily decanted and conserved in cold room+4° till purification.

4. Purification of the Serum

(*a*) Dilute half of the serum in physiological solution.

(*b*) Add 600 ml of serum to 1/2, 400 ml of ammonium sulphate, 50 g per 100 ml. Shake. Let it rest one night at room temp.+4°.

(*c*) Centrifuge in mugs for 20 minutes at 2800 t/mn. Collect the precipitate and dyalise it at 0° for 5 days against distilled water, of which the volume is at least 10 times the volume of the dialysed liquid, and is changed 5 times.

On the 6th day dyalise for 6 hours against a 8 g% solution of sodium chloride. After the dialysis, the absence of ammonia is verified.

(*d*) Collect the liquid, filter it on EKS amiante plaque. Note the volume and the titration in protein.

5. Distribution

The sterile purified serum is aspetically distributed in 1 ml sterile ampoules.

Contrary to the other biotherapics of which the pharmaceutical forms are doses and granules, the Anti-colibacillary serum is prepared in drinkable ampoules in dilutions 3 DH, 5 CH, 7 CH, 9 CH.

It is in fact the classical serum of Vincent but the animal from which it is obtained is a goat which is injected with two kinds of toxins :

1. One destroyed exotoxin at 75° which diffuses in the medium of the cultures of colibacilli after 2 to 3 days of incubation and which would be responsible for nervous disorders : fatigue, mental troubles, paralysis (neutrope toxins).

2. One endotoxin is the extract of the microbian bodies which are found in the 15 days old cultures and are destroyed by heat (90°). It is an enterotrope toxin.

CONTROL

It is submitted to a test of activity : When added the proportion of one hundredth and one millionth to cultures of colibacilli in nutritive bouillon, it should slow down the movement of the bodies of the bacilli and cause their agglutination.

The colibacilli cultures utilised should have the character near to those of which are used for the preparation of the lysate of Colibacillinum and it is good to verify the omnipotence of the serum on a sufficiently great varieties of stocks of pathological origin. The stock 113-3, cyanocobalamino-dependent is always agglutinated by Anticolibacillary Serum.

For Fortier-Bernoville who prefers much the Serum Anticolibacillary to the nosode Colibacillinum, preconised by L. Vannier, there would be in course of the passage in the animal a real dynamisation of the remedy. It is perhaps for this reason, Anticolibacillary Serum is, contrarily to other Nosodes, more often prescribed in lower dilutions : 3 DH, 5 DH.

HISTORY

Around 1930, the Colibacillosis attracted the attention of some clinicians. Thus *Albaran* admits of the "descending" infection by the blood system and *Heitz-Boyer* described the "syndrome entero renal" where the Colibacilli Escherisch, if it is the most frequent factor, is not alone but Bacilli of Friedlander, Proteus, Enterococcus, Staphylococcus may equally be the causes. This infection was first treated by vaccinotherapy then by serotherapy. It is *H. Vincent* who prepares an *Anticolebacillary serum.*

It is a serum coming from horses immunised by toxins, from several races of colibacillies, which produce some neurotropic toxins and an endotoxin. The serum is concentrated and de-albuminised.

It is why Fortier-Bernoville, having had some failures with Colibacillinum turns his mind towards the use of homoeotherapic *Anticolibacillary serum* of Vincent.

Here is what he writes in l'Homoeopathie Moderne of 15th Oct., 1934, p. 433.

Serum de Vincent : Diluted or not, it is, according to us, superior to *Colibacillinum*. Here are the rules that we have adopted for its use :

(*a*) *Acute case* : Try by mouth Serum Vincent 3 x, five, drops in some water three or four times during twenty-four hours. The results are often appreciable.

When there is the necessity to act soon, use the pure serum by mouth or by rectum, preferably by sub-cutaneous injection in order to avoid the accidents from serum.

It is M. Martiny who used first the Vincent serum by mouth (so it is ordered in ampoules the non-purified product, *i.e.* not de-albuminised by the use of formol, one or two ampoules a day in sugared water).

Results are remarkable and often very rapid on fever and on general acute phenomena.

We have also obtained very beautiful results using it by rectum (perhaps more rapid because of the absorption directly by the hemorrhoidary veins). One or two ampoules a day are prescribed to be used by a small douche after evacuating washing.

(*b*) *Chronic cases* : The *Vincent serum* may be used in all dilutions, from 3 x to 1,000 centesimal, either progressively, or concurrently.

The lower dilutions act better on physical, digestive, urinary troubles and on colibacilluria.

The medium and the high act electively on the nervous and mental symptoms : Asthenia, weakness, discouragement, diminution of activity. Thanks to S. Vincent 200 and 1000 (every ten to twelve days) and *Thuya* 200 and 1000 at the same time, associated with S. Vincent 30 (once every day when waking up in the morning) we have had fortunate results, and even three undeniable successes in psychoasthenic conditions (two personal cases and 1 case that we have followed with Professor Page of Montpellier).

Later on Kollitsch utilised even 10 DH of the Serum Anti-Colib, and thus it has entered in France in daily practice.

It is less or not known in Anglo-saxon countries where on the contrary, the nosodes of *Bach* and *Paterson* dominate the prescription.

In German countries, this medicine is being used since the publication of Materia Medica der Nosoden of Dr. O.A. Julian.

CLINICAL CORTICO-VISCERAL PROTOCOL
OR CLINICAL PATHOGENESIS

1. Generalities

Chronic asthenic conditions.

Allergoso states (Psoric)—tubercular conditions.

Great lability of the mind with the state of excitation or neurovascular inhibition.

Vaso-motor troubles of the peripheries, localised specially on the lower limbs.

2. Neuro-endocrino-psychic System

(a) *Psychic*

Anergy, loss of will power.
Doubt leads to scruple, scruple to phobia.
Phobia of crowds, of spaces.

Nocturnal anxiety.

Prostrated attitude, immobile, dumb, face with painful impression due to moral distress.

Mental confusion with difficult ideation and intellectual obnubilation.

(b) *Nervous* :

Perturbation of the *memory*, partial fixation.

Frontal headaches with vertigo and intense torpor.

Rachialgia ; myalgia.

3. Digestive Apparatus

Pasty tongue ; bad breath specially in the morning.

Dry, pasty mouth, need for cold drinks which ameliorates.

Intestinal gurgling, with spasmodic pain in the large intestine.

Swollen gall bladder, painful with sometimes sub-febrile condition and chill.

Atonic constipation.

Verminosis.

4. Cardio-hemo-vascular System

Hypotension and tendency to collapse.

Moderate cyanosis of ankles which are swollen during the day.

Thermoregulation : Moderate fever with chill.

5. Respiratory Apparatus

Irritation of the throat which is red, sensitive.

Spasmodic cough with stickly mucous secretions.

Pain in the throat while breathing deeply with spasmodic cough.

6. Organ of Senses

(a) *Nose* :

Pain in the root of the nose.

Purulent nasal discharge when bending the head forward.

Aggravation by humid cold.

Pain in the sub-orbitary hole, of the canine fossa, of the middle of the lower bone.

(*b*) *Eyes* : Conjunctivas painfully sensitive.

Ocular balls are painful with a sensation of coldness.

(*c*) *Ears* : Painful congestion of the tympanum which is of deep amber colour ; sometimes a line of transparent liquid surface is seen.

7. **Uro-genital Apparatus**

(*a*) *Urinary* :

Frequent micturition, urgent, imperious.

Burning of the meatus of the urethral canal.

Turbid, alkaline urines.

Oxaluria.

(*b*) *Genital—Man* :

Slow, difficult erection.

Clear diminution of the libido.

Sometimes pain in the urethra after ejaculation.

Small testicles, soft, painful.

Woman :

Yellow, irritating leucorrhoea.

Clear diminution of the libido.

Painful sensitiveness in the vaginal cul-de-sac.

Bilateral pains of the ovarian region.

8. **Loco-motor System**

Pains in the shoulders, better by movement.

9. **Modalities**

Aggravation : In humid cold.

Amelioration : By rest and by heat.

Laterality : Right, but not significative.

POSOLOGY

Dynamisation : 3 DH, 5 CH, 9 CH, 15 CH, 30 CH.

But this biotherapic has the particularity to be supplied in the form of liquid dilutions, in drinkable ampoules.

In acute cases, the Serum anti-colibacillary 3 DH is used.

—either by mouth, one ampoule every two to three hours.

—or by rectum, 3 ampoules by douche and to be retained taking the precaution to give beforehand an evacuating douche.

In chronic cases may be used 3 DH, one ampoule morning and evening for entero-renal troubles ; 7 CH, 9 CH or better 30 CH one dose a day for psychic troubles. (O.A. Julian)

Finally in acute genital affections, in acute cases, it is necessary to use the medicine as described above. If as a consequence, there is a sub-chronic stage it is 7 CH which is advised.

POSITIVE DIAGNOSIS

Cortico-somatic lability with the tendency of neuro-vascular obnubility.

Energy, doubt, scruples, phobias.

Loss of memory ; frontal headache.

Gastro-intestional dystonia.

Laryngo-tracheal irritation.

Micturitional troubles ; diminution of libido (male and female).

Salpingo-ovaritis.

DIFFERENTIAL DIAGNOSIS

Colibacillinum (See article).

The tuberculins : T.K., T.R. (See articles).

Folliculostimuline : Preconised by L. Fouché in SC. and IM injections, in 7 CH, 2 to 3 times a week. It is an excellent remedy of acute and chronic Colibacillosis.

It is also necessary to mention here the homoeotherapics : *Silicea* and *Anacardium orientalis*.

CLINICAL DIAGNOSIS

1. Generalities

Allergoso-tuberculinosic states.

Jacquelin-Burnard broken down condition.

2. Neuro-endocrino-psychic System

Depression neurosis.

Melancholy.

Schizophrenia (in the beginning).

Cyclothymia ; aprosexia.

Characterial troubles of children.

Part amnesia of fixation.

3. Digestive Apparatus

Gastro-enteritis.

Angiocholitis ; biliary lithiasis.

4. Cardio-vascular System

Hypotonia.

Acrocyanosis.

5. Respiratory and Sense Organs

Laryngo-tracheitis.

Ethmoidal frontal sinusitis.

Conjunctivitis.

Otitis of babies.

6. Loco-motor System

Scapulo-humeral arthrosis.

COMMENTARIES

Anti-colibacillary serum introduced by Martiny and Fortier-Bernoville in the isotherapic "Arsenal" is surely a useful remedy.

As some question regarding the School which separated L. Vannier from the authors mentioned above, the result was that Léon Vannier has ignored the Anticolibacillary serum and he did not mentioned in his Materia Medica while Martiny and Fortier-Bernoville, on the contrary, have denied the therapeutic action of Colibacillinum.

Thus we have two remedies : *Colibacill.* and *Ser. Anti-colib.* as two clinical biotherapics because they have not been proved according to the method of Hahnemann.

And it is regratable, because it is possible that their therapeutic importance might have been better defined.

Regarding the Anticolibacillary serum, the following remarks are, however, to be noted :

If one wishes really to obtain a serious therapeutic action in *an acute or subacute salpingitis*, in a *pyelitis, pyelonephritis* or *cystitis*, acute or subacute, the serum Anticolibacillary is to be prescribed in 3 DH, 1 ampoule every hour. To be espaced after 24 or 48 hours when the amelioration is manifested. The failures result for non-observation of this rule. It is for this reason at the beginning, when the prescriptions failed that one had to fall back to dosage or to allotherapic.

In chronic cases, regarding mind : *melancholy, anxiety neurosis, depressive neurosis, stupor stages*, it is the 7 CH, 9 CH but rather 30 CH twice daily are strongly advised. (O.A. Julian)

In the case of *hyponutrition* with ancrexia, micropolyadeno-pathies, tics, verminosis, in children, the 7 CH twice daily will surely give good results.

Without forgetting *the colibacillary otitis of babies* and of which the local symptom remains dumb but the aspect (athrepsic) becomes evident.

There is 3 DH, 2-3 ampoules a day then 7 CH may equally give clear amelioration.

Similarly the dragging "primo-infectious" conditions may be treated with good results by Anticolibacillary serum in 3 DH and 7 CH.

Thus, we see that if one knows how to manipulate this remedy like Colibacillinum, it is possible that it will become useful to the patient without being injurious.

SERUM OF YERSIN

BIBLIOGRAPHY

Fortier-Bernovile :

Sérum antipestieux de Yersin. L'Homoeopathie Moderne No. 6, 15 mars, 1936, p. 398.

Barishac :

Idem, p. 386.

Julian O.A. .

Biothérapiques et Nosodes. Maloine, 1962, Paris.
Materia Medica der Nosoden. 2e ed. 1975. Haug Verlag. Heidelberg.

P. Vallery-Radot, J. Hamburger and F. Lhermitte :

Pathologie Médicale, Flammarion Médecine, 1971, Paris.

Ferron Azele :

Bactériologie, 1930.

Clarke J. :

A Dictionary of Practical Materia Medica, London, 1955, v. 3, p. 740.

STOCK

The biotherapic Serum of Yersin is derived from the anti-pest serum described in the Codex, 1949, p. 741, supplied by institute Pasteur.

This serum is obtained from animals which have been immunised by means of "killed" cultures or living cultures of plague bacilli, *Bacillus-pestis*.

The Yersin Bacilli secrete an exotoxin of proteic nature, thermolabile (killed at 70%) and with which one may obtain an anatoxin by addition of 4% of formol.

(551)

Anatoxin and microbe bodies also produce a serum of the same quality.

Trial : 0·1 ml of anti-pest serum is sufficient to protect against the infection in a rat inoculated 16 hours before with a dose of the culture of pest bacilli, capable of killing the witness animals within a time which varies from 48 to 60 hours.

HISTORY

According to Fortier-Bernoville, it is Barishac who proposed, for the treatment of grave or a typical forms of influenza, this remedy in dynamisations 6 and 30 CK (4 CH and 7 CH).

There exists no pathogenesis according to the experimental method of Hahnemann.

CLINICAL CORTICO VISCERAL PROTOCOL OR CLINICAL PATHOGENESIS

Grave toxic-infectious state, either cutaneous (bubo) or pulmonary.

Septicemias accompanied with icterus and hepatic micro-abscess.

Mesenteric adenitis.

Acute gastro-enteritis with lesions of ileum.

Acute enteritis of young children.

Nodulous erythema.

POSOLOGY

Dynamisations : 4 CH, 5 CH, 7 CH, 9 CH.

At Nelson, London, may be had Pestinum 30-200.

DIFFERENTIAL DIAGNOSIS

Mimosa pudica : (Matière médicale d'Homoeopthérapie by O.A. Julian and Collab, Paris, Le François, 1971). Thoracic pain, dry cough, irritation of naso-pharyngeal and laryngeal mucous, frequent irritating stools with colic. Better by not bath.

Amorphophallus Rivieri : General ill feeling with great weakness, gastro-intestinal troubles with weakening diarrhoea, foetid stools.

CLINICAL DIAGNOSIS

Severe form of influenza, of pulmonary type with hyperthermia ; respiratory troubles, soft thick, rosy expectorations, presence of sub-crepitant rales in the base of lungs.

Acute entero-colitis.

Summer gastro-enteritis.

Acute toxicosis of babies.

Lymphoid terminal ileitis of Arnulf and Buffart.

Crohn's, regional ileitis.

Influenza of gastro-intestinal form.

Pseudo-typho meningitis of milkmen.

Meningitic syndromes of influenzal origin.

Encephalitis lethargica.

Parkinson's disease (?).

SPENGLER

(Immunising body of Spengler)

(C.J. Spengler)

BIBLIOGRAPHY

Vannier L :

Les tuberculiniques et leur traitment homoeopathique.

Doin, Paris, 1958.

Cartier Fr. :

Thérapeutique des voies réspiratories.   J.B. Baillére et Fils.
Paris, 1930, 2e ed.

Julian O.A. :

Biothérapiques et Nosodes.   Librairie Maloine, Paris, 1962.
Materia Medica der Nosoden. K. Haug Verlag, Heidelberg,.
1975, 2e ed.

Consult :

General Bibliography.

HISTORY

Spengler started from the idea (completely different from
all those ideas given out up to that time) that the hematies play
an essential part in the phenomena of immunity and that the
immunising substances are accumulated principally in the
stroma of these hematies from animals artificially immunised.

STOCK

It is therefore necessary to put the latter in liberty by the
dissolution of the total blood that is obtained by projecting
immediately in a solution of 3% lactic acid, a certain quantity
of blood collected by puncturing with syringe in the marginal
vein of the inoculated rabbit.

For inoculating the rabbits C. Spengler inoculates them at first in the plain muscle with a small quantity of human B.K. This method of inoculation is selected taking into account of the fact that the muscle and the tissue are the most favourable to the multiplication of tubercular bacilli. This blood may be mixed with that of other rabbits immunised against different other microbes. The rabbits may be prepared even by auto-vaccins (B.K. and other microbes taken from the patient to be treated). Spengler *calls them complete antitubercular immunising bodies.*

The mother tincture of blood is at 1/100,000. It is a colour-less liquid very slightly acid, does not become turbid while diluting and contains some traces of methemoglobine.

For therapeutic use, dilution is made in the following anti-septic vehicle :

> CINA..................... 5g
> Phenic acid.............. 5g
> Lactic acid...............3g
> Distilled water......1,000g.

Successively seven dilutions are made with each tenth of the mother tincture, in the vehicle ; these dilutions are numbered I-VIII. Since the mother solution is already at 1/100·000, *i.e.* 5 D, the therapeutic dilutions go from 6 D to 12 D.

Spengler attributes to this immunising bodies a lytic power face to face with B.K. and an antitoxic power face to face with tuberculin.

Measurement of a Lytic Power

The mother solution is injected to a rabbit and after 24 hours is inoculated with a small quantity of B.K. virulent, under the skin of the ear. If the bacilli are absorbed it is the proof of the lytic effect. Calmette strongly criticised this test estimating that the bacilli are not dissolved but carried and channelled through the lympth.

Control of the Antitoxic Power

Spengler simultaneously injected a cobaye with 1 ml of dilution at 1/1000,000 of the mother solution and a mortal dose of Tuberculin. If the animal resists then the dilution used had one antitoxic unit, *i.e.*, 1 million of units for the mother solution.

The immunizing treatment of Davos is carried out as follows. One injection every 10 days :

1st inj.........1 ml No. VI	6th inj............1 ml No. 1
2nd............1 ml No. V	7th...............0·2 ml mother solution
3rd............1 ml No. IV	8th...............0·5 ml mother solution
4th............1 ml No. III	9th ....0·8 ml mother solution
5th............1 ml No. II	10th ....1 ml mother solution

There would be some interesting results.

Roepke denies them, estimating the effects of that therapeutic comparable to those of distilled water.

But *Sophie Fuchs-Wolfring* (Revue de la Tuberculose, fev. 1912) and Castaigne and Benazet (Journal de Med. Franc, 15 juillet, 1914) have seen some undeniable clinical ameliorations.

Paul *A. Meckel* of Bad-Godesberg (Germany) continues to prepare the vaccin *"Spenglersan"* and of which the indication resides in the different forms of osseous and visceral tuberculosis. The field of therapeutics has been extended to a number of other infections in consequence of modifications and addition to the original product (vascular troubles, varicose ulcers, cancers...)

The Nosode of Spengler and the Spenglarsan are not found in the French pharmaceutical market. Therefore they cannot be prescribed.

CLINICAL PATHOGENESIS

1. Paleness of the face, skin, and mucous membranes.
2. Thermic elevation before menses.
3. Great fatigued state.

DIFFERENTIAL DIAGNOSIS

Ferrum phos. Congestive headache, epistaxis, dry painful cough, fever, congestion of the lungs or intestines, articular or otitic or abscess.

Ferrum met. : Anemia, slow digestion, hyperthermia, alternating redness and paleness.

Natrum mur. : Emaciation, anemia, headache, median fissure of the lower lip, desire for salt, sensitiveness to cold.

Kali carb. : Fatigue, slow digetion, hydric retention, swelling of the internal angle of the upper eyelids.

CLINICAL DIAGNOSIS

Tubercular conditions.

Beginning of tuberculosis.

Anemia.

Fre-menstrual fever.

POSOLOGY

None of the laboratories of France or of foreign lands prepare the Biotherapic Spengler.

In Germany the Spenglersan-Meckel is found. 53 Bad Godesberg 1 in colloidal and injectable form.

STAPHYLOCOCCINUM

BIBLIOGRAPHY

Julian O.A. :

Biothérapiques et Nosodes. Librarie Maloine, 1972, Materia Medica der Nosoden, 2e ed. K.F. Haug Verlag, Heidelberg, 1975.

P. Vallery-Rodot, J. Hamburger and F. Lhermitte :

Pathologie medicale-Flammarion, Medicine, 1959.

Ferron Azédé. : Bacteriologic. Azele Ferron, 1970.

Fasquelle R. : Elements de Bactériologie-Médical, Flammarion, 1959.

Cartier Ft. : Traité complet de Thérapeutique Homoeopathique. t.2, Baillere et Fils, Paris, 1929.

Lammason Fr. :

Traitement homoeopathique des manifestations aigues du zona et ses rapports avec la varicelle. Annales Hom. Fr. 1968, No. 6, p. 447.

STOCK

The biotherapic *Staphylococcinum* is prepared from a culture without addition of antiseptic from a mixture of many stocks of Staphylococcus.

The lysated suspension corresponds to 10 milliards in a cm^3 of *Pyogenes aureus, Staphylococcus*.

The trade presentation is a box of 3 ampoules of 1 ml to be used after homoeopathic dilution.

TECHNIQUES OF PREPARATION

1. Stock Utilised

Two stocks of *Staphylacoccus pyogenes aureus*, Marcy No. 435 and No. 436. These stocks have the characters of the classical type. They are checked for their morphological, bio-chemic characters and from an antigenic point of view.

Cocci in mass Gr+produce a homogeneous turbid bouillon.

Special characteristic of the stock 435 : Mix hemolysin gradu-ally and it spontaneously autolyses, quite completely in 5 days at 37°. This autolysate is very lightly hemolytic and non-toxic.

Special characters of the stock 436 : Hemolysine completes autolysis in 4 days at 37°. This autolysate is very slightly hemolytic and non-toxic.

They are conserved in lyophilised condition.

2. Culture Medium

(*a*) Maceration of chopped meat.....................500 g.
Water...1000 cm³.

Leave in contact for 34 hours, then filter after having heated in the stove for 30 minutes at 100° and 30 minutes at 110°.

(*b*) Add :
Peptone.......................................13 g.
Sodium chloride........................... 5 g.
Powder Gelose............................. 30 g.

Dissolve on autoclave at 100° for 30 minutes.
(*c*) Adjust the PH at 7, 2 by addition of soda.
(*d*) Put on autoclave at 110° for 20 minutes.
(*e*) Distribute in tubes, in Roux boxes.
(*f*) Sterilise at 110° for 20 minutes.

3. Inoculation of the Cultures

The two lyophilised stocks are put in solution then inocu-lated on slanting tubes of the medium described before.

After 24 hours of culture in an incubator at 37°, the colonies are examined to be sure of the characteristic types of these cultures and of the purity of the stocks.

The culture of each tube is washed in volume of 5 cm³ of solution of 9% Sodium chloride, then taken up by pippette for inoculating on Roux boxes containing 1,200 cm³ of the same medium.

The Roux boxes are placed in their turn in the incubator at 37°.

After 48 hours of stay in the incubator the boxes are individually examined in order to be assured of the purity of the colonies.   Now 25 to 30 cm³ of sterile distilled water is added to each.

After the suspension of the microbe culture by manual balancing the bacterian suspension obtained is collected by vacuum aspiration in a sterile recipient. This suspension is adjusted at 20 milliards of germs in cm³ by addition of sterile distilled water.

The suspension thus obtained is heated at 60° for one hour then placed immediately afterwards in refrigerator at +3, +5.

4. Lysate and Obtaining of Endotoxins

The killed suspension is placed in the incubator at 37° for 5 days. It is then centrifuged in sterile tubes at a speed to 6,000/t.mn for a time sufficient to obtain a complete sedimentation of the lysated bacterian debris. The floating suspension of endotoxins is then collected, submitted to a filtration on seitz EKS filters and conserved in the refrigrator at +3°+5°.

5. Dilution

To the suspension of endotoxins is added an equal volume of sterile distilled water which brings thus to the concentration of 10 milliards of germs in a cm³.

6. Distribution

The vaccin suspension may now be distributed aseptically in ampoules.

CONTROL

The products thus obtained undergo the following tests :

(*a*) *Neutrality* : The PH of the lysate should be between 7 and 7,2.

(*b*) *Sterility* : Inoculation on bouillon or gelose should not produce any culture.

(*c*) *Non-toxicity* : The injection subcutaneously of 1 ml of lysate should not cause any accident.

(*d*) *Activity* : It consists in the research of the hemolysing property of the lysate using standard hematines of rabbit.

CLINICAL CORTICO-VISCERAL PROTOCOL
OR
CLINICAL PATHOGENESIS

1. Generalities

Pre-diabetic conditions.

Allergoso-mesenchymatosic conditions (Psoro-sycotic).

Syndrome of acute septicemia : Oscilliating fever with great chill, general condition is weakened, splenomegalis.

2. Neuro-endocrino-psychic System

Radiculitis.
Myelitis.
Meningitis.
Abscess of the brain.

3. Cardio-hemo-vascular System

Endocarditis : Extinction then veiled but hard, reappearance of the first apexian sound or of the second sound at the base ; later on the durable organic sounds of valvular insufficiency.

Pericarditis : Pericardiac rubbing. Myocardia : dull noises, tensional fall and arythmias.

4. Respiratory Apparatus

Disseminated pulmonary condensation, miliary, disseminated or multiple abscesses.

Purulent pleural exudations.

5. Uro-genital Apparatus

Pyuria.

Peri-nephritic phlegmon.

Prostatitis.

Acute prostatic abscess.

6. Loco-motor System

Spondylitis.

Osteitis.

Osteomyelitis.

7. Skin

Follicular pustule.

Abscess of the nasaJ fossa.

Abscess of the eyelids (styes).

Sycosis of the moustache.

Folliculitis of the integument.

Hydrosadenitis of the armpits.

Anthrax. Ecthyma.

Panaris. Onyxis. Perionyxis.

Purpura, vesiculo-pustular.

POSOLOGY

Dynamisation : 4 CH, 5 CH, 7 CH, 9 CH.

DIFFERENTIAL DIAGNOSIS

Rajania-subsamarata (O.A. Julian-Matiére médicale d'homoeotherapie). High fever, prostration, neuro-hemo-vascular congestion, swelling of the neck and of the parotidian region, circumscribed inflammation of the skin with tumefaction or ulceration. As well as classics : *Rhus veneta* or *vernix* : *Anagallis arvensis*.

CLINICAL DIAGNOSIS

Furuncle. Impetigo.

Panaris. Anthrax.

Osteomyelitis.

Peri-nephritic phlegmon.

Zona (Lamasson).

CLINICAL CASES

Here are the clinical observations of F. Lamasson published in the Annales homeopathiques françaises No. 6, 1968, p 3/477.

Case 1 : Ophthalmic zona

Mme A. L......33 years. On the morning of the 10th April the patient feels an extreme pain above the left upper eyelid. Very rapidly, there appeared, at the end of three hours. three oval patches with regular contours, situated on the upper eyelid and on the left side of the forehead. These rosy patches are of 8 to 15 mm in diameter. Six hours after there are some functional symptoms ; on the patches appeared some vesicles having clear content. The pain is intolerable. There is not yet corneal anaesthesia. The diagnosis of ophthalmic zona was evident. We immediately gave a dose of *Staphylococcinum* 9 CH.

The 11th April in the morning *i.e.* to say 20 hours afterwards the starting of the disease and 12 hours after the dose of *Staphylococcin* 9CH, the pains completely disappeared. The vesicles persisted. We perscribed *Rhus tox* 4 CH, granules every two hours.

From that time, the evolution of vesicles was towards drying with such a rapidity that on the 12th April on the morning there persists only, on the temporal region, a light redness which disappeared in 'the evening. The total evolution did

19 F

not go beyond 50 hours. On the 14th April, we advised the patient to stop using *Rhus tox* 4 CH. There remained no pigmentation, and the most interesting phenomenon is that there was no anaesthesia of the frontal or palpebral zone affected by zona.

Case 2 : Left intercostal zona

M.G.B......23 years complains since yesterday evening a smarting sensation on the left hemithorax ; the pain begins above the point of the shoulder blade, crosses the axillary line at the height of the mammary line and stops on the sternal manubrium.

By examination we noted the extreme cutaneous hyperesthesis of that region and the presence of several red patches, which were of oval shaped covered with vesicles with a clear content.

The topography and the characteristic of these cutaneous elements led us to the diagnosis of herpes.

Stayphylococcinum 9 CH, one dose to be taken in the same evening, two hours after the dinner.

Rananculus bulhosus 4 CH, two granules every three hours because of the left laterality and the seat of the eruption.

The next day 13th November, pains stopped in the morning, towards 11 o'clock. The red patches have become pale, the vesicles sank down.

On the 14th November in the evening, the eruption completely disappeared, having consequently, taken a duration of three full days.

Case 3 : Zona of the sciatic nerve behind the knee

Mme Tar....68 years. On the 21st June, 1939, this patient felt a smarting on the posterior face of the calf, and under the left heel.

On 22nd June there appeared some oval red patches on the posterior face of the calf. These patches were of 12 to 30 milimeteres, their borders are regular, their surface is covered with papulovesicles having clear content. The smarting is particularly great, and it is this symptom and the appearance of the eruptions which forced the patient to come to consult us. The topography, the character of the eruption and the pains led us to the diagnosis of zona. We prescribed :

Staphylococcinum 9 CH : One dose to be taken immediately.

Rhus tox 4 CH :   2 granules every 3 hours from tomorrow morning.

The functional troubles stopped completely on the 24th June in the morning. The vesicles are dry, replaced by small crusts which were falling down. On the 26th June, the skin became normal, no pigmentation persisting, no pain inspite of the age of the patient—68 years.

Case 4 :

We were taking rest for some days in the Basse-Nomandie, in April 1931, when called to see a young man of 20 years who was suffering from a herpes since one week.

The seat of the lesions were on the left side of the face. Some vesicles and the ulcers in patches, extending to the integument, forehead, nose, the cheek, the upper lip. The mucous of the left nostril and the upper part of the palate were also attacked. The left eyelid of the patient was swollen and had two vesicles on the ciliary border. He was complaining of the light but except the conjunctiva the rest of the eye was unaffected.

The fever was rising up to 38·8°, and the beating of the pulse which is normal at 50 in this person, rose upto 70. He was suffering also from insomnia and nausea for which he could not take food for 24 hours, and violent headache "like electric shocks", very painful to the trajectory of the attacked nerve.

The young man was taking 1 g of Sulphate of quinine, divided into four doses daily, while the external medication was limited to a cleaning of the lesions with a bit of cotton imbibed in ether.

Wh₂t would a homoeopath have done having no special remedy with him ?

An Isopathic was prepared exactly according to the process utilised by Father Collet in Asia Minor. On a sterilised gauge we collected some erosions and some saliva flowing from the ulcer of the left side of the palate. The gauge is put into glass of water for 5 minutes then a 6th centesimal was prepared by hand. The last one is made in 95° alcohol.

In the afternoon, the patient took 3 doses of the Isotherapic every half an hour. In the evening he complained of slight exacerbation of pains and could not sleep before the morning, which did not happen to him since two nights.

On the day of 8th August, the day following the taking of the Isopathic, the pains calmed down, the nausea disappeared. Suddenly the patient was feeling much better, but the lesions remained as before. He was advised to take the Isopathic three times in a day and that he should stop Sulphate of quinine.

The 9th August : The sleep was good, there was only a vague headache, a kind of fatigue, said the patient in the attacked area. The ulcers reduced to half and the oedema of the lid almost disappeared. Three more doses of the Isotherapic.

The 15th August : Before coming back to Paris, we went to see the patient. Crusts on the face were thick, and hard and healthy, those of the parts the most attacked have begun to fall off. The palate and the nostrils are normal. The neuralgia has not reappeared any time during the week that we saw the patient.

We have not seen again that person, whom we came to know, only on our way, not knowing even his name. The ulcers were becoming cicatrised very rapidly, but the fact which struck us was the disappearance of the neuralgia within the 10 first hours which followed the adminstration of the Isopathic and which did not reappear any more during the eight days when we saw the patient again.

The action of an Isotherapic used on the 8th day, *i.e.* to say in a time when the well indicated remedies caused only temporary amelioration of the pains and the eruption, is a supplementary example of everything that one may expect of Isotherapics in acute cases and specially in virus diseases. It is the most dangerous experiment for the Isopathic then to use precisely at a time when the patient was in the most violent state of the disease, in the full period of evolution and the disappearance of pains within a few days in this condition is a remarkable success regarding to the activity of the Isotherapic.

STAPHYLOTOXINUM

BIBLIOGRAPHY

Consult the biliography of Staphylococcinum.

STOCK

The biotherapic Staphylotoxinum is nothing but the ana-toxins of Staphylococcus obtained by the combination of formol and of the heat on the Staphylococcus toxin. This toxin is the filtrate on the bougie L-3 and amiant of a culture of Staphylo-coccus stock Nelis 72. Toxin is titrated :

(*a*) For its necrosing effect : 1/2,000 mililitres of toxin should cause by intradermal injection a patch of oedema of 0·5 cm with a black crust of 2 mm diameter.

(*b*) For its lethal action : the injection of 0, 2 to 0, 4 ml to a rabbit should develop some grave cerebral symptoms : sinking of the hind paws, inclination of the head, convulsions of the front paws, restlessness and death.

(*c*) For its hemolytic effect, using a standard suspension of hematies of rabbit. The toxin is transformed into anatoxin by the technique of Ramon and Richou : addition of formol in the proportion of 3, 9 and 5 ml/l and maintaining the liquid for-molated at 37° for ten days.

CONTROL

(*a*) *Sterility* : The inoculation on bouillon or better on gelose should not follow in any culture.

(*b*) *Non-toxicity* : By sub-cutaneous injection of 1 ml to rats of 20 g each should not cause any accident. The rabbit should tolerate without damage the injection of the product.

(*c*) *Activity* : It is estimated by the method of initial floccu-lation by a standard antistaphylococcic serum.

It should be noted that the word "Staphylotoxinum" meant before the regulations on Biotherapics the simple filtrate of culture of Staphylococcus.

CLINICAL PATHOGENESIS

Staphylotoxinum (Staphylococcic antoxin) has not been the object of an experimentation according to the methodology of Hahnemann.

Its use is indicated as a complementary to Staphylococcinum and with the same indications, by its anatoxic specificity.

The presence of alpha hemolysine is a character, essential of the stocks, having the pathogenic potential in man.

Clinical indications :

Contractions.

Purpura.

Convulsions.

Hemophilia.

Alimentary intoxication.

POSOLOGY

Dynamisations : 4 CH, 5 CH, 7 CH, 9 CH.

STREPTOCOCCINUM

BIBLIOGRAPHY

Julian O.A. :

Biothèrapiques-Nosodes. Maloine, Paris, 1962.

Materia Medica der Nosoden. Haug Verlag, Ulm Donau, 1960.

Boericke. :

Materia Medica and Repertorium. Verlag Grundlagen und Praxis.

Margarethe Harms Leer. lre ed. Allemande, 1972, p. 468.

Materia Medica with Repertory, 9th ed. Boericke and Tafel, 1927, p. 541.

Sevaux F. and Emar. A. :

Contribution a l'étude de l'action biologique des dilutions homoeopathiques : Streptococcinum 7 CH and 9 CH. l'Homoeop, Fr., avril, No. 4, 1959, p. 197-206.

Julian O.A. and Collab :

Matiére Médicale d'Homoeothérapie 1971. Le Francois, 91, bd. St-Germain, 75006, Paris.

Fasquelle R :

Eléments de bactériologie Médicale, 1959. Méd., Flommarion.

Ferron Azele :

Bactériologie, 1970.

Pommier De Santi :

Etude théorique et pratique d'un nouveau nosode de la sycose : Le Strepto-Enterococque. Rev. Fr. d'Hom., No. 4, 1950.

J. Hui-Bon-Hoa :

Streptococcinum et Staphylococcinum. Revue de livres, in Annales Hom. fr., novembre, 1963.

Guillaume :

Streptococcinum. Annales Homoeop. fr. No. 2, février, 1969.

Steinschneider R. :

Complication de la Scarlatine. Suppl., Vie Medicale, mars, 1970 (II).

Guillame and Zissu :

Nosodes et Biothèrapiqus mineurs en pratique courante. Ann. Hom. fr., 1960, No. 2, p. 143.

STOCK

The streptococcus was discovered by Pasteur in 1879.

The biotherapic streptococcinum is prepared from the lysate obtained without the addition of antiseptic from culture prepared from a mixture of many stocks of Streptococcus, supplied by the Mèrieux Institute.

It is the question of a lysated suspension corresponding to 10 milliards of Streptococcus, per cm^3 pyogenus Rosenbach, and is supplied in the form of 1 ml ampoules from which the homoeopathic dilutions are made.

1. Stock Utilised

Two stocks of pyogenus Rosenbach Streptococcus, Mercy Nos. 433, 434. These stocks have the character of the classical type. They are checked for their morphological, biochemic and antigenic characters.

Cocci in short chains and in medium chains Gr+, producing in bouillon some flakes which sediment without disturbing the medium and on gelose some five white colonies.

2. Medium of Culture

(*a*)   Maceration of chopped viande   500 c.

   Water   1,000 m³

Leave in contact for 24 hours then filter after having heated on the autoclave for 30 minutes at 100° and 30 minutes at 100°.

(*b*)   Peptone   12g

   Sodium chloride   5g

   Glucose   10g

   To be added to the liquid (*a*).

(*c*) Adjust the PH at 7, 2 by the addition of Soda.

(*d*) Distribute two litres in bottles of 3 litres and in tubes of 20 cm³.

(*e*) Sterilise at 110° for 20 minutes.

3. Inoculations and Culture

These two stocks which are lyophilised are inoculated in tubes of glucosed bouillon and on a tube of gelose with blood which helps to control the purity and the hemolytic power.

After 24 hours of culture at 37° and microscopic examination, it is inoculated in phials of glucosed bouillon. It is cultivated 48 hours at 37°.

After microscopical examination of each phial the culture is centrifuged aseptically and the residues are taken in physiological water and centrifuged again. The residues of the second centrifugation are taken in distilled water so as to have a concentration of 20 milliards per cm³.

The suspension thus obtained is heated at 60° for one hour and then placed immediately in the refrigerator +3° +5°.

4. Lysate and the Getting of the Endotoxins

The bacterian suspension is transferred to a recipient of resistant pyrex glass. It is then congealed at a temperature of —30° to —40° for 24 hours. Then the suspension is left to be decongealed and left at least at + 20° during 24 hours.

The operation of congealation and decongealation should be done again for 3 times, *i.e.*, in total four operations.

Then centrifuged in sterile tubes at a speed of 6,000 t/mn for a time sufficient to obtain a complete sedimentation of the debris of the lysated bacteriae. The floating suspension of endotoxins is then collected, put to a filtration on Seitz filtre and conserved in refrigerator at $+3°, +5°$.

5. Dilution

The suspension of endotoxin is added to an equal volume of water, distilled and steriled which thus brings at a concentration of 10 milliards of germs in a cm^3.

6. Distribution

The vaccin suspension may then be distributed aseptically in sterile ampoules.

Control

(*a*) *Sterility* :

The inoculation on bouillon or better on gelose should not be followed by any culture.

(*b*) *Non-toxicity* :

By subcutaneous injection of 1 ml to some rats of 20 g, there should be no accident. The rabbit should bear without damage the injection of 5ml of the product.

HISTORY

The clinical pathogenesis has been established by F. Sevaux and A. Emar in 1958 (L'Homoeop. fr. 1959, p. 197).

A study by Dr. Gosh according to the report of J. Hui-Bon-Hoa, Ann Homeop. fr., November 1963, shows the differential interest of Strepto and Staphylococcinum.

Then a very interesting clinical work of Dr. Guillaume (Ann. H. Fr., 1969) completes the picture of the clinical pathogenesis of Streptococcinum.

Finally we add, our own clinical experience.

CLINICAL CORTICO-VISCERAL PROTOCOL
OR CLINICAL PATHOGENESIS

1. Generalities

Subject with tears, weeping without reason.

Multiple intolerance : Noise, light, least current of air caused by the moving of a person.

Exaggerated obsequiousness.

Hopeless of his cure, hopeless of his condition.

2. Neuro-endocrino-psychic System

1. *Psychic :*

Depressed, obsessional condition : Thinks that he will become mad.

2. *Nervous :*

Vertigo while rising and while lying down.

Sensorial troubles.

Auditive hallucinations (hears cry for help).

Visual hallucination (sees the room full of flies).

Cenestopathies : Sensation of vibrations in the vertebral column and in the limbs.

Tenacious migraine with vomiting of bile.

Pain of the whole head as if it is going to burst.

Choreiform movements.

Epileptiform attacks.

Agitated sleep with dreams (violence, scuffles).

Paresthesia of lower limbs.

3. Digestive Apparatus

1. *Mouth, tongue, pharynx :*

Feeling of having salty lips.

White tongue with the tip red, without papillies in the front and in the back part.

Gums painful when chewing, Alveolo-dental pyculeoa.

2. *Stomach, intestines, abdomen* :

Nausea with vertigo and vomiting of bile.

Sudden pains of the oesophagus after meals radiating to the back.

Dull, deep pain in the epigastric region.

While lying down cannot bear the weight of hand on the abdomen.

Pain in the appendix.

4. Cardio-hemo-vascular Apparatus

Carmping pain in the precordial region.

Sensation of weakness of the heart.

Pain of the point of the heart.

Electric perturbation of the heart : Focal blocks, partial right, sided blocks, elongation of the R.P. espace., early sign of R.A.A. crocheting of the R and of S in V2, crossing of the T wave. The wave T in the horizontal vector is not closed, subdenivellation or denivellation below of ST, all the electric varieties of coronary insufficiency. It seems to act in anginoid conditions with anemia more than angor with hypercholesterolemia. (F. Sevaux)

5. Respiratory Apparatus

Adenopathies of the neck.

Big, infected, purulent tonsils.

Red angina, with or without dysphagia, with or without temperature.

Persistent pain and redness of the supports of the throat, of the palatal vault, of the uvula.

Acute and chronic laryngitis.

6. Organ of Senses

(a) *Nose* : Serous nasal discharge, muco-purulent with nasal crusts. Sinusitis with headache ; fever with headache.

(*b*) *Eyes* : Troubles of vision with ocular hypertension.

Ocular fatigue with the need of wearing spectacles.

(*c*) *Ears* : Otalgia specially if the person is lying down on the left.

Intermittent puffs of wind in the ear (right).

Otitis and mastoiditis.

7. Loco-motor Apparatus

Articular pains with hydrarthrosis.

Pain of the backbone.

Acute pain on the clavicles.

Inflammatory muscular pain.

Rheumatism of small articulations of the wrist, of the hand, with local redness, sometimes with hydrarthrosis.

8. Skin-Phanera

Loss of hairs.

Cutano-mucous erythrosis.

Scarlatinal from exanthema.

Vesiculo-pustulous eruptions.

Erysipelatoid patches of the limbs.

Cellulitic patches.

Fibrinous dermatitis, oedema of the face.

9. Modalities

Aggravations : By consolation. By humid weather.

Amelioration : In the beginning of movement, then better after some movements in open air.

POSOLOGY

Dynamisation : From 4 CH to 9 CH.

For psychotic conditions 30 CH.

POSITIVE DIAGNOSIS

Weeping, obsequious, intolerance to noise.

Depressive with migraines, vertigo and myocardiac asthenia.

Audio-visual hallucinations.

Muscular asthenia, cardiac and nervous asthenia.

Articular rheumatism specially of the small joints.

Exanthema and erythrosis of the skin, face and legs in particular.

DIFFERENTIAL DIAGNOSIS

Ailanthus glandulosa, Belladona, Arsenic alb., Rhux tox., are the classical homoeotherapics for streptococcic syndrome.

Anhalonium : (Peyotl) for visual and auditive hallucinations, general and cardiac myasthenia.

Think equally of *Enterococcinum, Streptococcus faecalis, Pyrogenium.* (Guillaume)

Among the modern homoeotherapics we may mention : *Achyranthes calea, Paronichia illecebrum, Anhalonium.*

CLINICAL DIAGNOSIS

1. Generalities

Infectious conditions with leucopenia and proteinuria.

Streptococcus anginas.

Erysipelas.

Acute articular rheumatism (A.A.R.), (adjuvant treatment). According to Zissu and Guillaume it is necessary to prescribe *Poumon histamine 7 CH* in order to check all allergic reaction.

2. Neuro-endocrino-psychic System

Cancerophobia. Maniac depressive condition.

Migraine.

Sydenham's chorea.

Dupre's and Gelma's hallucinosis.

3. Digestive Apparatus

Alveolo-dental pyorrhoea.

Oesophagitis.

Depapilising glossitis.

Gastric manifestations of allergic origin (Renè Chevalier).

Chronic appendicitis.

4. **Cardio-hemo-vascular System**

   Post-infection phlebitis.

   Arythmias.

   Endocarditis (adjuvant treatment).

   Myocardiosis.

   Pericarditis (adjuvant treatment).

5. **Respiratory Apparatus**

   Chronic lymphadenitis.

   Chronic tonsilitis.

   Red anginas.

   Acute or chronic laryngitis.

6. **Sense Organs**

   Nose : Acute or chronic rhinitis.

   Sinusitis.

   Eyes : Uveitis of adult young persons for streptococcus infection.

   Ears : Acute or chronic otitis.

   Acute or chronic mastoiditis.

7. **Uro-genital Apparatus**

   Acute glomerulo-nephritis.

   Allergic nephritis of masugi.

   Degenerative epithelial nephritis.

   Interstitial nephritis.

8. **Loco-motor Apparatus**

   Arthritis and polyarthritis of small joints.

   Muscular rheumatism.

9. Skin, Phanera

Allergising erythrodermia.

Repeated eczema.

Desquamating dry eczema.

Chronic oedema of the lower limbs.

Streptococcic nodulous erythema.

Here are two case reports by F. Sevaux and A. Emar. l' Homoeop. Fr., April, No. 4, 1959, p. 200).

Case 1

M.D....28 years, comes to consult for a chronic oedema of lower limbs which he has since 13 years and which resisted all therapies. Vectography shows a clear crossing of the T belt in the horizontal vecto, indicating a coronary insufficiency well tolerated, of which it is easy to find the symptoms by questioning the patient. Some successive doses of *Streptococcinum* caused progressive lowering down of the rate of antistreptolysines which falls from 800 to 250 units, which suddenly rose up to 400 units in last March after an attack of influenza ; one new dose modifies the electro in the sense of an amelioration, the oedema of the lower limbs has almost disappeared. The treatment should be followed.

Case 2

Mlle E...comes to consult for pericardialgia and because she is losing her hairs. But, what dominates the picture are the psychic troubles complained of by the patient. In fact, although she had only a moderate fall of hairs, she does no more wish to go to her office, pretends that she looks ridiculous, that everybody mocks at her.

The antistreptolysines are at 640 units ; by vectography is noted the existence of a focal block, absence of the closing of T ; one dose of *Streptococcinum* 9 CH prescribed does not modify the electrocardiogram and the accentuation of the psychic troubles forced her to stop work, however the antistreptolysines rose at 1,480 units and that the sedimentation is clearly accelerated. New desensibilisation with *Streptococcinum 7 CH*, this time, normalised the sedimentation, the rate of antistreptolysines becomes less than 50 units but the [focal block persists in the vecto and haptoglobine is at 2 I.U., the C reactive protein is positive. The taking of one dose of *Streptococcinum 7 CH* associated with *Pneumococcinum 7 CH* normalised the electro by closing the T belt. The psychic troubles have almost totally disappeared and the patient took up again her work.

STREPTO-ENTEROCOCCINUM

BIBLIOGRAPHY

Pommier De Shanti .

The Strepto-enterococcus. Revue fr. d'hom, No. 4, 1950-1951, p. 165-173.

Julian O.A :

Biothérapiques et nosodes. Maloine, 1962.

Fallex Jean :

Une nouvelle form de sycose : the mycosycosis. Actes de la Sociétè rhodanienne d'hom, 4 e trimestre, 1955, p. 79-84.

STOCK

It is J. Fallex who first prepared a stock from the culture of blood obtained from some sanguin sacs irrigating the gums according to the technique of Vincent and Pretet regarding gingival Hemoculture.

It is a lysate of culture of Strepto-enterococcus or *Enterococcus proteiformis*, varieties of gingival origin of *Streptococcus faecalis* (See article Nosodes of Bach).

According to Pommier De Santi, the gingival origin is very important because "this germ which loses nine-tenth of its virulence in the intestine, has all its virulence the very moment it passes in the blood or comes in contact with the gums, *Saprophytes* of the mouth".

There does not exist a Hahnemannian pathogenesis.

(581)

CLINICAL CORTICO-VISCERAL PROTOCOL
OR CLINICAL PATHOGENESIS

1. Generalities

Allergoso-mesenchymatosic subjects (psoro-sycotic) suffering from different affections, but having on gums some congestive boils. The dominant is the chronic reticulo-mesenchymatose condition with arthritic manifestations, gonorrhoeal, colibacillary, tubercular.

2. Neuro-endocrino-psychic System

Asthenia, anemia, emaciation.

Vertigo, migraines.

Insomnia.

Myalgias.

3. Digestive Apparatus

Loaded tongue.

Redness of the pharynx.

Congestion of the gums, painful specially during teething of the babies.

4. Respiratory Apparatus

Chronic aphonia aggravated by tobacco and by humidity.

Redness of the larynx.

Chronic cryptic tonsilitis.

Pseudo-membranous tonsilitis.

Acute anginas with marked influenzal condition.

Vincent's angina.

5. Sense Organs

Nose : Chronic sinusitis, chronic purulent rhinitis, ozena.

Ears : Acute and chronic otitis.

6. Skin, Phanera

Eczema of the new borns.

Furuncles.

Repeated erysipelas.

7. **Modalities**

Aggravation : By humidity, by tobacco.

8. **Posology**

Dynamisation : Pommier De Santi indicates the M. Korsakoff, and the 30 CH.

9. **Differential Diagnosis**

Medorrhinum, Natrum sulphuricum, Argentum nitricum, Kali bichromicum, Hepar sulphur, Fekla lava, Lycopodium, Mercurius.

CLINICAL DIAGNOSIS

Chronic reticulo-endotheliosis.

Mycosycosis of fallex.

Gingivitis. Pyorrhoea.

Dental symptoms : Hyperesthesis, erpthrosis, adenopathy, hyperthermia, lymphitis.

Dental convulsions of babies.

Arthralgias. Myalgias.

Digestive migraine.

Chronic sinusitis ; purulent rhinitis. Ozena.

Acute or chronic otitis.

Eczema of the new borns.

TETANOTOXINUM

HISTORY

Introduced and used by Cahis of Barcelona towards 1930.

STOCK

Dilution of tetanic toxin.

This product is not commercialised and cannot be prescribed in France.

PATHOGENESIS

No experiment was done.

CLINICAL DIAGNOSIS

Inveterate bronchial affections.
Trismus.
Tetanus.
Parathyroidian synrdomes.

POSOLOGY

May be had of Nelson, London :
Tetanus-antitoxin 6 CH-30 CH
Tetanus-bacillus 6 CH-30 CH
Tetanus-toxin   6 CH-30 CH
Tetanus toxoid   6 CH-30 CH.

In Germany, *Reckeweg* with *Heel*—prepares the following Nosodes : Tetanus-anatoxin-Injeel +forte (D6), D12, D30, D200 (+an unique dilution (Einzel potenz) D200).

The clinical indications are : anaphylactic conditions, specially after the injection of serum (Stock from horse), all the spastic conditions, the muscular cramps, tetanus, dysfunction of the parathyroid gland, perturbation of calcic metabolism. Indications may equally be found in arthroses, neuralgias, spastic paresis and eventually in the multiple sclerosis and in Parkinson's disease.

(584)

TOXOPLASMA—GONDII

BIBLIOGRAPHY

Kollmer E.P. :

Elektro-akupunktur nach Voll. Haug-Verlag. 1962. Communication d'observations cliniques avec success thérapeutiques dans l'Encephalite (diseminé) with the Nosode Toxoplasma. Commentaire de Dr. Voll.

Voll R. : Medikamentestung, Fosodotherapie and Mesenchyment schlakung, 14 bd, Medizin literarischer, Verlag, Uelzen, Hambourg, 1965. Communications des Dr. Kunst et Schmitz-Harbauer.

Convreur L. :

La toxoplasmose et son avenir. Gezette Mèdiale de France, No 4, 25 janvier, 1974.

Modai J. :

Notions recentes sur la toxoplasmose. Gazette médicale de France, No. 4. 25-1-74.

Bickert P., Robineau M. and Veyssier P. :

Manifestations cliniques de la toxoplasmose acquise. Gazette médicale de France, No. 49·25.1-74.

Couvreur J. :

Comment je traite une Toxoplasmose. Gazette médicale de France, No. 4. 25-1-74.

Diagnostic sérologique actuel de la toxoplasmose.

Le test de Remington.

Gazette medicale de France, t. 82, No. 4. 31 janvier 75.

Demonts G. :

Toxoplasmose. E.M.C. Paris.

Maladies infectieuses 2 1267-8098-A-10.

Additif : 1st. ed. 4-1971-c-1-8098-2-10.

Askenasi J. :

Revue de presse Homöopathique de langue allemende.

Cahiers de Biothérapie, No. 4. sept. 1975, concernant l'article :

Traitement par Nosodes par le Dr. Schmitz-Harbouer, in, Klassische Homöpathie No. 2. mars-avril 1963.

P. Vallery Radot, J. Hamburger and F. Lhermitte :

Pathologie médicale Flammarion médecine, 1971.

Robert P. :

La toxoplasmose pour le médécin homéopath.

Les Annales Homéop. Fr., No. 1. jan-fev 1976, p. 21.

STOCK

Nicolle and *Manceaux* who in 1908, isolated this parasite from a rodent of the south of Tunisia, the Gondii.

Toxoplasma Gondii is an intracellular parasite and are found in three forms :

—Vegetative, cystic and oocystic.

We owe to Hutchinson the discovery of the evolutive cycle of toxoplasma and of which the *cat* seems to be the definitive host.

The infestation in intermediary host is done by ingestion of ripe oocystes or by the ingestion of visceral cysts.

The human toxoplasma has an origin *essentially alimentary* by the ingestion of meat of pork or of infected sheep.

There is also the *transplacental transmission* by the passage of toxoplasma in the foetal circulation of an infected mother.

There are three phases of the evolution of infection by toxoplasma :

1. A primary phase : In the histio-monocytary cells, which are necrosed burst and are disseminated by the blood system or by the lymphatic system, and lodged in the ganglions, the striated muscles, the myocardia, the nervous system and in the eye.

2. The secondory phase : It is characterised by the destruction by antibodies of free forms and for the reparation of the lesions. The multiplication of toxoplasma however happens in the nervous system and in the eye.

The tertiary phase : It is characterised by the passage to the chronic stage specially on the surface of encephale, the eye, the striated muscles and the myocardia.

The biological diagnosis is done with the *dye test* (or test of Sebin-Feldman) and indirect immunofluorescence.

A more recent test, *the test of Remington* helps by indirect immunoflurescence to characterise the specific antibodies of the toxoplasma of the type IgM while even the habitual serological method puts in evidence only some antibodies of the type IgG.

The test of Remington gives a rapid indication during a recent toxoplasmic infection and for the diagnosis of the congenital toxoplasma.

STOCK

The stock is a lysate of Toxoplasma-gondii, diluted and dynamised according to the homoeopathic pharmacopoea.

We are obliged to Mme Binsard pharmacist-in-chief of Loboratoire Dolisos and to Mlle Noyer, assistant pharmacist, for the preparation of this "Isotherapic" and thus enabling us to introdnce it in our therapeutic.

HISTORY

The merit goes to R. Voll and his school of Organometric Electroacupuncture to have, since 1955. attracted the attention on multiple manifestations of toxoplasmosis.

The diagnosis is done, thanks to the medicinal test, with the Diatherapuncture.

It is confirmed by the biological tests of the laboratory then can be treated successfully by the biotherapics.

Reckeweg preconises toxoplasminum (or Nosode Toxoplasmosis) as therapeutic in the retoxic phase in the course of the decrease of the Homotoxicosis (See Ch. 5. Pharmocodynamics).

There exists no experimental pathogenesis according to the methodology of Hahnemann.

CLINICAL CORTICO-VISCERAL PROTOCOL OR CLINICAL PATHOGENESIS

1. Generalities

Subjects with cyclic depression.

Carbo-fluoric, luetic type.

Tuberculinic state (O.A. Julian).

Precancer or precancerous state.

Predisposition to repeated spontaneous *abortion* (luetosis). *Embryopathies.*

Children with retarded development, physical or intellectual.

Children having the tendency to repeated rhino-pharyngitis, (O.A. Julian). Retarded growth.

Isolated, persisting, non-suppurative adenopathies of the peripheries, with tenacious *asthenia.*

Syndrome of Mononucleose infection of young children with a sub-febrile state, discrete adenopathy, eosinophilia and reaction of Bunnel-Davidson *negative.*

Mesenteric adenitis.

Septicemia neo-natal with icterus, hepato-spleno-megaly, purpuric or morbiliform erythema.

General toxoplasmosis in subjects under immuno-suppressors.

2. Neuro-endocrino-psychic System

(*a*) *Psychic* :

Psyco-motor retardation.

(*b*) *Nervous* :

Intense headache, intolerable with hypertonia.

Meningo-encephalitis : Somnolence, torpor, epileptiform convulsion in babies.

Acute lymphocytary meningitis of young children.

Myelitis of children or of adults.

Hydrocephaly.

Motor deficit : Hemiplegia, paraplegia.

Convulsive attacks of children.

Bravais Jakson epilepsy.

(*c*) *Endocrines* :

Hypothalamus-hypophysary syndrome.

3. Digestive Apparatus

Persistent enlargement of liver, with increase of bilirubin.

Diffused abdominal pains, not well localised or peri-umblical.

4. Cardio-hemo-vascular System

Precordial pains, *palpitation*, *dysponea* by effort, *orthopenia*, cough.

Nocturnal polypneic attacks.

Tachycardia, sometimes arythmia, galloping sound with systolic murmur.

Hypotension. E.C.G : Hypertrophy or overcharging of the left ventricule, troubles of repolarisation (segment ST, wave T).

Sometimes troubles of rythme or of conduction : fibrillation or auricular flutter, articulo-auricular bloc of the branch, extra-systoles.

Familial cardiomegalies.

Myocarditis.

Thermo-regulation :

Adult : Hyperthermia, weak general condition, maculo-papulous exanthema, osteo-articular and muscular pains.

Adenopathies of the cervical glands.

Encephalitis with psychic troubles, convulsions, signs of deficit.

Stiffness due to meninges.

5. Respiratory Apparatus

Atypic pneumonia.

6. Sense Organs

Eyes : Iridocyclitis.

Simple chorio-retinitis.

Chorio-retinitis with uveitis.

Optic neuritis.

7. Uro-genital Apparatus

Genital, feminine : Abortion during the first three months.

Normal pregnancy but with a congenital toxoplasmosis.

Early menstruation.

8. Loco-motor Apparatus

Arthritis, Myositis.

9. Skin, Phanera

Gibert's rosy pityriasis.

Maculo-papulur or vesiculous exanthema. Purpura.

POSOLOGY

Dynamisations : 4 CH, 5 CH, 7 CH, 9 CH, in granules, tubes 7 CH, 15 CH, 30 CH in granule tubes or dose globules.

R. Voll uses toxoplasma in 60 DH, 100 DH, 200 DH, 400 DH (Muller-Goeppingen).

Reckeweg : Toxoplasmosis—Nosode inject.+forte (D 10), D 25, D 30, D 200 (Heel, Baden-Baden).

POSITIVE DIAGNOSIS

Cancer states. Tuberculinosic states (O.A. Julian).

Tuberculino-luetosic states (O.A. Julian).

Isolated, persistent adenopathies.

Tendency to spontaneous abortion.

Embryopathies. Myocarditis. Chorio-retinitis.

Gibert's rosy pityriasis.

DIFFERENTIAL DIAGNOSIS

Corcinosinum : See article.

Bunias orientalis (Julian O.A. Matére Médicale d'Homoeothérapie, 1971, Le Fransçois, 91, Bd. St.-Germain, 75006 Paris): Cancerosic subjects, adenopathy with pruriginous eruption, asthenia, emaciation, sub-febrile condition, pathological pregnancy with embryopathies : lean luetic children, congenital malformation.

CLINICAL DIAGNOSIS

1. Generalities

Tuberculinic conditions ; cancer conditions.

Tuberculino-luetic conditions.

Lymphadenitis.

Tubercular primo-infection.

Adenolymphitis, lympho-adenopathy.

Acute benign adeno-lymphoiditis (infectious mononucleosis).

Acute lymphocytosis (*infectious*) *or Carl Smitt's disease* ; rhinopharyngeal catarrh, diarrhoea, leucocytosis and symphocytosis, moderate fever, asthenia, Bunnel Davidson's reaction negative.

Jacquelin-Burnand syndrome of worn out condition.
Rubeola.

2. **Neuro-endocrino-psychic System**
Post infectious encephalitis of children.

Encephalo-myelitis.

Atrophic encephalopathy of the childhood.

Trisomia 21 (mongolism).

Micromelic nanism (See Homoeotherapic Nepenthes).

Achondroplasia of Parrot. Impuberism.

Beginning of hydrochephaly.

Chorea, epilepsy.

Multiple sclerosis.

3. **Digestive Apparatus**
Epidemic hepatitis.

Juvenile familial hepatitis or Wilson's disease.

Hanot Kiener's disease (diffused mesenchymatous hepatitis with nodular lymphomatosis).

Acute or subacute mesenteric lymphadenitis.

Crohn's disease.

Follicular and segmentary ileitis of A. Rachet and A.Busson.

4. **Cardio-hemo-vascular System**
Myocarditis, subacute, primitive of Tripier and Galla-vardin.

Endocrino-hepato-cardiac syndrome of Laubry.
Congenital cardiopathies.

Thermo-regulation :
Septicimia, collibacillary.

5. **Sense Organs**
Eyes : Iridocyclitis.
Choreoretinitis and uveitis.

6. Uro-genital Apparatus

Meno-metrorrhagia.

Repeated abortion.

7. Loco-motor System

Myositis.

Arthritis.

8. Skin, Phanera

Purpura.

Polymorphous erythema.

Nodulous erythema.

Bibert's rosy pityriasis.

9. Commentaries

Toxoplasma-gondii seems to have the characteristics of a remedy having polyvalent indications, of a polychrest but wanting a regular homoeopathic ally proved pathogenesis.

Toxoplasmose-diseases have the characteristics of an infectious disease and ubiquitary immunologic character because of its multiple local seats, the deep and slow action on the tissues, humoral modifications and the genetic repercussions.

During our time, it has the tendency to come to the foreground of the scene in this vast composit fresco which constitutes the old psora of Hahnemann and our Allergoso.

Allergoso, according to us (O.A. Julian) is structural, morphologic, dynamic and contradictional condition to put the organism in a condition containing a genotypic and peristasic code.

The genotypic code is polymorphous, toxinic, infectious traumatic.

This polyetiology leaves in the cell memory some informations whence results a contradictional cortico-visceral conditioning.

From then Allergoso represents a state of unstable structural equilibrium, of excitation and cortico-visceral inhibition which is in quantity and quality different on the tissues and cells or on organs.

The clinical expression shows some desperate, contradictory nosographic forms.

It is even the meaning of alternance and morbid metastasis.

The clinic describes a subject having alternate excitation and cortico-visceral inhibition with restlessness, anxiety, depression and hyperactivity.

*   *   *
*   *

(See Commentaries under Psorinum)

Thus renovated the etio-pathologic comprehension of this vast multiform state of our old psora, of our present allergy, It seems to have given out some clinically important syndromes of pathology constituting thus some clinical forms, which are always possible to be revised according to the progress of our knowledge of science in constant renewal.

In our opinion we may at present distinguish the clinical forms of psora or allergy as follows :

(a) The tuberculinism of Nebel, L. Vannier, Bernard.

(b) The canceronosis of L. Vannier.

(c) The toxoplasmosis that we have individualised.

(d) The allerginosis which is in the course of study and represents the cortico visceral damage, psychic-somatic which is the result of the aggression of "Polluants".

Thus we are able to define a specific new morbid entity, thr Toxoplasminosis and of which Toxoplasma-gondii is Its Isotherapic but not exclusively.

10. The Summaries of Two Clinical Cases

O. Clause (Mitgeteilte Krankheitsgeschichte and Therapieerfolg beim Encephalitis disseminata mittels der. Nosode.

Toxoplasmose in : E.P. Kollmer : Elektroacupuntur nach Voll., p. 168-174 avec une commentaire de R. Voll) relates a case in detail of Encephalitis disseminata, treated one and half years ago without any result in the department of neurology of a Faculty of medicine and of which the cure was obtained by the use of Toxoplasma D6.

The therapeutic diagnosis with the *diatherapuncturer* of Voll has fixed the point on the Triple Rechauffeur (reanimator) the indication of Toxoplasma.

Two years later the patient remained always cured.

R.V. Leitner (See Cahiers de Biothérapie, No. 4, Sept., 1975. Revue de Presse Homeopathique allemande du Dr. Askenasi.), Berlin, reports a case of billious migraine which Allopathy could not cure. With Diatherapuncturer of Voll it was noted : Irritation of dental cavities, tonsils, maxiliary sinuses ; Meridian Spleen-Pancreas, kidney, bladder.

The prescription is a pluralist one : *Dental granuloma D4 +Gangrenous* pulp *D6+Meningococcinum D30, Toxoplasmosis D60, Colitis, D2, Hepatitis D 3,* and *Nephritis D 3.* After the second injection very clear improvement.

But two months later very strong attack of migraine and it is on the point of liver the diagnosis of Toxoplasmosis D4 was diagnosed which cured the case and the Sabin-Feldman test became normal.

Here is a 3rd case of Dr. Schmitz-Harbauer :

The first case where the Toxoplasmosis was used was a case of young girl of 15 years with an arterial tension of 140/80, a bradycardia, some extrasystoles and a systolic murmur. Cyanosis of the lips was very marked on her face. She complained that her hands and feet are icy cold.

The mother spoke of a general weakness, bad results in the school, with loss of confidence on herself, headaches, and a contradictory mentality.

Some abdominal pains give one to think of chronic appendicitis. The mother also said that the girl could not bear cold. I decided at first to rectify her alimentary hygiene with an appropriate hydrotherapy and 10 drops of *Aurum D12* every day. Two weeks later, there was a slight amelioration but not very conclusive : that amelioration was about constipation and abdominal troubles.

The patient received a dose of *Toxoplasmosis* sub-cutaneously in D15 and a week later D20, two weeks later D30 and 3 weeks after D60. Inspite of the reticence against the injections, the patient informs a very sensible amelioration from the second injection. Six weeks of treatment ameliorated the tension, the chilliness, cyanosis and the general condition.

.TUBERCULINUM (T.K.)

(TUBERCULINUM CRUDUM)

BIBLIOGRAPHY

Allen H.C. :

Materia Medica of the Nosodes. Boericke and Tafel, Phil., 1910.

Cartier Fr. :

Thérapeutiques des voies respiratories. Bailliére and Fils, Paris, 1920.

Vannier L. :

Les Tuberculiniques and leur traitment homoéopathique Doin, Paris, 1958.

Julian O.A. :

Biothérapiques et Nosodes. Maloine, Paris, 1962.

Materia Medica der Nosoden. Haug Verlag, Heidelberg, 1960, 2e. ed 2 1975.

Kent J.T. :

Arzneimittelbilder. Tr. Allen ande par E. Heits, 1958, Haug, Ulm/Donau.

Kent J.T. :

Tuberculinum Bovinum. Trad. fr. du Dr. H. Perichon-Bestaire. In Annales hom. fr., 1968, p. 630.

Schmidt P. :

Tuberculinum Bovinum (Kent). Groupement Hahnemannien de Lyon. X ser., No. 6, 1973, p. 259-261.

Jobin and Wright :

Tubercul. Bovin. Groupement hahnemannien de Lyon X, ser. No. 8, 1973.

Birot R. :

Pathogénésie de Tuberculinum T.K. Les Annales Hom. fr. Juin, 1955, p. 427.

Vannier L. :

Les Tuberculines diluées. (1) T.K., (2) T.R., Cours de C.H.F., du 28 janv., 1947.

Bloss W. :

Behaendlung mit Tuberkulinen. Zeitschrift für Klassishe Homeöopathie ; Bd. 17, 1973, Heft 4 et. 5.

Pischel :

Kongessbericht über die 123 Jahres versammlung : interventions de O.A. Julian ; Pischel ; Imhauser.

Allgemeine Hom. Zeitung No. 1 et 3, 1972.

Vannier L. :

Les Tuberculines diluées. Bulletin du C.H.F. 1960, p. 269.

Chiron :

Les Tuberculines diluées. Les Annales Hom. fr. No. 7, juillet 1973.

Tyler M.L. :

Homoeopathic Drug Pictures. The Homeop. Pubg. Co. London, 1952.

Boericke W. :

Pocket Manual of Homeopathic Materia Medica. Phil., 1927 et la traduction allemande de 1972.

Renard L. :

Bacillinum Burnett et Tuberculinum bovinum. L'Hom. Moderne, No. 20, 1936, p. 677-689.

Clarke :

Tuberculinum Kochi. Zeitschrift des Berliner Vereins Hom. Aerzte. Bd. 10, S. 169.

Nobel :

Zeitschrift des Berliner Vereins Hom. Aerzte. Bd. 19, S. 295, et Matiére Medicale de la T.K. L'Hom. Mod. 1937, No. 2, p. 71.

Hering C. :

The Guiding Symptoms of our Materia Medica. Phil. 1891, Gregg Press, 1967.

Clarke J. :

A Dictionary of Practical Materia Medica, London, 1955, v. 3, p. 1460.

HISTORY

There is a confusion as regards the authors who are consulted. Because the Tuberculine of Koch cannot be introduced in Nosodotherapy before its discovery by R. Koch (1843-1910). Koch's Bacilli was discovered in 1882.

In 1638 Robert Fludd professor of anatomy advised in a book entitled "Philosophia Myosaica (Goudae, 1638, folio. 149, column 2) : *Sputum rejectum a pulmonica post-debitam praeparatidenem curat phtisin*, the use of the expectoration of a tuberculous patient.

According to Cartier, *Martino*, a portugues homoeopathic doctor residing at Rio, who died in 1854, preconised *Tubercina* before Compton Burnett.

Swan, homoeopathic doctor of New York, prepared in 1886 a trituration of an expectoration of a tuberculous subject, in sugar of milk and named this substance *Tuberculinum*, which in reality corresponds to *Bacillinum* which is a lysate of the expectoration of a tuberculous subject containing some B.K. verified under microscope.

He treated with this product a case of tuberculosis and the case was reported in *The New Organon*, July 1879, p. 342, 439, 449.

Bicgler published at the same time a case regarding a tubercular meningitis which he cured with the same Tuberculinum (Org. vol. 2, p. 439 ; Hom Phys. v. 2, p. 187).

Then it is *Burnett* of London, who utilised, *Bacillinum*, prepared from a fragment of a tuberculous lung, between 1885 and 1890 and published in 1890, (21st November) a brochure entitled "The new cure of consumption by its own virus."

He related 54 cases of tuberculosis treated by Bacillinum.

In the 2nd. ed. of 1892, Burnett said that one should never use Bacillinum beyond 30 CH "and when I am afraid to cause some constitutional troubles, I never go beyond 100th".

With the appearance of Koch's Tuberculine and its allopathic use, appears first its injurious effect.

Also *De Keghel*, a Belgian homoeopath published at first an essay on the pathogenesis based on the toxicology, which appeared in 1892 in the v. 5 of the *Union homoeopathique*.

In 1893, *Clarke* published a more complete pathogenesis regarding the action of Tuberculine on tuberculous or nontuberculous patient. This work appeared in the Homoeopathic World XXVI.

Between 1890-92 *Pierre Jousset* tried, without success, the normal doses, then more ˙weak doses of tuberculine by injecttions (l'Art médical, 1890-91).

In 1892 he published in the Art Medical five favourable cases of renal tuberculosis treated with dynamised Tuberculine.

On February, 1912 appeared a study concerning the treatment of pulmonary tuberculosis by Tuberculine, by *Harlan Wells* in the *Journal of the American Institute of Homoeopathy*.

To commence with he used the 6D, then 5D, then 3D 1/10th of cc by injection, repeated according to the reaction of the patient.

The case reports began to multiply as Young and Clarke of England, Pinard and Olivey Gros of Spain, Younann of Calcutta, Snow of United States and Kunkel of Germany reported their cases.

Cartier in July 1894 had publisned in the Hahnemannian monthly the cure of a capillary bronchitis with hemoptysis in a patient of 80 years, treated in Höpital Saint-Jacques.

In 1895 Mersch of Brussels published in the Journal Belge d'Homoeopathie a pathogenesis of Tuberculinum based on 41 bibliographical references and toxicologic symptomatology on healthy man.

It was in 1902, Antoine Nebel of Montreux, then of Lausanne, published in the Zeitschrift des Berliner Vereins Homöopathischer Aerzte "The Symptomatology of Koch's Tuberculine".

In this article all the symptoms observed in patients suffering from tuberculosis after the injection or absorption of Tuberculine were stated.

In a second article "Effects medicamenteux de la tuberculine" (Medicinal Effects of Tuberculinum), Nebel related the results obtained with 7 CH.

In March 1912, a teacher of Philadelphia, published in the "Homoeopathician" a study of the pathogenesis of Tuberculinum.

Vannier Léon and Nebel created a great impulse for the study and use of Tuberculines. They even formulated the pre-tubercular states, known as *tuberculine or tuberculinism.*

Then, our contemporaries contributed to the study of the remedy. Their names are to be found in the general and special bibliography.

STOCK

The biotherapic Tuberculinum is prepared from the crude tuberculine described in the supplement of 1954 of the Codex,. p. 113, supplied by Pasteur Institute.

CRUDE TUBERCULINE
(OLD TUBERCULINE OF KOCH)

Tuberculinum crudum.   Tuberculinum pristinum :

The crude Tuberculinum is the product, without the addition. of any aseptic, obtained from a liquid culture medium on which is developed *Mycobacterium tuberculosis.*

The microbian stocks used belong to the human and the bovine type, as well as for the use on men and on animals ; however some crude tuberculines may as well be prepared with stocks obtained from birds for the diagnosis of the affections due to aviary bacilli.   These stocks are selected and watched over periodically in order to be sure of their activity.

The culture medium is some bouillon prepared with some meat of excellent quality, glycerinated at about 5% or a medium chemically defined, as for example that which is described in the article *Vaccin B C.G.* (See article V.A.B.)

The culture of the bacilli is grown at 37°·38° for several weeks ; it should produce abundant flocculences.   The culture it then sterilised by heating at 100° for one hour, concentrated by evaporation to the tenth of the initial volume.

The final product is cleared by filtration.

Characters : Syrup-like liquid, transparent, of yellow or brown colour having the characteristic smell of honey.

Trial : 1st trial, *sensibilisation*.   Intradermic injection to new cobaye, repeated three times at an interval of a week of 0.1 cm³ of a solution of crude tuberculine at 5% should not sensibilise the animal face to face with an injection and the same dose and n the same conditions.

2nd trial, *toxicity* : The injection of 0.5 cm^3 under the skin of a cobaye (normal), should neither kill the cobaye, nor produce in it any serious symptom.

3rd, trial for *activity* : Some cobayes having white furs, weighing at least 400 g are tuberculised by a culture of *Mycobacterium tuberculosis* var. *hominis* or *bovis* 2 to 3 weeks old of normal virulence by injecting subcutaneously in the thigh with 1 cm cube of a bacterial suspension of isotonic chloride solution containing from 0.01 mg to 0.001 mg of bacillies in a centimetre cube. After one month, confirm by a trial on two cobayes, that the animals respond by an inflammatory reaction of at least 8 mm diameter to the injection of 10 I.U. of tuberculine in an 0.1 cm cube in the skin, after shaving off the hair. If this trial is not positive, it should be repeated after two weeks.

When the cobayes show that degree of sensibility, proceed for the comparative experiment on 8 cobayes, eliminating at least from that trial, the animals who have bad state of health (soft, lustreless skin).

Prepare some dilutions in some isotonic chloride solution containing in the volume of 0.1 cm^3. 5, 10, and 20 I.U. of standard tuberculine, as well as a series of dilutions, estimated to correspond to the sample prepared for the trial. Give the injections as described above under the shaven skin at the volume of 0.1 cm^3. The effective region is the flank, between the shoulder and the hip avoiding the abdominal wall. Give the injections at distances of 2 cm one after the other injecting the quantity estimated to corresponding to the standard tuberculine and to the sample on the same level from one to the other of the vertebral column.

It is essential that the dose injected should be 0.1 cm cube in all the cases. The syringes should be precise, air-tight, and carefully cleaned. They should be reserved for this use only and should never be used for highly concentrated dilutions of tuberculines.

Proceed by the reading of the results, preferably at the 30th hour, *i.e.* to say when the inflammation is the maximum, then after the 2nd or the 3rd day to observe the eventual late hemorrhagic or narcotic effect. Measure the diameter of the inflammatory reaction, evaluate the quality of reactions (erythema, papule, hemorrhagic zone, or narcotic effect) and determine thus what quantity of the sample has caused, in proportion and in gravity, some reactions equivalent to those caused by first or the second dose of the standard tuberculine.

The action of the crude officinal tuberculine would be equal to that of a standard preparation of tuberculine titrating 100,000 international units in a cm cube. If it is more, make it equal to the titration of the standard by addition of an appropriate volume in equal parts of distilled water and of officinal glycerine.

If it is less, it should be rejected.

Preservation : The crude tuberculine can be preserved for a long time (more than 10 years) distributed in steriledair-tight glass recipients and kept in a cold place.

Conditions of use : The crude tuberculine is used for the research of allergic condition in man, either in crude state (cutireaction) or, for want of purified tuberculine, in diluted form (intradermal reaction).

The most used dillutions are at the rate of 1/200 or 1/1000.

Composition of tuberculine : This stock is particularly studied by Boquet in France and Seibert in America as regards its proteinic composition. The solution proteins of tuberculous bacilli have in fact a very high reactional activity as defined by Seibert. This author has put in evidence three types of proteins A, B and C characterised by their electrophoretic mobility for A and B. The molecular weight of these proteins vary from 8,000 to 32,000 ; and their reactional activity is in direct relation to this weight. These molecules, though relatively small for some proteins, are liberated in the medium of culture by a process of autolysis of tuberculous bacilli. Corper and Laporte have shown that it is in the old Tuberculine of Koch, *i.e* to say in the stock of our Tuberculinum that these proteins are the most abundant and have the most high molecular weight.

By the side of these specific proteins, are found some different and common substances such as polyosides, nucleic acid, peptones, glycerine, salts.

Pharmacological Study

Tuberculinum is the first biotherapic subjected to out general experimental study on animals. This work was carried between 1955 and 1957 by M. Tetau and S. De Luna (Experimental data on the action of Tuberculinum. *Problems of homoeopathy*, 1958, Lab. Dolisos). Its origin was out of fortuitous case ; some cobayes having served for the purpose of non-toxicity test of Tuberculinum 7 CH and 9 CH were tuberculised in order to use them for some experimental research having no other purpose besides this nosode. These cobayes were abnormally resistant to the tuberculous infection, which incited the researchers to undertake some experiments on new cobayes. 48 cobayes of 500 to 600g were used and received during 15 days a daily injection according to the following table :

Group A	8 cobayes	Tuberculinum 5 CH
Group B	8 cobayes	Tuberculinum 7 CH
Group C	8 cobayes	Tuberculinum 9 CH
Group D	8 cobayes	Tuberculinum 12 CH
Group E	8 cobayes	Tuberculinum 30 CH
Group F	8 cobayes	Sterile physiological serum

After these 15 days all these cobayes received 0.5 ml of a suspension of B.K. The cobayes of the group F (witnesses) and of group D and E (Tuberculinum 12 CH and 30 CH) all died within less than 2 months. On the contrary the cobayes of the groups A and C receiving Tuberculinum 5 CH and 9 CH died at different times from 2 to 4 months and the cobayes of the group-B 7 CH, of which none died at the beginning of the 3rd month and outlived up to 5 months.

This experiment shows the activity of Tuberculinum in homoeopathic dilutions administered as preventive in the experimental tuberculosis of the cobaye.

It proved false the works of MM Desbordes and Paraf regarding B.C.G. and of Galy regarding the dilution of culture of tubercular bacilli.

Other Tuberculines

Many other products from the tubercular bacilli have been used in Nosodotherapy but none among them, so far as we know, was the object of a pathogenesic experiment.

Koch himself prepared numerous tuberculines. Over and above the old Tuberculine (Tuberculinum) and the Residual tuberculine, he prepared the Tuberculine B.E. (emulsion of B.K. dried and crushed finely in glycerine) and the Tuberculine A.F. (Phenol K).

Other tuberculines were prepared by Klebs, Maragliano, Hirschfelder, Beranek (Oxytoxin). Landmann (Tuberculol), Rosenbach. Siebert and Roemer (Tubolytin), Vaudremer (this was made atoxic by the mixture of a juice of *Aspergillus Nigar*, which dampers the process of making the tubercular bacilli avirulent), and so many other authors among whom we will here mention only Spengler who prepared a Tuberculine similar on all points to that of Koch's except that it contains exclusively bovine bacilli. It should not be confounded with the immunising bodies of Spengler.

The Tuberculine of Spengler was very near to Tuberculinum Bovinum which Kent got prepared specially by Boerike and Tafel.

There is no Hahnemannian pathogenesis of Tuberculinum.

PHARMACODYNMIC CORTICO VISCERAL
PROTOCOL OR CLINICAL PATHOGENESIS

1. Generalities

Nervous subject, irritated when waking up, immediately when he opens his eyes.

Displeased of everything, catches cold easily, unstable ; sweats by the least effort, specially on the forehead.

Mobility and variability of symptoms.

Bad temper, pale face or paleness and redness alternately, of the face of cheeks and nose.

The sclerotica of the eyes are blue, the skin is dry, rough and hot.

Supra-ciliary oozing pustules ; crust on the upper lip.

Labial herpes, specially of the children.

Afraid of dogs, specially black dogs.

2. Neuro-endocrino-psychic System

(a) *Psychic* :

Hypochondriac look, easily broken down and discouraged, weeping mood.

Bad temper, weakness, *somnolence during the day*, nausea with the sensation of being intoxicated and trembling.

Changing character, sees everything rosy or broken down, melancholic.

Everything seems to him strange, does not like to be troubled.

Weakness of the memory, aversion to intellectual work or on the contrary clear mind.

Forgetfulness.

Distaste of life, aggravated by music, torturing ideas at night.

Anxious in the evening.

Feels himself broken, beaten, fatigue of the eyes, pains in the bones.

Always desires to go somewhere.

Alternance of troubles, mental and pulmonary.

Feels himself forced to use insulting language, obscene and uses rough words.

Children, nervous, restless, move and run on all sides, *cannot remain quiet.*

Children with violent character, become terribly angry, are afraid of dogs, extremely sensitive for nothing.

Aversion towards some persons without reason.

(*b*) *Nervous* :

Headache with the sensation that the skull is tightly tied by a band of iron. Periodical headache, every *7 days or every 14 days* or while reading.

Chronic headache caused by humid weather, intellectual overwork, by digestive troubles, *by the smell of coffee.*

Headache better by movement and by pressing the head into the pillow.

Headache on the right eye and extending towards occiput.

Deep pain, sometimes violent, which forces the patient to tear his hairs and strike on his head.

Headaches of the student, of intellectuals, worse by the least intellectual effort.

Vertigo. Cramping pains in the legs.

Neuralgias. Myalgias. Paresthesias.

Bad sleep, restless, chill at the beginning of sleep, then insomnia from 3 a.m. The patient is restless, tosses over his bed with pains in the back, sometimes coughs which wakes him up, sensation of heat all over the body.

Dreams, wakes up with a sensation of agony, presentiment of a bad luck in the near future.

3. Digestive Apparatus

(*a*) *Mouth, tongue, pharynix* ·

Foetid breath.

Bad taste in the mouth, rancid or greasy, or a metallic taste.

Swollen gums, bleeding with ulceration.

The teeth are coated with a viscous. sticky matter.

Abundant tartars of the teeth.

Sensation of the teeth tottering.

Coated tongue, of berry colour.

Tongue with vesicles, which leave some painful small ulcers.

Small ulcers of lips and on the gums ; aphthe.

Pain in the throat, pharynx, more on the left with radiation to the ear and difficulty of swallowing solid foods.

(*b*) *Stomach, intestines, abdomen* :

Loss of appetite, with the sensation of emptiness in the stomach.

Nausea, cramping gastralgia, headache.

Disheartened at the sight of the foods or at the smell of foods.

Aversion to meat.

Desire for cold milk, sugars, sweets, dainties dishes of fat hams.

Hunger at night.

Gastric cramps, abdominal distension.

Vomiting with headache, cold sweats and general weakness.

Pain in the hepatic region which may be accompained with a subicteric state.

Hepato and spleno-megaly.

Morning diarrhoea between 3 to 5 a.m. with urgent desire for stools which are watery, blackish brown, in jets, or fetid smell.

Diarrhoea followed by sweats and great weakness.

Constipation with big hard stools, alternating with diarrhoea accompained by the itching of anus.

Involuntary stools while passing wind or during sleep.

4. Cardio-hemo-vascular System

Cardialgia, pain as if from a band, lancinating.

Palpitation in the morning or after dinner.

Palpitation at night, with cough during deep inspiration.

Arythmia, weak pulse, discrete, frequent, irregular.

Thermo-regulation : Hyperthermia, face red or violet, with alternate heat and cold, and great loquaciousness.

Sensation of cold in the chest, in the stomach with formication.

Chill : Afternoon accompanied by shivering, broken down condition, heat and sweats.

Great sweat, while the fever falls.

Fever with chills, specially when uncovering, intermittent, with hot sweats and need for uncovering.

5. Respiratory Apparatus

Throat :

Pain in the neck. Swelling of the glands of the neck, indurated or suppurated.

Swelling of tonsils and of the pharynx.

Swelling of the epiglottis which may bleed slightly.

Pain of the neck in the morning with dryness, burning and deglutition difficult.

Pains radiate from the left side of the throat to the ear while swallowing.

Difficulty to swallow solid foods.

Intermittent nasal voice, painful and temporary aphonia.

Roughness of the right vocal chord.

Swelling of the left vocal chord.

Slight pain in the left half of the larynx with difficult deglutition.

Swelling with oedema or ulceration of the larynx.

Aryepiglottic ligament swollen.

Aphonia, roughness, and dryness of the larynx.

Lungs, pleuras :

Need for fresh air, oppression, loss of breath.

Asthmatic dysponea when there is heat at night.

Light cyanosis, sensation of *pressure* in the thorax: chocking, better when one speaks with the patient.

Pain on the apex of the lung, in front and behind.

Rough noise above the shoulder blade, right.

Vesicular murmur augmented towards the point of the left shoulder blade and isolated rales.

Rubbing of left pleura.

Pain in the chest and in the sacrum.

Cough with sweat, causing sometimes a tearing pain in the rectum.

Irritating cough, specially in the evening, for which the patient cannot sleep.

Cough dry, hard, cutting, when there is chill.

Cough aggravated in a hot room, better in open air, by a cold wind.

Expectoration. thick, yellow, often greenish.

6. Sense Organs

Nose :

Redness and swelling of the nose, of the upper lip and of cheeks.

Epistaxis, ulcerations in the left nostril.

Furuncles of the nose with greenish pus.

Burning secretion, abundant, from the back of the nose.

Repeated coryza with sneezing, pains in the teeth and in the ears.

Sneezing while uncovering the hands.

Dragging cold, with purulent, thick and yellow discharge.

Eyes :

Swollen eyelids, while waking up.

Repeated styes of the right eye.

Crusts on the borders of the eyelids.

Herpes of the eyelids.

Pains, burning in the eyes, lancinating pains and the need for winking.

Bilateral conjunctivitis.

Marginal keratitis of the right eye, with redness of the conjunctiva, photophobia and pains.

Pains in the eyes when moving them, by turning them to sides.

Visual troubles : Vision of blue colour or of green colour, or a halo of colour.

Ears :

Chronic painless discharge from both ears, of bad or without smell.

Buzzing and the sensation of a foreign body in the ear.

Otalgia with facial paralysis.

7. Uro-genital Apparatus

Urinary :

Painful tenesmus while urinating.

Difficulty to urinate with need for effort during stools.

Frequent need for urinating. Urine turbid, brown-red, with froth, and a smell resembling cooked haricots.

Albuminuria with cylinders, hyaline and graunlar casts ; hematuria.

Pain and heaviness of the renal region, specially right.

Incontinence of urine.

Genital :

Male

Scrotum relaxed.

Painful swelling of the right testicle.

Hydrocele and epididymitis.

Swelling of the prostate.

Temporary erythema of the penis.

Augmented, excessive or violent sexual desire.

Female

Prolonged menses, for 20 days, abundant, dragging.

Bilateral ovarian pain, radiating to the lumbo-sacral region with difficulty to walk.

Menses, irregular or absent.

Late menstruation in young girls.

Vesico-vaginal relaxation.

Galactorrhoea before and during or after suppression of menses.

8. Loco-motor System

Constant desire for movement.

Aggravation of articular pains in *standing position.*

Pain of all the limbs, and of all the articulations.

Pain of the back and a sensation of wearing humid dresses.

Lumbo-sacral pain, worse by pressure, extending to the legs.

Drawing in the legs, in the muscles, in the articulations.

Sensation of being beaten in the bones, specially *before storm.*

Drawing in the shoulders ; analgesia and paresthesia of upper extremities.

Drawing in the heels and in the feet.

Jerking in the muscles while lying down or during sleep.

9. Skin, Phanera

Dry rough, hot skin.

Sensation of formication under the skin.

Chair de poule with chill.

Sweats which stains the linen yellow, after the very least effort, specially intellectual.

Violet oedema above the eye lashes, at the roots of hairs.

Pruriginous eczema, aggravated by water, in open air, *squamous, localised* specially behind ears, in the folds, on the integument.

Eczema with fissures, dry or oozing, with deep red look, painful.

Nodular erythema, subcutaneous, indurated, with sometimes bronze patches, punctiforms.

Scarlatinaform exanthema.

Acne and comedons.

10. Modalities

Aggravation :

By barometric changes.   During storm.   In humid cold.

In a closed room.

In standing position.

By physical work, specially by intellectual work.

After 3 a. m.

Amelioration :

In the open air. By wind. By walking.

Laterality :

Right but not absolute.

Characteristics :

Symptoms changing, periodic, passing from one organ to another, beginning and ending suddenly.

POSOLOGY

Dynamisations : From 4 CH to the 30 CH.

In Federal Germany dynamisations from 1000 DH to 1000 CH.

According to the indications of Reckeweg injectable ampoules are prepared : 8 DH, 1000 DH, and 10,000 DH and also a complex dilution of 12 DH+30 DH+200 DH. At Nelson of London : 6 CM., MM.

POSITIVE DIAGNOSIS

Unstable subject, changing, changes places and changes the places of objects.

Mobility and variability of symptoms.

Anxiety, emaciation, capricious appetite, unstable character, afraid of dogs.

Periodic headache, sweats, imperious morning diarrhoea, sensation of bruised, sensation in the bones, standing position painful.

Intermittent fever, hands hot, chill, nasal and raucous voice.

Aversion to meat, desire for cold milk, sweets and alcohol.

Dyspnoea, irritating cough, greenish expectoration.

Skin dry, rough, fissured and sometimes subcutaneous indurated nodules.

Acne and pustules of the face.

Troubles of libido with sometimes a clear augmentation or perversion.

DIFFERENTIAL DIAGNOSIS

Dynamised Micro-immunotherapy Nosodotheraphy) : Aviare, V.A.B. and Psorinum. (See articles)

Classical homoeopathy : *Sulphur, Phosphorus, Argentum nitricum, Abrotanum, Drosera, Iodum, Natrum muriaticum, Pulsatilla, Rhus toxicodendron, Rumex crispus, Silica.* This enumeration is not limitative.

New Remedies

Aqua marina. Emaciation, sweats, shivering.

Tormented, agitated, distracted.

Morning weakness, anxiety, epigastralgia and foetid breath, pain in the thorax, cough with watery expectoration.

Rusty taste in the back of the throat, dorsal pains or pains of the limbs. Perturbed libido.

Indium-met. Aortico-somatic weakness ; posterior cephalalgia, face pustulous, dorsalgia and cardialgia, increase of libido.

Histaminum hydrochloricum : Irritable, impatient, desire for walking, sensation as if the teeth are tottering, cardio-thoracic pains, burning pains of the scrotum and of the ovaries (left), redness and papulae of the skin.

CLINICAL DIAGNOSIS

1. Generalities

Allergic states (Psoric), allergose-tuberculinosic conditions.

Morbid alternances.

Chronic malaria. Malta fever.

Burnand-Jacquelin syndrome (extreme weakness, broken down condition).

Scrofulosis. Scrofulo-tuberculosis (attenuated form of tuberculosis of ganglions and of bones).

Lymphadenitis. Adenomegaly.

Fever of growth (plastic osteitis of growth).

Eruptive fevers : Rougeola. Rubeola. Scarlatina. Chicken pox.

Sixth disease (three days' fever of young boys or infantile roseola).

2. Neuro-endocrino-psychic System

Psychic :

Hypochondria, Beard's disease (neurasthenia).

Obsessional neurosis.

Anxiety complex.

Nocturnal fear.

Manic-depressive psychosis.

Mental anorexia.

Endocrine :

Dysthyroidia or thyroidian dysrythmia. (O.A. Julian)

Basedow's disease.

Nervous :

Periodic migraine.

Hortons' vascular headache (histaminic).

Student's headache.

Epilepsy. Hydrocephaly.

Somnambulism.

Insomnia during the second part of the night.

3. Digestive Apparatus

Late denition. Gingivitis.

Alveolo-dental pyorrhoea (Fauchard's disease).

Adenoiditis. Hypertrophy of the tonsils

Cortico-gastric dysrythmia.

Chronic enterocolitis.

Hemorrhagic recto-colitis.

Bacillary dysentery.

Chronic hepato colitis.

4. Cardio-hemo-vascular System

Cardiac dysrythmia.

Cardiothyreosis.

Acrocyanosis (Syndrome of Crocq-Cassirer).

Erythromelalgia (Syndrome of Weir-Mitchell).

Nodulous periarteritis.

Anemia of young girls (chlorosis).

5. Respiratory Apparatus

Chronic laryngitis ; dragging bronchitis ; bronchiectasis.

Bronchial tuberculosis.

Asthma

Cortico-pleuritis.

Spleno-pneumonia of Grancher.

Pneumoconiosis.

6. Sense Organs

Nose : Epistaxis.   Chronic coryza.

Relapsing furuncles.

Hay fever.

Nasal polypus.

Eyes : Blepharitis. Conjunctivitis. Herpes of the eyelids.
Repeated styes. Irido-cyclitis. Phlyctenular keratitis.
Interstitial keratitis.

Choroiditis.

Ears : Otospongiosis. Meniers vertigo.
Chronic suppurated otitis.

7. **Uro-genital Apparatus**
Chronic glomerulo-nephritis.

Nephritic syndrome.

Cystalgia. Hydrocele.

Pyelocystitis, chronic.

Chronic metritis and cervicitis.

Bowen's disease.

Satyriasis. Tribadisme.

8. **Locomotor System**
Arthroses. Repeated luxations.

Dislocating tuberculous rheumatism of Poncet and Leriche.

Deforming juvenile osteochondritis of the hip (disease of Perthes-Calve).

Plastic osteitis of growth of Poncet.

Dissecting osteo-chondritis or König's disease.

9. **Skin, Phanera**
Nodulous erythema.

Besnier, Boeck. Schauman's disease (benign lympho-granu-
lomatosis or coidosis sarcosis).

Juvenile acne. Couperosis. Comedon.

Atopic eczema. Herpetiform eczema.

Dysidrosic eczema. Varicose eczema.

Psoriasiform eczema.

Gibert's rosy pityriasis.

Urticaria. Pigmentary-urticaria.

10. Commentary

The biotherapic *Tuberculinum* is a "polychrest" biotherapic, in the sense that its field of action is vast and efficiency certain.

It is necessary to note that in the spirit of Homoeopathy abiding with Nebel, L. Vannier, Rouy, Fortier-Bernoville, as well as a new Homoeopath O.A. Julian, there is always the necessity of practising at first the technique of *cleansing* (Julian) or drainage (Nebel, L.-Vannier) before prescribing *Tuberculinum*.

The drainage of the liver, kidney, intestine and skin with some homoeotherapics in lower *dynamisations* or with the help of *phytogemmotherapy*, will help the Tuberculinum to exert its full therapeutic effect.

It is prescribed in 7 CH and 30 CH. the dynamisations that have a action without inconvenience.

But a mixture of dilutions may also be used as for example :

5 CH+7 CH+30 CH, which will help the remedy to act on the sphere of perturbation, localised and cellular not only up to the level of the molecular perturbations but also of the rhino-cephalo-cortical level.

Thus the Tuberculinum finds a general dimension, broader than its tubercular specificity.

Although a Hahnemannian type of pathogenesis has not yet been laid down, the portrait of Tuberculinum, from the clinical experiment, has become quite clear.

It is for this reason that its prescription is not limited alone in a tuberculous or paratuberculous syndrome but in the whole of a category of morbid processes for which the choice of Tuberculinum should be done by the help of analogical relation, or by the method of analogical reasoning.

CLINICAL OBSERVATION

Before closing, here is an observation of P. Schmidt of Geneva published in the Review Groupement hahnemanien de Lyon, 3rd. ser, cahier No. 5., p. 179-80.

Dermatosis of the face (Case of Koch's tuberculine, prescribed according to the proving) :

Mme..., 31 years, suffers since the age of 24 *i.e.*, since seven years from a very ugly eruption on her face, a polymorphous dermatosis, a kind of furuncluous acne with pyodermitis, treated by all sorts of ointments and remedies and by specialists..,without any result. She was always told, "It comes from the intestine". The patient pretends that these eruptions have come out after having swallowed by mistake a solution of Potassium permanganatum while gurgling with it.

The patient is chilly and very lean, always fatigued, *catching cold in every occasion*, is afraid of being alone, and since her infancy she is afraid of dogs.

Becomes angry very easily *and feels herself very irritable while waking up, mental and physical restlessness*, constantly changes occupation, does not like to complete a thing, likes storms, headache in the sun with vertigo, *every 15 days she suffers from her head and it is worse while reading.*

The patient does not like meat, but likes always to add more salt ; *she likes much cold milk. The first menses appeared only at the age 16.* At present suffering from dysmenorrhoea. Menses are very near to each other and continue for 6 days, with clots.

Constipation.

Has white discharges which flows only when she *walks.*

In her eyes one can see clearly from two sides a floating thread from one collarette to the other. She informed us no tubercular antecedant.

No other symptoms ; sleeps well, urinary functions normal.

The only remedy which has these characteristics is Tuberculinum. At that time I had only Koch's tuberculine. We gave her M one dose.

The eruptions aggravated for two days, some while discharges, and general uneasiness. But afterwards, spectacular
amelioration. She is no more weak, stools regular, menses
perfect, eruptions very much diminished ; but the headache
much more frequent.

Forty-five days after, we repeated that dose, and the husband
telephoned me for felicitating Homoeopathy. The eruptions
have completely disappeared, the skin of the face transformed,
and the general condition is ameliorated. The moral is excellent ; she has no more changing mood and finally her husband
described her as a housewife.

The patient went to Argentina, but continues her cure with
Tuberculinum 10 M twice, then 50 M twice ; these doses were
given in the course of two years in a very long interval. One
intercurrent dose of *Bryonia M*, for a fluxion of the left cheek,
result of dental troubles. I saw again the patient at the end of
these two years. She is a living advertisement of the value of a
nosode applied according to the Hahnemannian principles for
a disease which was lasting for seven years.

It is a beautiful case-report. It is to be regretted that this
master of Homoeopathy does not give what is due to Cesar,
because *Tuberculinum K.* is biotherapic-nosode, the integral
part of *Isopathy. It is not* prescribed according to the
Hahnemannian methodology of analogy, having no experimental research in this sense, but according to the *etiological*
analogical reasoning.

TUBERCULINUM RESIDUUM—T.R.

BIBLIOGRAPHY

Boericke W. :

Pocket Manual of Homoeopathic Materia Medica. Boericke and Runyon, New York. 192/, p. 655-659.

Homöopatische Mittel and ihre Wirkungen Materia Medica und Repertorium. Trod, allemande : M. Harms 1972, Verlag Grundlngen und Praxis-Margarete Harms, Leer Ostfriesland.

Cartier F. :

Thérapeutique des voies respiratoire. Baillére and Fils, Paris, 1920.

Vannier L. :

Les tuberculiniques et leur traitment homéopathique.
Doin, 1958.

Julian O.A. :

Biothérapiques et Nosodes. Maloine, 1962, Paris.

Materia Medica der Nosoden. Haug Verlag, Heidelberg, 1960, 2nd ed., 1975.

Julian O.A. and Collab :

Matière Mèdicale d'Homoeopthrapie, 1971. Le François Paris.

Vannier L. :

Les Tuberculines. Cours C. H. F., 28 janv., 1947.

Askenasi J. :

Tuberculinum Residuum. Cours de 2e annèe du Séminaire de l'Institut de Recherche et d'Enseignement, de la Société Médicale de Biothérapie, 1973.

Harlan Wells :

Une méthode pratique et favorable de traiter la Tuberculose Pulmonaire avec la Tuberculine. Journal of the 'American Inst. of Homoeopathy'.

HISTORY

The Residual Tuberculine was prepared by Robert Koch in 1897. Its use in Nosodotherapy has been rather the object of experimentations clinically by french homoeopathic doctors, Cartier, P. Jousset, Mondain, Humea and Revel, Chiron.

A. Nebel of Montreux carried out a very complete study and it is Léon Vannier who, by his practice and his teaching, will give a place of choice to Residual Tuberculine. But these are studies of clinical pathogenesis and it is alone O.A. Julian who had a Hahnemannian pathogenesis in 1960-61 on four persons (two men and two women) with the dynamisations 5 CH, 7 CH and 9 CH. Thus T.R. possesses the double quality : Biotherapic and Homoeotherapic.

STOCK

The Biotherapic Tuberculinum Residuum is obtained from the stock-solution in glyecrine containging the principles insoluble in water of Koch's bacilli making the object of visa 2222 SV 1770 of Merieux Institute and admitted by the Ministry of Health-Central Services of the Pharmacy, on the 1st July, 1958.

This product is presented obligatorily in the form of a phial of 2 ml having the following composition : glycerine solution containing the principles insoluble in water of Koch's bacilli (Mycobacterium Tuberculosis).

One ml of this solution contains the active principle corresponding to 0·20g of lysated bodies of the bacilli.

This visa is given to this product uniquely for the preparations of biotherapics (Homoeopathic nosodes) and cannot be sold for any other use.

TECHNIQUE OF PREPARATION

1. Collection of the Bacillary Mass

The human stock PN-DT and C of *Mycobacterium tuberculosis* and the stock of Bovine Vallée are utilised for the preparation of Tuberculine. These stocks are cultivated on Santon medium for 6 to 7 weeks at 37°. The cultures are then heated at 100° for one hour, then filtered. The portion remaining on the filter is preserved. This portion is constituted by microbian bodies serves for the preparation of residual tuberculine.

2. Preparation of the Residual Tuberculine

The bacillary mass is put to suspension in distilled water, and washed several times to eliminate all traces of the medium of culture. Then it is centrifuged. The crucible of centrifugation is heated at 15° and then decongealed in the ambient temperature. The congealation-decongealation is carried out 10 times successively in order to cause splitting and the resultant is a complete lysate of the bacillary bodies. The homogeneous chamois brown mass thus obtained is put to suspension in 20 to 30 times of its volume of water shaken at the rate of 60 jerks a minute on a mechanical shaker for one hour. Thus all the matter soluble in water is separated.

It is now centrifuged again in suspension in Glycerine at the rate of 400 gr. for 2 litres. The glycerinised suspension is submitted to a shaking for one hour at the rate of 60 jerks per minute, filtered on gauge and the opalsescent liquid of a sufficient thickness thus obtained constitutes the residual tuberculine.

PHARMACODYNAMIC CORTICO-VISCERAL
EXPERIMENTAL PROTOCOL OR PATHOGENESIS

1. Generalities

Subject pale, greyish colour, lips slightly violet.

The upper lip is some times splitted.

Emaciation inspite of a good appetite

Tendency to sclerosis, fibro-chondro-osteo-mesenchymatous.

Great weakness with the desire of sleeping.

Feels better in open air in stretched position.

2. Neuro-endocrino-psychic System

(*a*) *Psychic* :

Discouragement, "Spleen".

Undefined sadness.

(*b*) *Neurological* :

Heaviness in the skull with the need for open air.

Head, heavy ; troubled vision.

Should wink the eyebrows to see distinctly.

3. Digestive Apparatus

Bleeding gums.

Heaviness, bloating after meals.

Pyrosis with eructation and regurgitation of an acid liquid, burning.

Stools easy and abundant.

4. Cardio-hemo-vascular System

Congestion of the veins of the legs.

Slight heaviness and cramps of the legs.

5. Respiratory Apparatus

Dry cough with dyspnoea.

Rare expectoration, difficult to throw out.

Pain in the side.

6. Uro-genital Apparatus

Urine less abundant, with strong smell.

Dull pain, drawing on the ovaries.

7. Loco-motor System

Sensation of stiffness and ankylosis of the articulations.

Shoulders painful, stiff, movements limited and difficult.

Dorsal pains, aggravated by movements.

Pains of all the articulations, drawing with the sensation of being drawn and rigid, aggravated when waking up after a long rest.

Aponeurotic and ligamentary retraction.

8. Skin, Phanera

Dryness of the skin which looks unhealthy.

Fissure of the upper lip, third external part.

Acnes on back and shoulders.

9. Modalities

Aggravation :

Long rest.

Amelioration :

In open air, by movement, by regular physical exercise.

POSOLOGY

Dynamisations : From 4 CH to 30 CH.

The 7 CH, 9 CH and 30 CH, taken repeatedly and for a long time is to be advised.

POSITIVE DIAGNOSIS

Subject, weak, pale, greyish, fatigued.

Discouraged, heaviness in the skull, better by open air and by movement.

Digestive heaviness. Dry cough.

Pains of articulations and rigidness of the ligaments.

Dryness of the skin. Fissure of the upper lip, the external third part.

21 F

DIFFERENTIAL DIAGNOSIS

Sulphur iod : Tuberculinic auto-intoxication with tracheitis, adenopathies, itching eruptions.

Baryta carb : Vascular sclerosis with cortico-somatic slowness.

Calcarea flourica : Afraid of the future, internal inquietitude, febrility, impatient, discouraged or full of arduousness.

Spasms and contractions of the muscles, hairs thin, better by open air and by pressure.

Cobaltum nitricum : Emaciation, fatigue, paleness, general lassitude, frontal headache, vertigo, bone pains.

Acidum hippuricum : Broken down subject, fatigued, maculo-articular pains, papulous eruptions, hepatalgia, nausea and sub-icterus stage, better by open air and pressure.

CLINICAL DIAGNOSIS

1. **Generalities**

   Allergoso state (psoro), tuberculinosis.

   Arthritic diathesis.

2. **Neuro-endocrino-psychic System**

   Jacquelin-Burnad syndrome (broken down condition).

   Depression psychosis of tuberculars.

   Headache.

3. **Digestive Appartus**

   Cortico-gastric dystonia (of Cl. Bergeret).

   Peri-duodenitis.

   Peri-cholecystitis.

   Chronic fibro-adhesive peritonitis.

   Perityphlitis.

4. **Cardio-hemo-vascular System**

Varices, varicositis.

5. **Respiratory Apparatus**

Pulmonary sclerosis.

Chronic bronchitis.

Emphysema.

Fibrous tuberculosis.

Dry pleurisy.

6. **Uro-genital Apparatus**

Chronic salpingitis.

Chronic metritis.

Sclerosis of the neck.

7. **Locomotor System**

Periarthritis.   Arthrosis.

Spondylarthritis, ankylosing.

Tubercular rheumatism of Poncet and Leriche.

8. **Skin, Phanera**

Dupuytren's disease (aponervous retraction of the palms).

Volkmann's syndrome (Ischemic muscular retraction) tuberous acne.

COMMENTARIES

The biotherapic T.R. should be prescribed in a peresevering manner because it acts slowly.   It will act on an old immunological perturbation and it is for this reason that it will be very often indicated together with other homoeopathic remedies to cure a long lasting sclerosis.

Here is a case of Dr. J. Askenasi :

"Mme A...68 years, as a result of an R.A.A. happened at the age of 15, she has progressively and inexorably gone towards a state of chronic rheumatism, P.C.E.

In her familial and personal antecedants a tuberculous condition was found.

It is a very old case dating back a long time before the introduction of antibiotics and corticoids, and so the patient had a very simple treatment *viz* : aspirin and thermal stations.

She was lean, pale, fatigued, terribly deformed by repeated attacks of successive arthritis.

Nevertheless the lungs, the heart and the arterial tension were normal.

Years have only increased her pains and blocked more almost totally her articulations had specially of the right hip and the right knee with ligamentary rigidness. The right knee had deformed due to some exostosis and the soft deposit has become hard, which did not allow any flexion. Consequently not only walking but also sitting and lying down were problems.

This patient was for a long time in foreign land and only very lately and intermittently homoeopathic treatment was taken. From the very beginning of the treatment the serological constants were ameliorated.

This treatment consisted specially of the drainers in low dilutions and for a very longtime some unitary remedies in very high dilutions every fifteen days eased the changing of positions by the patient. The remedies are well known to the practitioners. The trio : *Sulphur, Causticum, Rhus tox* in 9 CH repeated at regular intervals.

Other remedies were not forgotten : *Rhododendron, Arnica, Lachesis, Bryonia, Ruta* etc.

The gouty attacks were treated by *Ledum palustre, Colchicum, Formica* etc.

A certain stability concerning ankylosis, the rigidness of the ligaments and appreciable reduction of the affects of aspirine were obtained.

But the most painful was the right sided gonoarthrosis which did not yield to habitual treatment.

On a Sunday, as it was the 15th day, she took *Tuberculinum residuum 9 CH*.

There was no violent reaction, as it...always happens with Sulphur, and to the astonishment of the patient and to all around her, her deformed right knee, painful with a enormous tophic puffiness with all the lines of the knee cap invisible since a long time, began to move slowly forming an acute angulation, which increased day by day to an angle sufficiently acute for flexion of a knee that has remained rigid since 10 years.

Unfortunatety I have lost sight of the patient, but above fact seemed to me really extraordinary and I could never forget for all the cases of chronic articular rheumatism the effect of *Tuberculinum residuum*.

V.A.B. (EX-B.C.G.)

BIBLIOGRAPHY

Julian O.A. :

Pathogenesie Hahnemannienne du B.C.G. Archives homoeopathiques de Normandie, No. 31, Septembre 1963. Pathogénésie du B.C.G., Zeitschrift für Klassische Homöopathie, No. 4., 7 Juillet, 1963.

Biothèrapiques et Nosodes. Ed. Maloine, Paris, 1962.

Materia Medica der Nosoden. Haug-Verlag Heidelberg, 1960, et Pathogenesie du B.C.G. Recherches théoriques et Partiques en Homoeopathie, t. 1. Ed. Maloine Peyronnet, Paris, 1965.

Traitement et Prophylaxie Homeo-Biothérapique des complications vaccinales. Cahiers de Biothérapie, No. 12, 1966 et No. 13, 1967.

Julian O.A. and Collaborateurs :

Matiére Médicale d'Homeotherapie. Librarie Le François. Paris, 1971.

Julian O.A.

Prevention et traitement Bio-Homeothérapique des complications vaccinales. Le François, Paris, 1973.

Askenasi J. :

Pathogenesie du V.A.B. Cours de 2e annee du Séminaire de 1, Institute de Recherche et d'enseignment de la Société Medicale de Biothérapie, 1973.

Pischel :

Kongressbericht über dia 123 Jahres versammlung : Communications de O.A. Julian, Pischel. Allgemeine Homöopatische Zeitung, No. 1, 1972.

HISTORY

The Biotherapi V.A.B. is obtained from the vaccin B.C.G. as described in the supplement of 1954 of Codex, p. 54, supplied by Institute Pasteur.

O.A. Julian undertook a Hahnemannian experiment of the pathogenesis in 1960-61, on six persons with the dynamisations : 5 CH, 7 CH, 9 CH.

This work and the experimental protocoles were published in the Archives homoéopathiques de Normandie, No. 31, September 1963.

Clinical experience of numerous homoeopaths, in France and in Germany has confirmed the therapeutic value of this Biotherapic.

At first it was prescribed under the name of B.C.G. A change came on the 10th February, 1971. On that date the *Syndicat des Pharmacies et Laboratories Homoéopathiques Spèciaux*, made a communication as follows :

"The Pasteur Institute have informed us that the name 'B.C.G.' was the object of a trade mark in 1933 and consequently, the name B.C.G. can no more be used by a third party.

"Following the interdiction which was thus done to us, we have obtained from the *Service Central de la Pharmacie et des Médicaments* the authorisation to replace the name of that patent by that of V.A.B. which we should prescribe in the place of B.C.G. and it is under the name of V.A.B. that this product will now be sold".

STOCK

Vaccin B.C.G.

Vaccinum B.C.G.

Vaccin Bilié Calmette Guérin.

The vaccin B.C.G. meant for protecting men and some animals against tuberculous infection, is prepared from *Mycobacterium tuberculosis var, hominis bovis.*, is constituted by a suspension of microbes coming from the subcultures of the artificially attenuated stock, described by A. Calmette & Guerin, under the name of Stock B.C.G. The latter has been obtained by reinoculating regularly 230 times in 13 years on potato impregnated by beef bile, glycernated at 5 : 100, the *Mycobacterium tuberculosis var. bovis* "Nocard Milk".

Preservation of the Stock

The stock of B.C.G. is preserved in such a way that its culture and biological characters remain stable. It undergoes every year three consecutive passages on boiled potato ; between this time it is preserved by inoculations, every two weeks, on potato in Sauton medium of which the formula is as follows :

        Asparagine.......................................4 g.

        Chemically pure glycerine.................60 g.

        Citric acid   ....2 g.

        Bipotass of phosphate ....0·5 g.

        Sulphate of magnesium ....0·5 g.

        Citrate of ferrum and ammonia.........0·05 g.

        Distilled water q.s.p ....1000 cm^3

        adjusted to pH 7, 2.

At each re-insemination on potato, the original stock of B.C.G. should undergo some cheeks which help to verify its purity, its inoculation and its allergising and inoculating power.

Preparation of the Suspension

From the culture on potato on Sauton medium 14 days old, by taking the flocculation, the first passage is done on the liquid Sauton medium.

The flocculation thus formed is taken on the 8th day of culture and inoculated again in the liquid Sauton menium. These are the cultures obtained from the second passage which are utilised to prepare the vaccin when 17 to 21 days old.

This fresh vaccin is prepared by suspension of microbe bodies in a liquid Sauton medium diluted by one-fourth, and a dry vaccin is the dry microbe bodies in congealed state as follows :

Fresh Vaccin

The flocculations are collected aseptically and finely divided. Some known quantities are put in suspension in the following liquid :

Sterile liquid Sauton medium	1 part
Sterile distilled water	3 parts.

These quantities vary according to the method of utilisation of the vaccin respectively. by cm^3 of suspension, of ·

75 mg for the vaccin used for cutaneous scarification.

5 mg for the vaccin used to administer by mouth.

1 mg for the vaccin used by intradermic way.

0·01 mg for the vaccin used by sub-cutaneous injection.

Dry Vaccin

The microbe bodies are dried in congealed stage in the following excipient :

Anhydrate glucose	50 g.
Distilled water q.s.p.	100 cm^3.

The quantities of microbe bodies present in each ampoule are such that the addition of an appropriate quantity of bi-distilled water will yield a microbian concentration identical to those of the fresh vaccin.

Trials : 1. *Sterility* : The B.C.G. vaccin should satisfy the sterility controls regards aerobi and anaerobi germs.

2. *Innocuousness* : Injected, subcutaneously or intraperitonially in the dose of 10 mg to cobayes of 250 g, it should not cause any general effect or any determined evolutive tuberculous affection.

MM. Desbordes and Paraf were entrusted by the Syndicate of Laboratories and Homoeopathic Pharmacies with the study of this Biotherapic. They stated that the solution of concentration 10^{-15} of B.B.G. had an immunising effect on the cobaye inoculated by B.K. and also observed that the cobayes lived longer by one month ; at the end of this period the animal was killed and the post-mortem examination revealed a very weak attack on the viscera and ganglions.

EXPERIMENTAL PHARMACODYNAMIC CORTICO-VICERAL PROTOCOL OR PATHOGENESIS

1. Generalities

Great fatigue with heavy head, diffused heaviness of the occipital regions.

Great chilliness, cannot make himself warm.

Isolated febricula, rare of short duration.

Head painful, face pale, distaste for cigarette.

Intellectual excitability with the tendency to exaggerate his cares.

Persistent asthenia.

Tuberculinic states of lean subjects, always fatigued and suffering from chronic constipation.

Phosphoric or carbo-phosphoric type, hypersensible, nervous ansiptos, restless.

2. Neuro-endocrino-psychic System

(a) *Psychic* :

Easily enervated, angry, depressed.

Every noise irritates.

Brain as if benumbed : difficult to find words, to undertake an intellectual work which makes him weak.

Anxiety, vertigo, feeling of an imminent death.

(*b*) *Nervous* :

Headache, towards the end of the afternoon and in the evening.

Restless sleep with erotic dreams.

Prolonged insomnia during the second part of the night.

(*c*) *Endocrine* :

Thyroidian symptoms, towards hyper.

3. Digestive Apparatus

(*a*) *Mouth, tongue, pharynx* :

Bitter mouth, pasty.

Saburrale tongue with yellowish while coating.

Nauseating condition, while waking up, while standing, better by eating.

(*b*) *Stomach, intestines, abdomen* :

Anorexia with a state of nausea or unceasing hunger.

Pricking pains in the liver, better by lying down.

Slow digestion, gastric bloating with the impression that he should vomit.

Troubles of intestinal transit, tendency to constipation.

Dry abdominal cramps.

4. Cardio-hemo-vascular System

Hypotension.

Precordial obstruction, situated between the two nipples, not influenced by rest, nor by movement.

5. Respiratory Apparatus

(*a*) *Throat* :

Adenopathy of the neck, simple or suppurated.

Slight pain during swallowing on the right tonsil.

Scraping and pain in the back of the throat.

(b) *Lungs, pleura* :

Inflammation of the pleura with relapse.

Hypertrophy of the mediastinal ganglion.

Rough cough, dry, fatiguing.

Pleurodynia.

6. Sense Organs

Nose : Sneezing and the sensation of intense coldness.

Nose dry, worse in a room, better in open and cold air.

Eyes : Conjunctivitis, red.

Eyelids swollen.

Ears : Acute, lancinating pain in the left ear.

7. Uro-genital Apparatus

Absence of libido.

8. Loco-motor System

Cervical pain, worse turning towards right, ameliorated by slow and continued movement.

Polyarticular pains, specially of the articulations.

Left temporo-maxillary pain, worse by mastication.

Cramps of fingers and left leg.

9. Skin, Phanera

Dryness of the skin and of the lips.

Ichthyosic appearance of the skin.

Painful sensitiveness of the integument, specially while brushing the hairs.

Cracks and fissures of the labial and anal commissures.

10. Biological Characteristics

Hyperleucocytosis.

Acceleration of the rapidity of sedimentation.

Arneth formula deviated to the left.

Increase of Vernes-Resorcine index.

11. Modalities

Aggravation : By noise, towards the end of the day, by exercises.

Amelioration : While eating, by stretching.

Laterality : Left.

POSOLOGY

Dynamisations : From 4 CH to the 30 CH.

POSITIVE DIAGNOSIS

Subject, asthenic, lean, hypersensible, constipated.

Chilly, cannot tolerate noises, headache with restless sleep.

Anorexia, persistent nauseating state.

Adenopathies, dry cough, fatiguing pleurodynia.

Stuffing of the nose frequent, red eyes, otalgia.

Dryness of the skin and fissures.

DIFFERENTIAL DIAGNOSIS

Drosera : Weakness, dryness of the throat, spasmodic cough, worse after midnight, cervical adenopathy, axillary and inguinal adenopathesis.

Calcarea phos. : Asthenic type, intellectual work makes weak, bone pains, diarrhoea after cold drinks dry, jerking cough, chest painful and sensitive to touch. Troubles of growth.

Natrum muriaticum : Emaciation, chronic headache, desire to be alone, depressed, medial fissure of the upper lip, sensitiveness to cold, feverish, dry cough, irritating. Asthenia at 10 a.m.

Aqua marina : Anxious, subfebrile, foetid sweats, cephalalgias. Thoracic pains, dorsal pains with cough and acquous expectoration or mucous expectoration, with the taste of rust. General weakness, vesicular eruptions.

Hedera helix : (See. O.A. Julian and Collab : Matère Médicale d'homoeotherapie, 1971, Le François, Paris.) lives in anxiety and inquietitude, better in the open air, loss of appetite or hunger pain, troubles of peripheric circulations, articular pains.

CLINICAL DIAGNOSIS

1. Generalities

Tuberculous conditions.

Burnand-Jacqulin syndrome (or "weakness" of Burnand attenuated form of an atypic tuberculosis, with general torpid toxemia, subfebrile condition, with slow evolution).

Becegitis.

Cattan and Mamou's disease or "Periodic" disease.

2. Neuro-endocrino-psychic System

School boys' or students' headache, of overworked intellectuals.

Dysthyroidia, with tendency towards hyperism (O.A. Julian).

Constitutional emaciation, specially of tuberculinics.

Depressive psychoneurosis.

Hypochondriasis.

Melancholia.

Insomnia of students.

3. Digestive Apparatus

Gastro-colitis.

Constipation.

Cholecystatonia.

4. Cardio-hemo-vascular System
Chronic hypotension with emaciation and hyposthenia.

5. Respiratory Apparatus
Chronic tonsilitis ; hypertrophy of tonsils, vegetations of tonsils.

Adenoidism. Adenopathy, chronic cervical adenitis.

Dry pleuritis. Sero-fibrinous pleuresy. Whooping cough of the terminal stage. Ganglionary tuberculosis. Repeated bronchitis.

Infantile asthma. Loeffler syndrome : labile infiltrates, with temporary eosinophilia of the blood.

Besnier-Boeck Schaumann's disease or benign lymphogranulomatosis.

6. Sense Organs
Nose : Chronic rhinitis, nasal polypus, repeated colds.

Eyes : Eczema of the eyelids, blepharitis, catarrhal conjunctivitis.

Interstitial keratitis.

7. Loco-motor System
Poncet-Leriche syndrome or atypic tuberculous rheumatism (inflammatory rheumatism, para-tubercular with diencephalic neuro vegitative troubles).

Calvé's disease (or osteochrondritis of the vertebra of children of 5 to 10 years).

Scheuermann's disease (painful dorsal cyphosis of children).
Vertebral epiphysitis.
Sever's syndrome.

8. Skin, Phanera
Nodulous erythema. Darier's tuberculide.
Keratosis of hairs of Brocq.
Leuckeratosis (or leucoplasis).
Peri-buccal rhagade.
Anal fissure.

COMMENTARIES

V.A.B. has proved itself in the clinic as a polychrest, of certain utility in all the paratubercular and somato-psychic states. It replaces well the Nosode *Marmoreck* (O.A. Julian).

In acute affections, it is prescribed in 4 CH or in 5 CH. frequently and sometimes alternated with *Aviaire*.

It complements very well *Eupatorium perfoliatum* or *Influenzinum* or *Yersin serum*.

Here is a case of Dr. J. Askenasi :

The child Vincent C., aged 6 years in October 1969, is a little blonde child with blue eyes, who had a good result for an ectopia of the testicles with a trituration in low dilution of *Testoterone 3x* and compound of *Calcareas*.

It is for this reason he was brought in a state of fatigue, nervousness and specially for a chronic tracheo-rhino-pharyngitis complicated by intermittents, for which his grandfather called him "Eternally catarrhal". His grandfather was a doctor of Eure. He was given all obligatory vaccinations. Ganglionary hypertrophy.

Punny child, nervous, angry and chilly, weighing 18 kg for 122 cm who has taken several cures at Bourboule without result ; habitual infantile diseases. Pediatrists were consulted, pneumologists and allergologists of the University centre of Caen detected after numerous tests a sensitiveness to dusts, furs, wools, streptococcus.

The vaccination of B.C.G. could not check frequent rhinopharyngitis.

Even different therapeutics such as antihistaminic, Lantigene, Denoral and even Corticotherapy in the forms of drops of Celestine, could not change anything in the condition of the child who proceeded towards a chronic asthmatic bronchitis.

During his colds which are renewed very often, the child seems to feel well in open air, unfortunately his tracheo-bron-chial affection increased with every cold and the antibiotheraphy repeated as usual.

The homoeopathic treatment was started with ordinary drainers in low dilutions of the type of *Ferrum phos.*, *Bryonia*, *Antim. tart.*, *Pulsatilla 4 CH*.

As regards high dilutions every 15 days the choice was relatively easy being given the tuberculous ground of the child : *Calcarea phosphorica* and V.A.B. (B.C.G.) for sufficiently long time.

The amelioration was at first slow, but now the child has no relapse of the rhino-pharyngitis, nor of bronchitis, since 2 years, not even in winter.

VACCINOTOXINUM

BIBLIOGRAPHY

Allen H.C :

The Materia Medica of the Nosodes. Boericke and Tafel, Phil., 1910.

Boericke W. :

Pocket Manual of Homoeopathic Materia Medica. Boericke and Runyon, New York, 1927.

Allen H.C. :

Key-notes and Characteristics of Materia Medica with Nosodes, Jain Publishing Co., New Delhi, 110055.

Boericke W. :

Materia Medica and Repertorium, 1st. ed. German, 1972, M. Harms Leer.

Clarke J.H. :

A Dictionary of Practical Materia Medica, v. 3, p. 1493, London, 1955.

Hui-Bon-Hoa :

Variolinum. Rev. de Livers anglais. Annales Hom. France, nov., 1963, p. 72/152.

Etude comparative de Variolinum et Vaccinum. Annales Hom. France nov. 1967, p. 76, 736.

Fortier-Bernoville M. :

Nosodes, l'Homoeopathie Moderene, No. 2, 15 janv., 1937.

Allen T.F. :

Encyclopedia, v. 10.

Henke :

    Allgemeine Homöop. Zeitg., Bd. 45, S. 373.

Le Normand :

    Hygea. Bd. 10, S. 68.

Schuklitsch. :

    Allg. Homöop. Zeitg. Bd. 4, S. 12.

Julian O.A. :

    Biothérapiques et Nosodes. Maloine 1962, Paris.

    Materia Medica der Nosoden. 2e ed. 1975, K.F. Haug, Heidelberg.

    Prévention et traitement bio-homeo-therapique des complications vaccinales. Le François, 75006, Paris.

Goldstein, Neff, Lane and Koplan :

    Réactions à la Vaccination antivariolique. Pediatrics, mars, 1975, p. 55, 342.

STOCK

The Biotherapic Vaccinotoxinum is obtained from the antivariolic vaccin described in the Codex 1949, p. 968, supplied by the Vaccin Institute.

Vaccin antivariolic or Vaccinum vaccinae or Jennerian vaccin :

The antivariolic vaccin is a preparation obtained from the shreds collected by scraping of an eruption on the skin developed in a hoofer five days after inoculation of the vaccin virus. These epidermic shreds, or "crude pulp", are carefully crushed and inacerated with 4 or 5 parts of glycerine at 75%. Thus the "prepared vaccin" is obtained. It is charged with foreign germs also and is as such sent to the Vaccinogenous Institute for bacteriological purification.

An antivariolic vaccin can be used only if it does not contain anaerobics or streptococcus, or more than 5,000 foreign germs in a cm³.

On the other hand its specific action should be such that 0.3 cm³ of a dilution 1/10,000 inoculated in a rabbit on the skin of 25 cm³ does not produce more than one pustule in a cm³.

The control of antivariolic vaccin preparations is exercised by the *Institute superieur de Vaccine* de l'Académie de Médicine.

The crude pulp, non-glycerinated, may be preserved for years (1 to 20 years) in a refrigerator where a temperature of 15°C is maintained.

The prepared vaccin, which is in a glycerinated medium, may, if it is preserved in the same temperature, retain its action for one year.

A prepared vaccin taken out of the refrigerator should be kept in a cold place and utilised within a maximum period of one month.

The commercial preparations of antivariolic vaccin should have a number of the origin and the date of expiry.

There does not exist any experimental pathogenesis.

CLINICAL CORTICO-VISCERAL PROTOCOL
OR CLINICAL PATHOGENESIS

1. **Generalities**

    Subject, nervous, impatient, restless.

    Sickly humour with restless sleep.

    Asthenia with the need of stretching and yawning.

    General weakness.

    The child wants to be carried.

2. **Neuro-endocrino-psychic System**

    (a) *Psychic* :

    Subject, weeping, anxious.

    Morbid fear of being attacked with small pox.

    Depressed condition with confusion and forgetfulness.

(*b*) *Nervous* :

Frontal headache as if the forehead is going to burst.

Non-reposing sleep.

Wakes up in the middle of night by a lightning-like pain in the frontal region or in the ocular cavities.

Pricking as if by needles on the right temporal region.

Sensation of ice water along the back.

Sensation of burning, tearing, pricking, cutting, and heat in the lower limbs.

Sensation as if the bones are broken.

Post zosterian neuralgia.

3. Digestive Apparatus

(*a*) *Mouth, tongue, pharynx* :

Tongue thick, yellow, dry with papilliae prominent through the coating.

Mouth and tongue dry.

Loss of appetite, cannot tolerate the smell and sight of foods.

Coffee has a sour taste.

(*b*) *Stomach, intestines, abdomen* :

Pains of the pit of the stomach with abdominal bloatedness.

Shooting pains in the hepatic region.

Pricking of the splenic region.

4. Cardio-hemo-vascular System

Precordial pain.

Erethism of the heart and of the arteries.

Thermo-regulation :

Chill, intense fever, coldness of the back, rapid pulse, intense headache, pains of the lower limbs, as if broken.

Sensation of coldness with tremblings.

Fever with great heat, thirst, restlessness, weeping.

Distaste for all foods.

5. Respiratory Apparatus

(a) *Throat* :

Dark red with painful swelling of the tonsils.

(b) *Lung, pleura* :

Short breath with pains in the epigastric region and oppression of the precordial region.

Pricking on the left of the thorax, on the false ribs.

6. Sense Organs

(a) *Nose* :

Sensation as if the nose is full of discharges.

Bleeding of the nose, preceded by a sensation of pinching high up in the nose between the eyebrows after breakfast.

Sensation of coldness in the throat extending towards the presternal region.

Swelling of the right parotid region.

Redness and swelling of the face.

(b) *Eyes* :

Eyelids and conjunctivas, red.

Asthenopia.

Orbitary pains and of the ocular globes as if they are going to burst.

Trouble of vision, veil in front of the eyes, specially in the morning.

Pricking pain in the internal angle of the left eye.

Eyes and the face, red with little eruptions on the face and on hands.

7. Uro genital Apparatus

(a) *Urinary* :

Nephritis, with hematuria and albuminuria. Oedema.

(b) *Genital* :

Abundant and very frequent menstruations.

8. Locomotor System

Back :

Dorsal pain, diminishing towards the lumbar region and radiating around the body.

Upper extremities :

Pain of the left arm, difficult to rise in the morning.

Pains of the wrists and the hands with the sensation of a current of hot air.

Rigidness, redness and trembling of the left arm.

Sensation of *numbness and burning of the 4th finger of the left hand.*

Lower limbs : Pains of the long bones as if broken.

Sensation of tearing in the left hip.

Painful sensation of the legs as if after a great fatigue.

Legs, heavy, painful, difficult to raise.

Sensation of chewing in the bones.

Sensation as if the bones have become short.

Pain and tightness of the knees.

9. Skin, Phanera

Face, red ; skin, hot and dry.

Small eruptions and red pustules on whatever part of the body, come up during heat.

Pustules of deep red colour, raised, round and elongated, containing a yellowish-green pus, and situated on the left side of the trunk, between the shoulders, on the *left shoulder, behind* *the right ear.*

Pustules like small pox, small peas-size, with a central depression and an indurated base, *prupriginous.*

Shooting, burning pain on the skin, particularly localised on the forehead and on the integument.

Milk crusts on the integument.

Cheloid on the cicatrices of the vaccin.

10. Modalities

Aggravation : All the symptoms aggravate in the morning, by humidity.

Ameliora : By movement.

Laterality : Left.

POSOLOGY

Dynamisation : 4 CH, 5 CH, 7 CH, 9 CH.

POSITIVE DIAGNOSIS

Weeping and anxious subject, of sickly humour.

Capricious children.

Bone pains : dorsal and of the upper and lower limbs with the sensation that the bones are broken.

Fronto-orbital neuralgic pains.

Fever with coldness in the dorsal region as if icy water is flowing along the back.

Nose with greenish yellow mucus, right parotid swollen.

Oliguria. Hematuria. Oedemas.

Skin, red, hot, burning vesiculo-pustulous eruptions.

DIFFERENTIAL DIAGNOSIS

Classic homoeopherapics : *Arsenicum album, Rhus toxico-* *dendron, Mezerum.*

Modern homoeotherapics. (Julian O.A. and Collab. Matiere Médicale d'Homoeothérapie, 1971, Le François, 91 bd St.-Germain, 75006, Paris).

Achyranthes calea : Congestive stage, acute, fever, dryness and burning of the skin and mucous membranes.

Decapetalum : Sulky mood, interior trembling, stuffing of the nose, rigidness of the neck, back, lumbo-sacrum.

Hoitzia-coccinea : Acute infectious condition, face red, high fever, oneuro-circulatory ; over excitation, congestion of the head, of eyes, of stomach, genital organs. Scarlatinaform or urticarial form eruptions.

CLINICAL DIAGNOSIS

1. Generalities

Prevention of small pox, desensibilisation of anti-variolic vaccination.

Chronic mesenchymatosis (Sycosis).

Zona.

2. Neuro-endocrino-psychic System

Depressive psychosis, characterical troubles after anti-variolic vaccinations ; post zosterian neuralgia.

Intercostal neuralgias.

Pains of the long bones (in luetic subjects).

3. Digestive Apparatus

Cortico-gastric dyspepsia.

Summer entero-colitis.

4. Respiratory Apparatus

Whooping cough.

Tuberculosis (adjuvant treatment).

5. Sense Organs

Eyes : Conjunctivitis, blepharitis.

Iritis, Phlyctenular keratitis.

Nose : Purulent, rhinitis.

Nasal polypus.

6. **Uro-genital Apparatus**

Urinary : Hematuria, interstitial nephritis.

Genital : Metrorrhagias, bleeding fibromas.

7. **Loco-motor Apparatus**

Polyarthrosis. Tendinitis. Infectious rheumatism. Neuro-trophic rheumatism of the upper limbs.

8. **Skin, Phanera**

Cheloids. Naevus. Zona. Chicken pox. Herpes.

Vesicular erysipelas. Juvenile acne. Pustulous acne. Impetigo.

Phlegmonous cellulitis. Eczema (acute) (post-vaccinal).

CLINICAL OBSERVATION

We reproduce here an article of E. Ducoeurjoly of Boulogne-sur-Seine, published under the title of "Vaccination and Zona" in l'Homoeopathie Française, 1973, No. 2, p. 101-104.

"The zona (herpes zoster, sacred fire, of St.-Antoine, erysipelous zoster) has a very bad reputation in the minds of the patients, who, having passed the age of 50, have known its effects, and in the mind of the doctors, who stumble against the unsolvable difficulties. In fact, the pains that accompany the eruptions of the disease, are generally excessive and more painful it is the more the patient is aged. These pains are of neuralgic type, paroxysmal and with a sensation of shooting, with an intense burning, constrictions, tearing and moreover of a tenacity almost hopeless. We must admit that our therapeutic means are poor. Continued electrisation, high frequency current, the radiotherapies, salicylated ionisation, U.V. rays, auto-hemotherapy, intravenous injection of ascorbic acid, anti-staphylococcic injections, antiviral chemotherapy, have given, in the course of my long practice, many cases of dissatisfaction.

It is perhaps better to recall here, that the medical literature indicates us the practice of gasserian radiocotomy of cervical ganglion in the treatment of the pains of herpes zoster in order to cure the effects of an ulcero-neurotic zona.

Homoeopathy has, also a word to say for treatment of the troublesome Zona. Numerous cases, collected during thirty years, have helped me to establish a therapeutic schema, always the same as the symptoms observed are always similar. The cases therefore do not merit being given in detail as they will tend to merely toll over the patience of the reader.

What is this schema of therapeutic ?

1. Local applications of an ointment made of *trypan blue* and *amyleine chlohydrate* on the vesicles under cotton wool every morning and evening.

The antiseptic, cicatrising and anesthesic action of this preparation on the dermatoses of neurotropic ultra-virus cannot be denied.

2. *Arsenicum album* 5 CH, 2 granules morning and evening every second day. This prescription is justified by the following symptoms :

Anxiety, restlessness, nightly aggravation, burning pain, aggravated by cold, ameliorated by heat in all forms, specially by local application of heat.

Vesiculo-pustular eruptions with ulcerative and necrosing tendency.

3. *Rananculus bulbosus* 5 CH, 2 granules morning and evening the next day.

Pricking pains, burning, aggravation by touch, by cold and humidity. Confluence of the vesicles having violet colour. Localised in intercostal spaces, and on temporo-orbitary region.

4. *Rhus toxicodendron 5 CH*. Replacing Rananculus, when the aggravation of painful symptoms is at night and when the patient feels better by movement with the instinctive need of moving or changing position.

5. Intramuscular injections daily of *Hydroxocobalamine* without any risk of toxicity.

6. And, since some years, *Vaccinotoxinum 7 CH*, one dose every day in the beginning, 9 CH every 4th day later on.

This biotherapic is the antivariolic vaccin, prepared from the shreds collected by scraping of an eruption of the vaccin. The majority of researchers side with the hypothesis of an ultra virus in the etiology of zona. The vaccin and the zona have some erythemato-pearly vesicles. In the present case the law of similitude should be respected totally.

Application of the above mentioned means might eventually be reproached. The vitamin B_{12} possesses a proved action on the neurotic painful symptoms. The associated action of Vaccinotoxinum seems then contingent. Two recent cases, in my opinion are concluding :

Case 1. 15th October, 1972, M.D.......52 years, shopkeeper, who has always enjoyed a good health, has a left sided opthalmic zona, with eruption on the forehead, on the upper eyelid and the nose. No reaction on conjunctiva. A satellite adenopathy accompany the eruption. The pains are atrocious, specially at night, and are slightly better by the use of aspirin.

The treatment is given according to my schema. On the 25th Oct., M.D.......brings, to his surprise, the good news of the disappearance of the pain after the third dose of *Vaccinotoxinum*. There remains in the frontal region, only a sensation of light spider's web. Our patient admits his aversion to all hypodermic injections, for the uneasiness at the first injection, and the decision that he has taken to stop all treatment by injections.

Case 2. M. T.......full of pathological past, who suffered from the bad effect of exogenous intoxication, slow, ethylic and of tobacco, has been treated since many years for an arteritis of the lower limbs. In 1970, some dyspnoeic troubles, with stubborn cough, led the clinicians to the diagnosis of cancer of the left lung, inoperable. Specific chemotherapy is rapidly abandoned because of the hematologic repercussion. The patient was given 24 sittings of cobalto-therapy. Since two years the tumor did not develop. Unfortunately a pericarditis, adhesive and constrictive, exists at the site of violent thoracic pains accompanied with breathtessness after effort. The patient refuses all intervention.

On 15th October 1972, the patient has a left sided intercostal zona with a vesicular red patch 10 cm wide and oozing going from the waist line to the vertebral column, and groans at night because of pain. I met with an unshakable resistence from this man who has become irritable because of his future. He refused all treatments but agreed however on the local applications of trypan blue and the use of one dose of *Vaccinotoxinum 7 CH*, every two days. In eight days the patient and the doctor were both glad on a considerable amelioration of pains. Our patient sleeps without any analgesic.

A conclusion is necessary

Vaccinotoxinum alone or associated to vitamin B_{12} seems to have good action in zona.

My colleague will have the dedicated duty to affirm or infirm the value of this judgment.

VARIOLINUM

BIBLIOGRAPHY

Allen H.C. :

The Materia Medica of the Nosodes, Phil., 1910, Boericke and Tafel.

Clarke J.H. :

A Dictionary of Practical Materia Medica, London, 1950, v. 3, p. 1503.

Julian O. A.

Biotherapiques et Nosodes. Maloine, Paris 1962. Materia Medica der Nosoden : 2e ed. Haug-Verlag, Heidelberg, 1975.

Consult also General Bibliography.

STOCK

Lysate obtained from the serosity of small pox pustule.

This Nosode has no legal existence in the French Pharmacopea.

Vaccinotoxinum may be used in its place.

CLINICAL CORTICO-VISCERAL PROTOCOL OR CLINICAL PATHOGENESIS

1. Generalities

General fatigue. Restlessness, anxiety. Morbid fear of contracting small pox.

Swelling of the eyelids and impression of becoming deaf.

2. Neuro-endocrino-psychic System

Occipital headache, violent, intolerable.

Sensation of a tight band around the head.

Sensation of ice water flowing along the back.

Vertigo. Lipothymias.

Impression of a ball in the throat.

Sees green when waking up.

Post zosterian neuralgia.

3. Digestive Apparatus

Foetid breath. Tongue covered with a dirty yellow or black coating.

Putrid coppery taste in the mouth.

Painful deglutition.

Any smell causes nausea.

Tympanism. Vomiting. Diarrhoea.

Bloody stools, brown, foetid.

4. Cardio-hemo-vascular System

Hypotension.

Lipothymia.

Thermo-regulation : High fever with intense radiating heat abundant sweats, bad smelling.

5. Respiratory Apparatus

Throat sensitive, as if chocked

Difficult deglutition.

Sensation of having a mass in the throat, on the right side.

Oppression.

Cough and expectoration of viscous mucus, thick bloody.

6. Uro-genital Apparatus

(a) *Urinary* : Bilateral renal pain always accompanied by a dorsal pain.

(b) *Genital* : Metrorrhagia, accompanied by lumbar pain.

7. **Loco-motor System**

Intense pain of the lumbo-sacral region.

Gripping pains of the back, radiating towards the belly.

Pains of the limbs and wrists.

Sensation of cold water, icy, flowing in jets along the back.

8. **Skin, Phanera**

Skin, dry and hot.

Face, dark red, purple.

Eruptions, scarlatinalform or morbiliform like nettle rash.

Varioliform eruptions of red round mascule which transform into papulae and then become papulo vesicular.

Petechiae.

9. **Modalities**

Aggravation : By movement.

Laterality : Right, not exclusive.

POSOLOGY

Dynamisations : At Nelson of London : 12 CH and C.M.

POSITIVE DIAGNOSIS

Anxious subject with purple red face, eyelids swollen and the impression of becoming deaf.

Violent occipital headache.

Dysphagia.

High fever with abundant, nauseating sweats.

Dorso-renal pain. Metrorrhagia.

Maculo-pustulo-vesicular eruptions, petechiae.

DIFFERENTIAL DIAGNOSIS

Vaccinotoxinum : See article.

Malandrinum : See article.

CLINICAL DIAGNOSIS

Chronic mesenchymatosis.

Preventive of small pox.

Chicken pox. Zona. Typhoid. Influenza.

Spring dysentery.

Rachialgia. Post-vaccination encephalitic affection.

Distant sequalae of an anti-variolic vaccination (Julian, O.A. Prévention et traitement bio-homeotherapique des complications vaccinales. 1973, Le François, 75006, Paris).

Hemorrhagic fibroma.

Pustular acne.

Tubercular lupus : Fortier-Bernoville had in a case remarkable success with 30 K.

COMMENTARY

The disappearance of this remarkable Nosode is to be regretted.

It may be replaced by Vaccinotoxinum.

In Germany with Heel, Reckeweg prepares Variolinum Injeel+forte (D 15), D 20, D 30, D 200 (plus some unitary dynamisations in D 15, D 200, D 1000, D 10,000).

GENERAL BIBLIOGRAPHY

Actes de la Société rhodanienne d'Homeopathie. 1956. Fascucule 2. Articles des Docteurs : *Martiny, J. Jarricot, Couturier, Lamasson et Dano.*

Actes de la Société Rhodanienne d'Homéopathie, 1938.

Boiteux : Sur le recours á l'Isopathie dans les affection á virus neurotrope, p. 126. *H. Duprat* : A propos de deux guerisons par l'Isopathie, p. 134.—*J. Jarricot* ; Surle recours á l'Isopathie : observations et réflexions, p. 139.— *Jaccard* : Les Nosodes et l'Homéopathie, p. 145.—*Pahud* : L'emploi des tuberculines eu thérapeutique hom., p. 153.

Aguilar (F.) : Pyrogenium—Quelques applications cliniques non habituelles, *l'Homéopathie Française,* 1924 - 1925, p. 635, 639.

Albahary (C.) : Maladies médicamenteuses d'ordre thérapeutique et accidentel, Edition Masson, Paris, 1953.

Alexandre : Colibacillose et Psychisme, *Archives Homéopathiques de Normandie,* 1959, n° 15, p. 799.

Allen (H.C.) : Keynotes and characteristics of the Materia Medica with Nosodes, Jain Publishing, New Delhi-110055, 1974.

—The Materia Medica of the Nosodes. Edition Boericke et Tafel, 1910, Philadelphia (U.S.A.).

Propagateur de l'Homéopathie. 1910 (juillet), p. 159 (Trad. (Duprat).

Allen (T.C.) : Encyclopedia of Pure Materia Medica. Tome VIII, p. 164.

—Diphterinum, *Homeopathy* 1935, p. 106.

PART III

REPERTORY

INDEX

Compiled by

Ratnakar V. Patwardhan

LIST OF REMEDIES WITH ABBREVIATIONS

Abbreviation	Name of Remedy
Anthr.	Anthracinum
Avi.	Aviary
Baci.	Bacillinum
Carc.	Carcinosinum
Diph.	Diphterinum
Hydroph.	Hydrophobinum
Infl.	Influenzinum
(Lues.) Syph.	Syphilinum, Luesinum
Malan.	Malandrinum
Malar.	Malaria
Hippoz.	Hippozaeninum, Malleinum
Medo.	Medorrhinum
Morb.	Morbillinum
B. Morg.	B. Morgan
Dys-Co.	Dysentery-Co.
B.Gaert.	B.Gaertner
B.Mut. (a,b,c)	(a) B.Mutabilis (b) Bacillus Faecalis (c) Cocal-Co.
Baci-7	Bacillus No.7
Syco.Co.	Sycotic Co.
Morg.G.	Morgan-Gaertner, Bacilli of . ..
Baci-10	Bacillus No.10.
Osc.co.	Oscillococcinum
Parot.	Parotidinum, Ourlianum
Paratyph.	Paratyphoidinum
Pert.	Pertussinum
Pneum	Pneumococcinum
Prot.	Proteus
Psor.	Psorinum
Pyro.	Pyrogenium, Putrescinum
Staphyl.	Staphylococcinum, Staphylotoxinum
Streptococ.	Streptococcinum
Tub. (TR, TR, VAB (Ex-BCg.)	Tuberculinum (All Tuberculinums)
Var (φ VAC.)	Variolinum, Vaccinotoxinum

INTRODUCTION

Nosodes are powerful homoeopathic medicine. However, it appears that there is no detailed reference book or a repertory available which will enable a prescriber to really put to use these nosodes with their full potential. A reference book is compiled and presented here so that information about nosodes becomes accessible, and hence can be prescribed with broader and finer basis.

This books gives a lot of information about nosodes. We have attempted here to pick out key-words, arrange them alphabetically like rubrics; and under them group all the remedies in which the words have occured in the "Materia Medica of Nosodes". The 'Key words' are thus all the words which individually or in a group or in a sentence constitute a meaningful homoeopathic information for a prescriber. But this book, although it is structurally similar to a repertory, does not really constitute one. It is a word index.

Here is an example to show how this book can be used. Suppose there is a patient who reports — "she has a brownish discharge before menses with blood." She further reports that her menstrual discharge is clotted in nature. Now, to arrive at the medicine one can use the various available rubrics from this Word Index. Supposing we use the following—1) Menstruation/Menses, 2) Brown/brownish, 3) Before, 4) Blood/Bloody and 5) Discharge. The common medicines arrived at are 1 Prot., Psor. and Tub. from O.A Julian's Materia Medica of Nosodes. Now the second symptom is Menses with clots. We have already looked up menses in the analysis above. Therefore only "clots/coagula" rubric remains to be looked into. This rubric "clots/coagula" has following medicines recorded: Prot. from O.A. Julian's "Materia Medica of Nosodes". Therefore, it is clear that Proteus and Ustilago are the two most important remedies that must be looked into for their suitability in this case. The prescriber can take this decision only after referring to the original works of O.A. Julian. In this process he can come across the sentence "inprotecus" in O.A. Julian's book which reads as follows "Brownish bloody discharge before the menses".

But this is not the only way this "Word Index" can be used because both the books analysed here give other clues like names of the diseases (diagnostic names) and other clinical descriptions like "Furuncles of the ano-vulvar region" or "Thoracic Panniculitis" or "Sciatica" and so on. All these words can be found in this Index under which are grouped the medicines found very useful. Therefore, even if one refers to this book with the clues of the kind given above, he can get his bearings.

However it will be evident that this work can never be used independently. It has to be used with original work the just as one goes from Repertory to the Materia Medica to confirm medicine before prescribing it.

It is therefore necessary to say a few more words regarding the use of this work.

Only available drugs have been taken here for analysis. Drugs like Marmorek and Flavus have been dropped as these are not available.

When searching for any indication like say "sleeplessness" in this work, it is also advantageous to look for other words relating to the root word, viz. `sleep' in this case. Also one must remember to see 'Foot' under "Feet", "Teeth" under "Tooth" etc.

By addition of suffix or prefix or by inflection, the meaning of a word may change entirely. But in this work word is used as an indicator and therefore anything that is spelt in a similarly way has been put together. That is why "Noise" and "Noisy" are put together here. However, where ever possible, similar or same word with different meanings has been shown in correct perspective.

Julian's book uses unfamiliar expressions — e.g., "Fissures of the joints of lips". Ordinarily, I suppose, we would say "cracks in the corners of the mouth". It has been made possible here to arrive at the same medicine no matter which expression is used by the prescriber. Similarly, "Phlebitis" is also grouped under "vein" here although the original book does not use the word 'vein' in the text.

Expression such as 'lips' may be in the rubrics as 'Lips' and yet in the alphabetical order it will appear before 'Lipoma'. This alphabetical anomaly must be kept in mind when referring to this work.

A rubric in this work may give several words with the same or similar meanings (symptoms) of the heading. It does not mean that all the synonyms are necessarily given as rubrics in this index. It is merely to help the reader to recollect the alternative expressions that may be used in any given context.

There is a card called the "Time". All the medicines which have symptoms or aggravations and ameliorations occuring at a particular time are grouped under this title.

A patient's symptom may be recorded as "non-reposing sleep" by a homoeopath. To be able to accommodate this expression a card has been added with a heading "Not-Negative-Non". While this card facilitates negation, it has necessitated the reference back to the "Materia Medica" all the more for confirmation of medicine to be prescribed.

The original expression "Hygrometric and meterological" which is rather unfamiliar has been added to the card "Weather/season". Therefore, when going back to O.A. Julian's book one must remember to revert to the expression of the author. Similarly, the following changes of expressions must be remembered: "Retroauricullar" means behind the ear, "Pollakuria" means frequent urination, "Cystalgia" means the bladder pain, "Peri-buccal-Herpes" means eruption around the mouth, etc. The language in O.A. Julian's book is rather strange and requires special application of mind to get at the correct meaning.

In this book it has been attempted to add the medicine under suitable rubrics so that even if an expression like "Eruption around the mouth" is used still the resulting medicine will be the same as that under "Peri-buccal Herpes."

In this work some medicines, supposedly having the same action and more or less the same source, have been grouped together under one name. These are as under:-

1. Putrescinum and Pyrogenium have been grouped under Pyrogenium.

2. Tuberculinum T K and Tuberculinum TR and VAB (Ex-B.C.G.) are grouped together under Tuberculinum.

3. Variolinum & Vaccinotoxinum have been grouped together under Variolinum (VAR)

4. Ourlianum is a nosode made from saliva of patient suffering from mumps. We have grouped it with Parotidinum which is a more familiar name.

This means if medicine that is to be considered is Tuberculinum as found in this "Word Index" then all Tuberculinums grouped under Tuberculinum, i.e., Tuberculinum TK, Tuberculinum TR and VAB (Ex-BCG) have to be looked into from O. A. Julian's "Materia Medica of Nosodes". Similarly, if Parotidinum comes up from the Word Index then both Ourlianum and Parotidinum have to be looked into from the original work. Same is the case with Variolinum and Vaccinotoxinum.

The word Hydrolipopexia occurs in O. A. Julian's book, the exact meaning of which can not be confirmed as the word can't be found in the dictionaries. "Lipopexia" however, means accumulation of fat in the tissue. Similarly, word Dysthermia or Disthermia seems to have gone out of use. Its meaning could not be ascertained from the dictionaries available at present.

The rubric called 'Pain' contains few remedies mainly because only when the pain is very specific it has been included in this rubric, otherwise this word occurs so often that it will be of no use in the process of elimination. All words qualifying 'pain' have, of course, been included in their respective alphabetical order in this work.

I wish to thank my friend Shri Mohan Shankar Dandge who has worked with me throughout the period when this book was being compiled.

Gole Colony **Ratnakar V. Patwardhan**
Nashik - 422 002

Abdomen: Baci., Baci.-7, Dys.-Co., Hydroph., Malar., Medo., Morb., Osc.co., Parot., Paratyph., Psor., Pyro., Streptococ., Syco.-Co., Syph., Tub., Var.

Ablution: Psor.

Abortion/Miscarriage: Morb.

Above/Top: Baci., Baci.-10, Malar., Morb., Tub.

Abscess (See Boil): Baci., Paratyph., Psor., Pyro., Staphyl., Syph.

Absent/Absence (See Negation/ Not) Not Present: Pneum., Tub.

Abulia (Absence of Will Power): Malar.

Abundant/copious (See Excessive, profuse) numerous/ Free/Plenty: Baci., Baci.-7., B. Gaert., Dys.-Co., Hippoz., Hydroph., Malar., Medo., Prot., Psor., Pyro., Syph., Syco.-Co., Tub., Var.

Accommodation/Accomodative: Diph.

Accompanied/Concomitant: Baci., Tub., Var.

Acetone/Acetonemia: B. Gaert., Dys.-Co., Malan., Syco.-Co.

Aching: Syph.

Acidity/Acidic/Pyrosis/Sour/ Heartburn: B. Morg., B. Gaert., Malar., Medo., Morgb., Prot., Psor., Syco.-Co., Syph., Tub., Var.

Acne: (Rosacea): Anthr., Baci., B. Morg., Carc., Syco.-Co., Tub., Var.

Acrocyanosis: B. Morg., Tub.

Acro-paresthesia: Prot.

Active/Action/Activity: B. Morg., Baci.-10.

Acute: Anthr., Avi., B. Morg., Diph., Dys.-co., Medo., Morb., Osc.co., Paratyph., Pneum., Pyro., Staph., Streptococ., Syco.-Co., Syph., Var.

Addison's Disease: Baci., Malar.

Adenopathy/Adenitis/Adenoma/ Adenoid/Adeno-/ Adenoiditis: Anthr., Avi., Baci., B. Morg., Baci.-7, Medo., Morb., Pert., Psor., Streptococ., Syph., Tub.

Adherent (See Sticky): Syph., Tub.

Adrenal Glands: Baci.

Aynamic (See Weakness): Anthr., Diph.

Aerophagia *(Swallowing of Air)*: Medo., Prot.

Aetiology/Etiology: Baci.

After/Antecedent/Post: B. Gaert., Malan., Malar., Medo., Morg-G, Parot., Pert., Pneum., Prot., Psor., Streptococ., Syco.-Co., Tub., Var.

Afternoon/Noon: Morg-G., Psor., Tub.

Agglutination (See Sticky): Syph.

Aggravation/Worse: Baci., B. Morg., B. Gaert., Baci.-7, Baci.-10, Carc., Diph., Hydroph., Malar., Medo., Morg-G., Osc.co., Pneum., Prot., Psor., Pyro., Streptococ., Syco.-Co., Syph., Tub., Var.

Aggressiveness/Assertive: Prot., Syph.

Agitated/Agitation: Streptococ.

Agony (See Grief etc.): Medo., Osc.co., Prot., Tub.

Agora-Phobia *(Open Spaces, Fear of):* B. Morg.

Agustia *(Loss of Taste)* **(See Taste):** Psor.

Air (See Open Air): Baci., Meco., Pneum., Psor., Pyro., Tub.

Albumen/Albumenoria/ Proteinuria: B. Muta (a),

Carc., Medo., Parot., Pyro., Streptococ., Syco.-Co., Tub., Var.

Alcoholism (Alcohol/Wine/ Drunkard/Beer/Liquor/Liquor/Whisky: Medo., Prot., Syph., Tub.

Algomenorrhoea (Dysmenorrhoea): Syco.-Co., Syph.

Alimentary (Pertaining to Food): Staphyl.

Allergic: Carc., Prot., Psor., Staphyl., Streptococ., Tub.

Allergoso: Staphyl.

Alone (Lonely): B. Morg., B. Gaert., Syco.-Co.

Along: Syph., Var.

Alopecia (Aerata/Baldness/ Calvitias): Baci., B. Morg., Morg.-G., Psor., Syco.-Co., Syph.

Alternating: Baci., B. Mut. (a) Pneum., Prot., Psor., Tub.

Alvelo-Dental: Psor., Streptococ., Tub.

Amenorrhoea: Meno.

Amnesia (See Memory/Forgetful): Medo., Syph.

Amylase: Parot.

Analgesia: Tub.

Anemia/Chlorotic: Carc., Malar., Medo., Syco.-Co., Streop-tococ., Tub.

Anergy *(Lack of Resoponse to an Allergen):* Pert., Psor.

Aneurism: Syph.

Anger/Angry/Rage/Chagrin/ Cross: Hydroph., Prot., Syco. Co., Syph., Tub.

Angina(See Heart)/Angio/ Anginoid: Diph., Morg-G, Paratyph., Prot., Psor., Streptococ., Syph.

Angulation: Syph.

Animals (Dogs/Birds/Black)/ Savage: Baci., Syco.-Co.

Ankilosis (See Joint, Stiffness): Tub.

Ankle: Medo., Psor.

Annexes: Baci.

Anorectal (See Anus & Rectum): Syph.

Anorexia (See Appetite): Baci.-10., Diph., Infl., Pert., Tub.

Anosmia (See Smell, Loss of Sense of): Avi., B. Morg., Medo., Syco.-Co., Syph.

Antecedant (Family): Carc.

Anthrax: Anthr., Malan., Pyro., Staphyl.

Anterior: Medo.

Anus/Ana/Ano: B. Morg., B. Gaert., Baci.-10, Infl., Medo., Prot., Pyro., Syph., Syco.-Co., Tub.,

Anxious (Anxiety): Anthr., Baci.-10, B. Morg., Diph., Dys. Co., Osc.co., Pneum., Psor., Pyro., Syco.-Co., Tub., Var.

Aortitis: Syph.

Apathy/Apathetic: Carc., Psor., Syph.

Apex: Tub.

Aphasia: Psor.

Aphonia (See Voice): Osc.co., Syph., Tub.

Aphrodisia/Nymphomania: Hydroph.

Aphthae (See Ulceration Cancer): B. Morg., Medo., Paratyph., Pneum., Prot., Tub.

Aponeurotic (See Tendon): Tub.

Appearance/Look: Psor.

Appendix/Appendicular/ Apendicitis: Morb., Osc.co., Pyro., Streptococ.

Appetite (See Annorexia): Diph., Malar., Medo., Paratyph., Psor., Syco.-Co., Tub., Var.

· **Axilla/Arm-pit:** Baci.-10, Prot., Staphyl.

B

Back/Backward: Baci., B-Morg., B. Gaert., Baci.-7, Carc., Dys. Co., Hydroph., Malar., Medo., Morg-G., Prot., Psor., Streptococ., Tub., Var.

Bacterial/Bacillary: Tub.

Bad/Difficult: Baci.-10, B. Morg., Diph., Dys.-Co., Hydroph., Medo., Morg-G, Pneum., Psor., Syph., Tub., Var.

Bad Effect of Drugs/Therapeutic/Damage/Iatrogenic Diseases (See Sequalae): Malan, Syph.

Balanitis *(Inflammation Glans Penis)* **(See Glans):** Prot., Syco.-Co.

Baldness/Calvitias/(See Alopecia & Pelade): Psor.

Ball (See Plug etc.): Var.

Band (Iron) **/Bandage/Ring/Corset:** Baci., Medo., Tub., Var.,

Barking: Hydroph

Barometric (See Weather): Tub.

Barre-Lieoli Syndrome: Psor.

Barthonian Glands: B. Morg.

Basal Metabolism: Medo.

Basedow's Disease: Diph., Pneum., Tub.

Bath/Bathing (See Wash): Medo., Pneum., Pyro.

Bear/Endure/Suffer/Tolerate: Hydroph., Osc.co., Paratyph., Psor., Streptococ., Var.

Beating/Beaten: Avi., Carc., Malar., Medo., Psor., Pyro., Tub.

Become/Becoming: Streptococ., Var.

Bed: Diph., Morg-G, Psor., Pyro., Tub.

Before: Carc., Medo., Morg-G., Pneum., Prot., psor., Syph., Tub.

Beginning *(See Words with precard pre)* **Starts/First/Commence/ensue:** Baci, B. Morg, Baci.-7, Malar., Prot, Psor., Syco.-Co., Syph., Tub.

Behind: Baci, Medo., Morb., Osc.co., Psor, Syco.-Co., Tub., Var.

Bending/Stooping: Hydroph., Medo., Pneum., Psor.

Benign: Medo., Tub.

Berry: Tub.

Better/Amelioration/Relieved:

Brain: Psor., Staphyl.

Bread: B. Gaert.

Breaking (Point at the)/Breakdown: Pneum., Psor.

Breath/Breathing: B. Morg., Baci.-10, Diph., Dys.-co., Medo., Morg-G., Psor., Pyro., Syco.-Co., Syph., Var.

Bright/Flash/Brilliant: B. Morg., Hydroph.

Brine: Medo.

Brittle/Crumbling: Psor., Syco.-Co.

Broken/Shattered: Medo., Pert., Pyro., Tub., Var.

Bronchi-Ectasis: Baci., Psor., Tub.

Bronchitis/Bronchial/Bronchitic : Avi., Baci., B. Morg., Baci 7., Diph., Dys.-Co., Hippoz., Infl., Malar., Morb., Osc..co., Paratyph., Pert., Pneum., Prot., Psor., Tub.

Broncho-Alveolitis: Infl.

Broncho-Pneumonia: Avi., B. Morg., Infl., Paratyph.

Broncho-Pulmonary: Avi.

Bronchorrhoea: Diph.

Bronze: Tub.

Brows (See Eye Brows): Morg.G.

Brown/Brownish: B. Morg., Baci.-10, Malar., Medo., Morg-G., Prot., Psor, Pyro, Syph., Tub., Var.

Brucellosis/(See Malta Fever: Malar

Bursting/Burst: Streptococ., Var.

Business: Psor.

Busy/Busy-body/Work: Medo., Osc.co., Psor.

Butter: B. Morg., B. Gaert., Prot., Syco.-Co.

Bruises/Laceration: Osc.co., Pyro., Tub.

Burning/Pyrosis/Burnt/ Scorched/Scalded: Anthr., B. Morg., B. Gaert., Dys.-Co., Hydroph., Malar., Medo., Morg-G., Paratyph., Pneum., Prot., Psor., Pyro., Syco.-Co., Syph., Tub., Var.

Buttock: B. Morg.

Button: Baci., Psor.

Buzzing: Morg-G., Psor., Tub.

C

Calamity/Catastrophy: Medo.

Calculate/Mathematics: Syph.

Calves/Calf: Prot.

Cancer/Cancerous (See Malig-

Cheek/Malar: Baci., Dys.-Co., Malar., Morb., Pyro., Syco.-Co., Tub.

Cheerful/Rosy/(See Joy Happiness, etc.: Tub.

Cheese: B. Morg., B. Gaert., Syco.-Co.

Cheloid/Keloid: Var.

Chemosis: Pert.

Chest (See Thorax): B. Gaert, Dys.-Co., Malar., Morg-G., Psor., Pyro., Tub.

Chicken Pox (See Varioli Form): Syco.-Co., Tub., Var.

Chilblains: B. Morg., Syco.-Co.

Children/Child/Babies/Infants: Avi., Baci., B. Morg., B. Gaert, Carc., Diph., Dys.-Co., Hydroph., Infl., Medo., Morb., Paratyp., Pneum., Prot., Psor., Pyro., Streptococ., Syph., Syco.-Co., Tub., Var.

Chills/Chilliness: Avi., Baci., Baci-7, Diph., Infl., Osc.co., Psor., Pyro, Staphyl., Tub., Var.

Chin: Prot., Psor.

Chlorosis: Tub.

Chocolate: Baci.-10, Hydroph., Prot.

Choked/Stuffed/Blocked (See Congestion/Gagging): Osc.co., Syco.-Co., Syph., Tub., Var.

Chole-cystitis: B. Morg., Morg. G., Paratyph., Prot., Pyro., Tub.

Cholera: Psor., Pyro.

Cholesterolemia: Streptococ.

Cholitis: Morg-G., Tub.

Chorea/Choreiform: Dys.-Co., Streptococ.

Choroiditis: Tub.

Chronic/old: Baci., B. Morg., B. Gaert., Baci.-7, Carc., Diph., Dys.-Co., Hydroph., Hippoz., Infl., Malan., Medo., Morg-G., Streptococ., Syco.-Co., Syph., Tub., Var.

Cicatrical/Cicatrices: Pyro., Syph., Var.

Circulatory: Avi.

Clairvoyance: Medo.

Clammy: Medo.

Claudication: Prot.

Claustrophobia (See Closed Space etc.): Dys.-Co., Morg-G.

Clavicles: Streptococc.

Clear/Clearing: Tub.

Climbing/Mounting/Ascending/ Upstairs, Going: Pneum., Prot.

Close/Clench/Closed: Baci.-7., Prot.

Closed Room/Indoors/Room/ Closed Space/(See Claustrophobia): Dys.-Co., Malar., Pneum., Prot., Psor., Pyro., Streptococ., Tub.

Clots/Coagula: Prot.

Cloth/Linen/Pillows: B. Morg., Tub.

Coated/(See Cover): Medo., Pyro., Tub., Var.

Coccyx/Coccygian: Baci.-10, Medo.

Coeliac disease (See Intenstine): B. Gaert.

Coffee: Malar., Psor., Pyro., Tub., Var.

Coition: Pneum.

Coldness/Colds/Cool: Baci., B. Gaert., Baci.-7, Diph., Hydroph., Infl., Malan., Malar., Medo., Morg-G., Osc.co., Pneum, Prot., Psor., Pyro., Syco.-Co., Syph., tub., Var.

Coli-Bacillary: Paratyph.

Colic/Colicky: Paratyph., Psor.

Colitis: Dys.-Co., Malar.,

Paratyph., Tub.

Collapse/Faint: Medo., Pyro.

Colon: Morg.-G., Syco.-Co.

Colopathies: Prot.

Colour: Osc.co., Prot., Psor.

Combing: Dys.-Co., Psor.

Comedones/(See Acne): Tub.

Compelling/Forcing/Obliging/ Must: Pneum., Tub.

Company: B. Morg., B. Gaert., Morg.g., Prot., Syco.-Co.

Compete: Dys.-Co.

Complaint/Fretful/Grumbling: Morb.

Complication: Avi., Pyro.

Compress/Impacted/Squeezing: Psor.

Concentrate/Concentration: Syph.

Concomittant (See Accompanied): Medo., Psor., Var.

Condensation: Staphyl.

Condition: Streptococ., Tub.

Conduct/Passage: Baci., Morg. G., Syco.-Co.

Condyloma (See Growth): Medo.

Confluent: Morb.

Confused/Confusion/Cloudy (See Obnubilation): Medo., Pert., Var.

Congestion/Congestive/Stopped/ Engorement/Replition: Avi., B. Morg., Hippoz., Infl., Morg. G., Osc.co., Paratyph., Prot., Psor., Pyro., Syco.-Co., Syph., Tub., Var.

Conjunctiva/Conjunctivitis: Avi., B. Morg., Dys.-Co., Infl., Morb., Osc.co., Paratyph., Psor., Syco.-Co., Syph., Tub., Var.

Connective/Connectivosis/Connective Tissue: B. Gaert, Medo., Staphyl.

Conscience: Pert.

Conscious/Consciousness/ Awareness/Knowledge: Pyro.

Consolation: Carc., Streptococ.

Constant/always/Steady/ Persistant/Continuous/Permanent/Incessant/: Avi., Baci., B. Morg., Diph., Hydroph., Malar., Medo., Paratyph., Pneum., Psor., Pyro., Syph., Streptococ., Syco.-Co., Tub.

Constipation/Bowels Inactive: Baci., B. Morg., B. Gaert,

Baci.-7, Carc., Diph., Malar., Medo., Morg-G, Osc-co., Paratyph., Pneum., Prot., Psor., Pyro., Syco., Syph., Tub.

Constitution/(See Diathesis): Carc.

Constriction/Incarcerated/Contraction: Carc., Dys.-Co., Hydroph., Malar., Morg-B., Prot., Psor.

Consumptive/Consumption/(See Phthisis & Tuberculosis): Hippoz.

Contraction/Contracted/(See Constriction): Staphyl., Syph., Tub.

Contrarity: B. Morg.

Control: Hydroph.

Contused (See Injury): Prot.

Convalescence: Prot.

Conversation: Carc., Medo.

Convulsions/Convulsive/ Eclampsia: Avi., Hydroph., Morb., Pert., Prot., Staphyl.

Cooking: Syco.-Co., Tub.

Copper/Coppery: Medo., Syph., Var.

Cornea: B. Morg., Morg-G., Syph.

Corner/Angle: B. Morg., Malar., Morg-G., Psor.

Coronary (See Heart): Prot., Streptococ.

Corpo-pedal: Prot.

Corrosive/Acrid/Excoriating: B. Morg., Baci.-10, Hippoz., Morg-G., Syco.-Co.

Cortico-Gastric: Diph., Morg-G, Pneum., Prot., Psor., Syco.-Co., Tub., Var.

Cortico-Medular: Medo., Syph.

Cortico-Pleuritis: Tub.

Cortico-Somatic: Prot.

Cortico-Tube rositis: Prot.

Cortico-Visceral: Psor.

Coryza: Diph., Hippoz., Infl., Medo., Morb., Morg-G., Syco.-Co., Syph., Tub.

Cough/Coughing: Avi., Baci., B. Morg., B. Gaert., Baci.-10, Carc., Diph., Dys.-Co., Hydroph., Hippoz., Infl., Malar., Medo., Morb., Morg-G., Osc-co., Paratyph., Pert., Pneum., Prot., Psor., Pyro., Syph., Syco.-Co., Tub., Var.

Cover/Covering/Covered/ Sheath: Psor., Pyro., Var.

Coxarthrosis: Hydroph., Psor.

Cracked/Fissured/Chapped (See Rhagades): B. Morg., B. Gaert., Baci.-7, Dys.-Co., Morg-G., Malan., Prot., Psor., Pyro., Syph., Tub.

Cramps/Crampy/Catch/(See Spasm): Baci.-7, Medo., Osc.co., Pneumo., Prot., Psor., Streptococ., Tub.

Cranium (See Skull): Malan.

Cranky/Fretful/Peevish: Morb.

Craze: Baci.

Crossing-Street: B. Gaert.

Crowd: B. Morg., Dys.-Co.

Crusts/Scabs/Sordes: Diph., Malan., Morg-G., Psor., Streptococ., Syph., Tub., Var.

Crying (See Weeping)/Cries: Morg-G., Pert., Psor., Syph., Streptococ., syph., Var.

Cucumber: Prot.

Cutano-Mucous (See Skin): B. Morg., Streptococ., Syph.

Cutting: Medo., Tub., Var.

Cyanosis: Avi., B. Morg., Pert., Psor., Tub.

Cylindrical: Tub.

Cyst/Cystic/Cystitis/Cystalgia/ (See Bladder/Kyst): B. Morg., Dys.-Co., Morg-G.,

Paratyph., Prot., Psor., Syco.-Co., Syph., Tub.

D

Dainties/Cakes/Pastries: Tub.

Dance/Dancer: Carc., Prot.

Dandruff/Scurf: Dys.-Co., Medo.

Danger/Dangerous: Psor.

Dark (Coloured) High Coloured/ (See Black): Infl., Malar., Medo., Psor., Pyro., Var.

Day/Day-Time: Baci., Medo., Pneum., Psor., Syph., Tub.

Dazzling: Psor.

Deafness/Hypoacusia/Hard of Hearing): B. Morg., Baci.-7, Medo., Osc.co., Psor., Syph., Var.

Death/Dead/Dying: Anthr., Pneum., Prot., Psor., Syco.-Co.

Decomposing: Anthr.

Decrease/Diminish/Reduce/ Lessen: Syco.-Co., Syph.

Decubital/Eschar/Bed-sore (See Ulcer): Pyro.

Deep/Profound: Baci., Carc., Malar., Psor., Streptococ., Syph., Tub.

Defective/Deformed/Impaired/

Irregular: Baci., Syph.

Deficient/Deficit/Lack/Insufficient: B. Gaert., Carc., Pert., Pneum., Psor.

Deformation: Medo., Prot., Tub.

Deglutition (See Swallowing): Diph., Hydroph., Syco.-Co., Tub., Var.

Dehydration: Paratyph., Psor.

Dejection (See Sad/Gloomy, etc.): Pyro.

Delirium: Anthr., Malar., Pyro.

Delirium-Tremens/Mania-a-potu: Hydroph.

Deltoid: Morg-G., Syph.

Demineralisation/Demineralised: Diph., Psor.

Dental/Dentition/Dentitional: Baci., B. Morg., Carc., Tub.

Dented/Cupuliform: Syph.

Denutritional State/Malnutrition: Baci., Paratyph.

Depapillising/Glossitis (See Tongue): Streptococ.

Depressed/Morose/Depressive State (See Gloomy): Baci., B. Morg., B. Gaert., Baci.-10, Carc., Diph., Dys.-Co., Hydroph., Infl., Medo., Morg-G, Paratyph., Pneum., Prot.,

Disease/Illness: Hippoz., Malar., Medo., Pneum., Psor.

Disseminated: Pneum., Staphyl.

Diskinesia (See Aggravation by Movement): B. Morg.

Dislike, Disinclined (See Averse) : Carc., Prot., Psor., Syph., Var.

Dislocation/Luxation/Displaced/ Sub-Luxation: Psor., Tub.

Disordered/Disturbance: Osc.co., Pyro., Syph.

Displeased/Out of Humour: Tub.

Disrhythmia: Prot., Tub.

Dissecting: Tub.

Disociated: Pyro.

Distention/Fullness/Repletion/ (See Bloated): Dys.-Co., Morg-G., Pneum., Psor., Pyro., Syco. Co., Tub.

Disthermia/Dysthermia (Fever): Diph., Morg-G., Pneum., Psor.

Disthyroidia (See Dysthyroidea): Infl.

Distinguish: Pyro.

Distonia/Dystonia (Postural Defect caused by disease of the basal ganglia): Medo., Syco.-Co.

Distracted: Baci.

Dogs: Tub.

Dorsalgias/Dorsum/Dorsal/ Dorso: Baci., Baci.-7., Carc., Pneum., Psor., Syco.-Co., Syph., Tub., Var.

Double: Prot

Down/Below/Downward/Descending: Pneum., Psor.

Dragging/Protracted (See Drawing, Long): Avi., Medo., Prot., Syph., Tub.

Drained: Pyro.

Drawing/Pulling/Drawn (See Dragging): Malar., Psor., Tub.

Dreams/Unreality: Baci., Medo., Psor., Pyro., Streptococ., Syco.-Co., Tub.

Dress (Clothes): Baci., Psor., Tub.

Drink/Drinking: Carc., Hydroph., Malar., Medo., Prot., Psor., Pyro.

Drip: Prot.

Drops: Medo., Prot., Psor.

Dry/Parched/Dryness: Avi., B. Morg., B. Gaert., Dys.-Co., Infl., Malan., Malar., Medo., Morg-G., Osc-co., Pert., Pneum., Prot., Psor., Pyro., Streptococ., Syph., Tub., Var.

Dull/Lustreless/Dim: Malar., Paratyph., Psor., Staphyl., Streptococ., Tub.

Duodenum/Duodenitis: Dys.-Co., Prot., Tub.

During (See While): B. Morg., B. Gaert., Dys.-Co., Pneum., Prot., Psor., Tub., Var.

Dysentery: Hydroph., Tub., Var.

Dys-function: Medo.

Dysidrosic/Dyshidrosic (See Sweating): Tub.

Dysmenorrhoea: Baci., B. Morg., Dys.-Co., Medo., Morg-G., Pneum.

Dysparunia/Prinful coitus: B. Morg.

Dyspepsia: Morg-G, Var.

Dysphagia Deglutition Painful (See Swallowing): Hydroph., Streptococ., Var.

Dysphonia: Syph.

Dyspnoea/Breathlessness/Short of Breath/Gasping: Avi., Diph., Medo., Psor., Tub.

Dysthyrodia (See Disthyroidia Dysthyroidea: Psor., Tub.

Dysuria (See Urination, Painful): Hydroph., Psor.

E

Ear/Auditive Conduit: Baci., B. Morg., Dys.-Co., Malar., Medo., Morb., Osc.co., Psor., Pyro., Strepptococ., Tub., Syco.-Co., Syph., Var.

Early: Medo., Prot., Psor., Syph.

Earthy: Medo., Syph.

Easy/Least Efforts/Fast/Quick: B. Morg., Medo., Prot., Syco.-Co., Tub.

Eating/Meals/Prandial/Breakfast/Supper: B. Morg., Baci.-10, Dys.-Co., Morg-G, Paratyph., Pneum., Prot., Psor., Streptococ., Tub., Var.

Ecchymosis/Petechia (Subcutaneous Bleeding): Morb.

Ecthyma (Ulcerative Impetigo): Staphyl.

Ectopia (Abnormality of Position): Syph.

Eczema: Baci., B. Morg., Dys.-Co., Malan., Medo., Morg-G., Psor., Streptococ., Tub., Var.

Eggs: B. Morg., B. Gaert., Baci.-10, Carc., Morg-G, Prot., Psor., Syco.-Co.

Elbow: Baci.-10., Carc., Medo., Morg-G., Psor., Syph.

Electric/Electrified: Streptococ.

Emaciation: Anthr., Avi., Baci., Diph., Paratyph., Psor., Syph., Tub.

Embarassed: Dys.-Co.

Emission: Morg-G., Pyro.

Emotion/Emotive: Pert., Pneum., Prot.

Emphysema: B. Morg., Pneum., Psor., Tub.

Empty/Emptiness: Tub.

Encephalitic/Encephalopathy, Encephalitis: Infl., Paratyph., Pert., Pyro., Var.

Encephalo-Myelitis: Paratyph.

End/Termination/Last: Prut., Psor., Tub.

Endocarditis: Diph., Staphyl., Streptococ.

Endocrine Glands: Psor.

Engrossed: Pyro.

Entering: Pneum.

Entero colitis/Enterisis: Infl., Malar., Paratyph., Psor., Pyro., Syco.-Co., Tub., Var.

Enuresis (See Incontinence): Hydroph., Medo., Morg-G., Psor., Syph.

Ephydrosis (See Sweating): Prot.

Epidemic: Malan.

Epidermis: Morb.

Epididymis: Tub.

Epigastrium/Epigastric: B. Morg., Dys.-Co., Morg-G., Psor., Streptococ., Var.

Epiglottis: Tub.

Epilepsy (See Convulsions)/ Epileptoid/Fits: Hydroph., Paratyph., Pert., Prot., Syph., Streptococ., Tub.

Epistaxis (See Nose+Blood): B. Morg., Diph., Medo., Morg-G., Paratyph., Pert., Psor., Syco.-Co., Tub.

Epithelioma: Syco.-Co.

Epithelium: Streptococ.

Erethism (See Excitement): Var.

Erosion: Syph.

Erotomania: Hydroph.

Erratic: Paratyph.

Eructation/Belching: Baci.-7, Morg-G., Prot., Psor., Syco.-Co., Tub.

Eruption (See Exanthema/ Pimples: Baci., B. Morg., B. Gaert., B. Mut-a., Baci.-7, Malan., Medo., Morb., Morg-G., Paratyph., Pneum., Prot., Psor., Streptococ., Syph., Tub., Var.

Extending/Extension/Irradiating (See Radiant etc.)/spreading/towards: Baci., Malar., Medo., Morb., Pert., Psor., Streptococ., Tub., Var.

External/Outer: Prot.

Extra-systole: Dys.-Co.

Extremities/Legs & Feet/Hands & Legs (See Limbs): Avi., B. Morg., Baci.-7, Diph., Morg-G., Pyro., Streptococ., Syph., Tub.

Exudation (See Discharge, Oozing etc.): Staphyl.

Eyes/Eye Balls (See Occullar Occular Globes): B. Morg., B. Gaert., Baci.-10, Carc., Dys.-Co., Malar., Medo., Morb., Pneum., Prot., Psor., Pyro., Syco.-Co., Syph., Tub., Var.

Eyebrows: Var.

Eyelashes: Tub.

Eyelids/Lids: Baci., Baci.-7, Dys.-Co., Medo., Morg-G., Psor., Pyro., Staphyl., Syco. Co., Syph., Tub., Var.

F

Face/Facial: Aci., B. Morg., Baci.-7, Carc., Dys.-Co., Malan., Malar., Medo., Morb., Morg-G., Pneum.,

Psor., Pyro., Streptococ., Syph., Tub., Var.

Fall/Falling: B. Morg., Malar., Prot., Staphyl., Streptococ., Syph., Tub.

False (Pseudo): Diph., Malar., Pneum., Prot., Psor., Var.

Fan/Fanlike/Fanned: Medo., Pyro.

Fat (See Obesity): B. Morg., B. -Gaert., Baci.-7, Baci.-10, Carc., Dys.-Co., Morg-G., Prot., Syco.-Co., Tub., Var.

Fatigue/Tired/Weakening/Fatiguing/Wornout/All Gone - Sensation/Exhausted (See Weak.): Baci., Baci.-7, Carc., Diph., Infl., Malar., Medo., Parat., Pneum., Prot., Psor., Pyro., Streptococ., Syco.-Co., Syph., Tub., Var.

Fear/Afraid/Phobia/Frightened/Dread/Terror/Threatened/Alarmed: B. Morg., B. Gaert., Carc., Dys.-Co., Hydroph., Malar., Medo., Morg-G., Osc.co., Paratyph., Pneum., Psor., Pyro., Syco.-Co., Syph., Tub., Var.

Feather: Pneum.

"Feels as if . . . ": Baci., B. Morg., Malar., Psor., Pyro., Tub.

Focal/Focus: Pneum., Prot., Streptococ.

Folds/Folding: Baci., Baci.-10, Malar., Medo., Psor., Syco.-Co., Tub.

Follicullar/Folliculitis: Staphyl.

Following/Followed by/then/Succeeded: Pneum., Pyro., Tub.

Fond: Psor.

Food/Ingesta: Malar., Medo., Prot., Tub., Var.

Forearm: Malar

Forehead/Frontal Eminance): Avi., Malar., Pneum., Psor., Syph., Tub., Var.

Foreign/Foreign Body: Tub.

Forgets/Can't Recollect/Vanishing of Thought (See Amnesia): Medo., Psor., Syph., Tub., Var.

Formiction/Numbness/Insensibility/Tingling/Pins & Needles: Tub.

Forward: Medo., Psor.

Fossa: Baci.-10, Morg-G., Staphyl.

Frequent/Often/Now & then: Baci., B. Morg., Dys.-Co., Malar., Medo., Morg-G., Osc.co., Paratyph., Pneum., Prot., Syco.-Co., Tub., Var.

Fresh:Tub.

Fried: Baci.-10.

Frigidity: Baci.-7, Medo., Pneum., Psor., Syph.

Front: Tub.

Frontal/(Frontal Eminance)/Forehead/Sinciput: Avi., B. Morg., Baci.-10, Dys.-Co., Hippoz., Medo., Osc.co., Pneum., Prot., Psor., Syph., Var.

Frost: Syco.-Co.

Frothy/Form/Foamy: Hydroph., Tub.

Frozen: Malar., Prot.

Fruits: Carc., Medo.

Fulgurating: Syph.

Fuliginosities, Sooty: Pyro.

Full/Complete/Whole: Psor., Pyro., Streptococ.

Fungus/Ringworm/Tinia Athlete's Foot: Psor.

Furious: Syph.

Furuncles: Anthr., Baci., B. Morg., B. Gaert., Malan., Prot., Pyro., Staphyl., Tub.

G

Gall Bladder (See Cholecystitis): Baci.-10, Malar., Morg-G.

Gallactorrhoea: Tub.

Ganglion: Anthr., Avi., Psor.

Ganglionary Primo Infection: Anthr., Avi.

Gangrene: Anthr., Pyro.

Gas/Aerogastria/Aerophagia/ Aetocholia: Morg-G., Pneum., Prot., Pyro.

Gastric/Gastritis/Gastralgia: Baci.-7, Diph., Dys.-Co., Malar., Medo., Pneum., Prot., Pyro., Streptococ., Tub.

Gasteroenteritis/Gastrointestinal: Anthr., B. Gaert., Baci.-7, Infl., Osc.co., Pyro.

Gay/Joyful/Well Disposed (See Cheerful/Rosy): Hydroph., Medo., Psor., Tub.

General/Generalised: Avi., Hydroph., Malar., Morb., Paratyph., Psor., Pyro, Staphyl., Syco.-Co., Tub., Var.

Genital: Baci., Baci.-10, Psor.

Gestures: Syph.

Gingivitis (See Gums): Tub.

Girls: B. Morg., Tub.

Glairy: Medo.

Glands: Anthr., Baci., Hippoz., Medo., Morg-B., Tub.

Glans/Corona Glandis (See Balanitis): Syco.-Co.

Glomerulo(Nephritis): Streptococ., Tub.

Glossitis (See Tongue)/ Glossodynia: B. Morg., Streptococ., Syco.-Co., Syph.

Glottis: Medo., Pert.

Glue/Gelatinous/Glued/Glueye: Medo.

Glycosuria (See Diabetes): B. Morg.

Gonarthrosis: B. Morg., Baci.-7, Dys.-Co., Morg-G.

Gonorrhoea: Medo., Syco.-Co.

Gout: Baci.-7, Medo., Psor.

Gradual (See Slowness): Syph.

Grammer: Syph.

Granular: B. Morg., Tub.

Grave: Anthr., Hippoz.

Great (See Intense): B. Gaert., Carc., Malar., Medot., Prot., Psor., Pyro., Staphyl., Tub., Var.

Green/Greenish: Baci., B. Morg., Baci.-10, Medo., Prot., Psor., Tub., Var.

Grey/Greying/Greyness: Medo., Syph., Tub.

Grimace: Carc.

Gripping: Var

Groin/Loin: B. Morg.

Growth/Lump/Grown: Baci., Medo., Syco.-Co., Syph., Tub., Var.

Guillaum-Barre: Diph.

Gums (See Gingivitis): Baci.-10, Carc., Morb., Morg-G., Prot., Psor., Streptococ., Tub.

Gushes/Flashes: Baci., Malar., Medo., Psor.

H

Hacking: Malar.

Hair: B. Morg., Medo., Morg-G., Prot., Psor., Streptococ., Syco. Co., Syph.

Half (Semi. . .): Psor.

Hallucination/Illusion: Baci., Medo., Pyro., Streptococ.

Halo: Psor., Tub.

Ham/Hamstrings: Tub.

Hammering: Prot.

Hand/Hands (See Arms): Baci., B-Morg., B. Gaert., Baci.-10, Carc., Dys.-Co., Malan., Malar., Medo., Morg-G., Osc.co., Prot., Psor., Syco.-Co., Syph., Tub., Var.

Hard/Hardness: Anthr., Malan., Morg-G., Prot., Pyro., Tub.

Haricots: Prot., Tub.

Harsh/Rough: Diph., Morb.

Hasty/Hurry: Medo.

Hay-Fever: B. Morg., Tub.

Hazy/Cloudy/Blurred/Glausy/ Veiled: Malar., Var.

Head (See Scalf): Baci., Malar., Medo., Pneum., Psor., Pyro., Streptococ., Syco.-Co., Tub., Var.

Headache: Avi., Baci., B. Morg., B. Gaert., Baci.-10, Carc., Diph., Dys.-Co., Hydroph., Infl., Malan., Malar., Medo., Osc.co., Paratyph., Pneum., Prot., Psor., Pyro., Streptococ., Syco.-Co., Tub., Var.

Health: B. Morg.

Hearing/Heard: B. Morg., Medo., Osc.co., Streptococ., Syco.- Co.

Heart: Baci.-7, Cars., Medo., Paratyph., Pneum., Prot., Pyro., Streptococ., Syph., Var.

Heat/Heated: Baci., B. Morg., Baci.-7, Carc., Diph., Malar., Medo., Morg-G., Osc.co., Prot., Psor., Pyro., Syco.-

Hunger/Hungry: Medo., Pneum., Prot., Psor., Tub.

Hyaline (Cylinders, Casts): Medo., Tub.

Hydrarthrosis: Paratyph., Streptococ.

Hydrocele: B. Morg., Tub.

Hydrocephalic/Hydrocephale: Baci., Tub.

Hydrogenoid: Medo.

Hydrolipopexia: Infl.

Hydrosadenitis: Staphyl.

Hydrosis: Prot., Psor.

Hyper (See High): Pert., Prot., Psor., Streptococ.

Hyperamylasemia: Parot.

H y p e r e s t h e s i a (Hypersensitiveness]: B. Gaert., Hydroph., Syco.-Co.

Hyper-Salivation/Ptyalism (See Sialorrhoea): Hydroph., Syph.

Hyper-Secretion: Morg-G., Syco. Co.

Hypertension/Blood Pressure: B. Morg., Baci.-7, Streptococ.

Hypertonia: Syph.

Hypertrophy: Dys.-Co., Medo., Morb., Prot., Psor., Syco.-Co., Syph., Tub.

Hypochlorhydria (Deficiency of Hydrochloric Acid): Diph.

Hypochondria: Malar., Morg-G., Pneum., Tub.

Hypochondriasis: Pneum., Tub.

Hypofunction: Psor.

Hyporesistivity: Psor.

Hyposthenic: Baci.-7, Psor.

Hyposystole: Baci.-7.

Hypotension: Baci.-7., Diph., Infl., Psor., Var.

Hypothalamus: Medo.

Hypothermia: Pyro.

Hypothrepsia: B. Gaert.

Hypothyroidism: Baci.-7, Psor.

Hypotonia: Osc-co., Psor.

Hysteria (See Epilepsy): Prot.

I

Ice/Icy: Medo., Var.

Ichorus/Corroding: Anthr.

Ichthyosis: Syph.

Idea/Ideation/Notion/Imagine: Baci.-7, Medo., Osc.co., Prot., Psor., Pyro., Tub.

Idiocy/Idiot: Baci.

Iliac/Ilium/Ileo-cecal: Baci.-10, Malar., Syco.-Co.

Intelligent: B. Gaert.

Intense/Furious/Vehement/Terrible: Anthr., B. Morg., Malan., Medo., Prut., Psor., Paratyph., Var.

Intercostal: Morg-G., Syco.-Co., Var.

Interest: Carc.

Intermittent (See Malaria, Paludism, Ague): Infl., Prot., Psor., Streptococ., Tub.

Internal (See Inner): Malar., Var.

Interstitial/Subserous: Streptococ., Tub., Var.

Intertrigo: Syco.-Co.

Intenstine/Enteritis/Bowels/Intestinal: Baci., B. Morg., Baci.-10, Malar., Morg-G., Osc.co., Paratyph., Pyro.

Intolerable/Intolerace (See Intense): Anthr., Psor., Streptococ., Var.

Intoxication: Staphyl., Tub.

Intracranial: Prot.

Intuitive: Syph.

Involuntary: Hydroph., Psor., Pyro., Tub.

Irido-cyclitis: Syph., Tub.

Iritis: B. Morg., Var.

Irregular: Dys.-Co., Hippoz., Paratyph., Pert., Psor., Pyro., Tub.

Irritable/Irascible/Cross/Vexed/Humourless: Baci., B. Morg., B. Gaert., Baci.-10, Hydroph., Medo., Morg-G., Prot., Psor.

Irritant/Irritation: Anthr., Avi., Baci.-10, Dys.-Co., Medo., Morg., Morg-G., Psor., Syco. Co., Syph., Tub.

Ischemia: Prot.

Itching (See Pruritus, Prurigenous): Baci., B-Gaert., Malan., Malar., Medo., Morg-G, Prot., Psor., Syph., Tub.

J

Jaquelin-Burnard Syndrome: Avi., Diph., Infl., Pert., Tub.

Jaundice/Icterus/Sub-Icteric: Osc.co., Tub.

Jaws: Dys.-Co., Malar.

Jealousy: Morg-G.

Jerking/Jarring: Baci., Per., Pyro., Syph., Tub.

Jets: Tub.

Joints/Flexions/Sockets/Junction/Arthrosis/Arthro: B. Morg., Baci.-10, Medo., Morg-G, Paratyph., Psor., Strepto-coc., Syco.-Co., Var.

Lethargy: Morg-G.

Leucopenia: Infl., Streptococ.

Leucorrhoea: B. Morg., B. Gaert., Baci.-10, Medo., Morg-G., Prot., Syco.-Co, Syph.

Libido: Tub.

Lichen-Planus: Syph.

Lie: Medo., Syph.

Life: Pneum., Tub.

Lift/Lifted: Psor., Syph.

Ligament: Tub.

Light *(Alco with Respect to weight)/Lamp/Glare/Luminous:* B. Gaert., Baci.-7, Hydroph., Prot., Psor., Streptococ.

Lignous: Anthr.

Like/Similar to/As if, Feeling: Baci., Psor., Pyro., Streptococ., Tub., Var.

Limbs (See Extremities): Diph., Infl., Malar., Paratyph., Pyro., Streptococ., Tub., Var.

Linear: Syph.

Lips: B. Morg., B. Gaert., Dys.-Co., Malan., Malar., Medo., Morg-G., Prot., Psor., Streptococ., Syco.-Co., Tub.

Lipoma: Baci.-10.

Lipothymia: Infl., Osc.co., Var.

Liquid/Fluid/Fluent: Anthr., Hydroph., Pneum., Psor., Pyro.

Lithiasis (Stone Formation): B. Morg., Morg-G.

Liver (See Hepatic): Baci.-7, Malar., Paratyph., Pneum., Pyro.

Livid (See Blue): Pyro.

Localised/Location/Site: Medo., Morb., Paratyph., Pyro., Streptococ., Tub., Var.

Lochia: Pyro.

Long (See Protracted)/Prolong: B. Gaert., Baci.-7, Malar., Paratyph., Pneum., Psor., Syco.-Co., Syph., Tub., Var.

Loose/Looseness: Psor.

Loquacity (See Talking)/Speaking: Hydroph., Pyro., Tub.

Loss of/Lost/Diminution/Lack of: B. Morg., Carc., Diph., Dys.-Co., Hydroph., Malar., Medo., Morg-G., Paratyph., Pneum., Psor., Syco.-Co., Streptococ., Tub., Var.

Loud/Raucous/Aloud: Tub.

Lower/Lowering/Inferior/Low: Diph., Dys.-Co., Infl., Malar., Paratyph., Psor., Streptococ., Var.

Meat (See Mutton): B. Morg., Carc., Syph., Tub.

Meatus: B. Morg., Syph.

Median/Mid/Central (See Middle): Baci.-7, Malar.

Medulla: Medo.

Megaly/Enlargement: Malar., Morb., paratyph., Staphyl., Tub.

Melaena: Prot.

Meibomian Glands: Prot.

Melancholic/Morose: Hydroph., Prot., Psor., Tub.

Membrane/Pellicle: Diph.

Memory: Medo., Pneum., Psor., Syph., Tub.

Menace: B. Morg.

Menier's Disease: B. Morg., Prot., Syph., Tub.

Meningial/Meningitis/Meningio: Avi., Infl., Parot., Paratyph., Pert., Prot., Pyro., Staphyl.

Meningism: Morb., Prot.

Menopause/Climaxis/Climacteric: B. Morg.

Menorrhagia: B. Morg., Psor.

Menstruation/Menses: Baci., B. Morg., Dys.-Co., Medo., Morg-G., Pneum., Prot., Psor.,

Pyro., Syco.-Co., Syph., Tub., Var.

Mental/Psychic (See Mind)/ Mentally: Baci., Baci.-7, Carc., Medo., Pert., Pyro., Syco-co., Tub.

Mesenchyma/Mesenchymatosis/ Mesenchymatosic/ Mesenchymatous: B. Gaert., Medo., Osc.co., Paratyph., Staphyl., Var.

Mesenteric: Baci., Morb.

Metallic/Metal: Tub.

Metastasis/Mobility of Symptoms: B. Mut (a) Prot., psor., Tub.

Meteoropathy: Psor.

Meticulous/Particular: Carc.

Metritis: Medo., Prot., Psor., Syco.-Co., Tub.

Metrorrhagia: B. Morg., Var.

Microbe: Syph.

Microadenophthy/Micropolyadenopathy: Avi., Diph.

Middle/Centre (See Median): Var.

Midnight/Middle of the night: Malar., Medo., Syph., Var.

Migraine: B. Morg., Carc., Pneum., Prot., Psor., Streptococ., Tub.

Mustaches: Staphyl.

Myalgias: Tub.

Mucosis (See Fungus): Psor.

Myelasthenia: Prot.

Myelitis: Diph., Paratyph., Pert., Staphyl.

Myocarditis/Myocardic/ Myocardiosis: Diph., Infl., Morg-G., psor., Staphyl., Streptococ.

Myopia: Baci.

N

Naevi: Carc.

nails/(See Onyx)/Including the Metallic Nail: B. Gaert., Carc., Medo., Morg-G., Prot., Psor., Syco.-Co.

Names: Medo., Syph.

Nape (Of the Neck): Pneum.

Narrowing: Syph.

Nausea/nauseating/Disgust/ Qualmish: Baci., Baci-10, Carc., Diph., Hydroph., Ma- lar., Medo., Paratyph., Pneum., Prot., Psor., Pyro., Streptococ., Syco.-Co., Tub., Var.

Navel/Umbilicus/Naevus: B. Morg., Var.

Neck/Cervix: Baci.-7, Baci.-10, Diph., Hydroph., Malar., Medo., Morb., Pneum., Prot., Psor., Streptococ., Syco.-Co., Syph., Tub.

Necrosis: Syph.

Needs (See Desires/Craves Wants): Medo., Psor., Pyro., Tub.

Needle: Morg-G., Osc.co., Var.

Neglected: Psor.

Neon: Pneum

Nephritis/Nephrosis: Diph., Morg-G., Prot., Pyro., Staphyl., Streptococ., Syco.- Co., Tub., Var.

Nerves/Neurological/Nervous System: Diph., Syph., Staphyl.

Nervous (i.e. of Nerves):B. Morg., B. Gaert., Dys.-Co., Hydroph., Malar., Medo., Pert., Pneum., Prot., Stretococ., Syco.-Co., Syph., Tub., Var.

Nettle Rash (See urticaria): Var.

Neuralgia/Neuritic Pain: Dys.- Co., Medo., Morg-G., Pneum., Prot., Psor., Syco.- Co., Syph., Tub., Var.

Neurasthenia/Beard's Disease: Prot., Tub.

Paratyph., Streptococ., Syph., Tub.

Obstinate/Stubborn/Intractable: Carc., Osc.co., Paratyph., Prot., Psor., Streptococ.

Obstruction/Stoppage/Blockage (See Chiced) Incarcerated: Aci., Medo., Osc.co., Prot.

Occipital/Occiput: B. Morg., Malan., Malar., Psor., Pyro., Syph., Tub., Var.

Oculo/Occular (See Eyes): Dys.-Co., Infl., Morb., Osc-co., Psor., Streptococ., Syph., Var.

Oedema: Baci.-7, Infl., Medo., Morg-G, Streptococ., Syco.-Co., Tub., Var.

Oesophagus/Oesophagitis: Diph., Hydroph., Streptococ., Syph.

Oil/Greasy/Oily: Baci.-10, Medo., Psor., Syco.-Co., Tub.

Old Men/Old Persons: Carc., Diph., Psor.

Oldness (See Sense/Mummified: Baci.-7, Prot., Psor., Syph.

Oligomenorrhoea: Pneum., Syph.

Oliguria: Baci.-7, Infl., Var.

Onion: Prot.

Onychophagia [Nail Bitting): Medo.

Onychorrhexia: Syph.

Onychosis (See Nails): Medo.

Onyxia/Onyxophagia/Onyxis (See Nails): B. Gaert., Baci.-7, Staphyl., Syco.-Co., Syph.

Onyxurosis: B. Gaert.

Oozing (See Discharge): B. Morg., Malan., Medo., Morg.-G., Prot., Psor., Tub.

Opacity/Cataract: Morg-G., Syco.-Co.

Open: Tub.

Open-air: Malar., Pneum., Psor., Streptococ., Tub.

Oppression: Carc., Prot., Psor., Tub., Var.

Opthalmia: Medo.

Optic: Morb.

Orbital (See Eye Ball): Dys.-Co., Var.

Orchitis: Parot.

Orgasm: Pneum.

Orifices: Psor., Syco.-Co.

Oscillating (See Undulating): Avi., Staphyl.

Osteitis: Staphyl., Syph., Tub.

Osteo-Arthritis: Dys.-Co., Paratyph.

Papule/Pustule: B. Morg., Prot., Syph.

Papulous: Morb., Morg-G., Psor., Var.

Paralysis/Paralytic: Diph., Hydroph., Malar., Pert., Syph., Tub.

Parasitosis/Worms/Verminosis/ Helminthiasis/Oxyuris: Carc., Medo., Prot., Syco.-Co., Syph.

Paratyphoid: Paratyph.

Parenchymatous: Syph.

Paresthesia: Streptococ,, Tub.

Paretic (See Paralysis)/Paresis: Baci.-10, Diph., Pert., Pyro., Syph.

Parotids/Parotitis: Anthr., Hippoz., Parot., Paratyph., Var.

Part/Parts: Pyro.

Partial/Partly: Streptococ.

Passing: Tub.

Pasty (See Viscous, Thick): Malar., Prot.

Patches (See Spots): B. Gaert., Morb., Streptococ., Tub.

Patrarquerie (See Jaquelin Bernard Syndrome): Diph.

Pectoris/Pectoral: Morg-G.,

Prot., Syph.

Peduncular: Medo.

Pelade (See Alopecia Areata): Prot., Syph.

Pelvic/Pelvis: Dys.-Co., Malar.

Pemphigus: Syph.

Penis: Syco.-Co., Tub.

Pepper: Malar.

Perception: Avi., Morb.

Perforation: Prot., Psor., Syph.

Peri . . . /Circumscribed: B. Gaert., Baci.-7, Baci.-10, Pyro., Straphyl., Streptococ., Syco.-Co., Tub.

Periarthrosis: Medo.

Peri-Buccal: Paratyph.

Pericardial/Pericardiac: Medo., Staphyl., Streptococ.

Perineum: B. Morg., Dys.-Co., Medo.

Perinephritic: Staphyl.

Periodical/Rhythmic: B. Morg., B. Gaert., Dys.-Co., Psor., Pyro., Syco.-Co., Tub.

Periostitis/Periosteum: Dys.-Co.

Peritonium/Peritonitis: Medo., Tub.

Periumbilicus (Navel, Around

the): Malar.

Pernicious: Carc.

Persons: B. Morg., B. Gaert., Dys.-Co., Syco.-Co., Tub.

Personality: Pyro.

Perspiration (See Sweat): Baci., Malar., Medo.

Perturbation: Streptococ., Syph.

Perversion: Tub.

Pessimist: Paratyph., Psor.

Petechae (See Haemorrhage)/ Ecchymoses: Var.

Phallus: Medo.

Pharyntitis/Pharynx: B. Morg., Dys.-Co., Infl., Medo., Paratyph., Prot., Syco.-Co., Syph., Tub.

Phlebitis (See Veins): Paratyph., Prot., Streptococ.

Phlegm, (See Mucus): B. Gaert., Dys.-Co., Malar., Medo., Morg.g., Pert., Prot., Psor., Pyro., Staphyl., Syco.-Co., Var.

Phlegmon/Phlegmonous: Anthr., Pyro., Staphyl., Var.

Phlyctenary/Phlyctenular [Minute vesicle or Boil]: B. Morg., Morb., Syph., Tub., Var.

Phosphenes: Prot.

Phospho-Fluoric: Pneum., Syph.

Photophobia: Morg., Psor., Syco.-Co., Syph., Tub.

Phrenic (Diaphragm): Pyro.

Physical: Baci.-7, Tub.

Pianist: Prot.

Pigmentary: Tub.

Pinching: Var.

Pit: (of Stomach, Throat): Carc., Var.

Pitchy/Tar-like: Psor.

Pityriasis: Baci., Psor., Tub.

Places: Baci.

Plaque: Morg-G.

Plastic: Pub.

Play: Diph.

Pleuritis/Pleural, Pleuricy/ Pleuro: Diph., Dys.-Co., Infl., Morb., Paratyph., Pyro., Staphyl., Tub.

Pleurodynia: B. Morg., Dys.-Co., Morg-G., Syco.-Co.

Plexalgia: Medo.

Plug/Blunt Pressure/Block or Cork/Ball.: Dys.-Co.

Pneumoconiosis: Tub.

Pneumonia (Bronchopneumonia): Avi., Carc., Paratyph., Tub.

Pneumopathy: Carc., Paratyph.

Pockets: Medo.

Pointed: Baci.-10, Medo., Streptococ.

Poison: Pyro.

Pollakuria/Frequent Urination/ Polyurination: Baci.-10, Medo., Morg-G., Syco.-Co., Syph.

Pollution: Osc.co.

Poly: Baci.-7., Medo., Morg-G., Paratyph., Pert., Pneum., Staphyl., Syco.-Co., Var.

Polyarthritis/Polyarthrosis/[See Joints]: Diph., Streptococ., Var.

Poly-Morphous: Psor.

Polyneuritis: Diph., Pert., Syph.

Polypnoea: Avi., Morb.

Polypus: B. Gaert., Infl., Medo., Morg-G., Syco.-Co., Syph., Tub., Var.

Polysinusitis: Infl.

Poncet-leriche (Rheumatism, Type of): Baci., Tub.

Pork: Psor.

Position: Carc., Psor.

Post: Dys.-Co., Medo., Paratyph., Parot., Prot., Psor.

Potato: Malar

Pre . . . . : B. Gaert., Malar., Morg-G, Pneum., Psor., Staphyl., Syco.-Co., Var.

Precancer: B. Gaert., Carc., Paratyph., Syco.-Co.

Precede: Var.

Precordialgia/Precordium: Dys.-Co., Morg-G., Pneum., Prot., Streptococ., Var.

Predisposition (Diathesis (See Tendency, Repeated): Carc., Infl., Pert.

Pregastrial Region: Diph.

Pregnancy/Parturition: Hydroph.

Premature: Baci.-7., Medo., Syco.-Co., Syph.

Premonition/Presentiment: Psor., Tub.

Presbyopia: Diph.

Pressive/Press/Pressure/Compress/Pressing/Squeezing: B. Morg., Malar., Morb., Osc-co., Prot., Psor., Pyro., Syph., Tub.

Prevention/Preventive/Prophy-

Pupils: Syph.

Purple: Var.

Purpura (See Ecchymosis): Staphyl.

Purulent: Morb., Osc.co., Paratyph., Prot., Psor., Pyro., Staphyl., Streptococ., Syph., Tub., Var.

Pus: Baci., Morb., Psor., Pyro., Tub.

Pyelitis: Morg-G., Prot.

Pyelo: Morg-G., Paratyph., Prot., Tub.

Pyloric: Dys.-Co.

Pyohemia: Pyro.

Pyorrhoea: Morg-G., Psor., Streptococ., Tub.

Pyoria: Staphyl.

Q

Quarrelsome: Psor.

Quiet/Calm., Still: Pyro., Tub.

R

R a b i e s / H y d r o p h o b i a / Lyssophobia: Hydroph.

Rachialgia: Var.

Rachitis/Rickets: Baci., Syph.

Radiant/Irradiating/Emanation/ Radiates (See Extending):

Var.

Radiculitis: Staphyl.

Raising/Elevating: Syph., Var.

Rales: B. Morg., Morb., Paratyph., Syco.-Co.

Rancid: Tub.

Rapid (See Also Violent Fast)/ Hasty: Carc., Diph., Hydroph., Malar., Psor., Pyro., Var.

Rare: Hydroph.

Raynaud's Disease: Prot.

Reabsorption (Resorption): Paratyph.

Reaction/Response: Morg-G., Prot., Psor.

Read/Reading: Malar., Tub.

Recent: Medo.

Recessive/Recede/Receding: Syph.

Recovery/Cure: Streptococ.

Rectorrhagia: Psor.

Rectum/Rectal/Recto: Dys.-Co., Medo., Morg-G., Paratyph., Psor., Pyro., Syco.-Co., Tub.

Red/Redness (See Inflammation, Erythema, Erythrosis)/ Strawbery: Avi., B. Morg., B. Gaert., Diph., Dys.-Co.,

Ringing/Humming/Singing (In the ear): Psor.

Rising (See Climbing): Prot., Streptococ.

Rolling: Malar., Prot.

Root/Base: Avi., Baci., B. Morg., Dys.-Co., Malar., Morg-G., Medo., Staphyl., Syco.-Co., Tub., Var.

Rope: Psor.

Rosela: Tub.

Rosy: Morb., Tub.

Rotten: Psor.

Rough/Roughness: Morb., Psor., Tub.

Round/Circular/Circinate/Oblong (See Oval): B. Gaert., Baci.-7, Morg-G., Syco.-Co., Var.

Rubbing/Brushing/Massaging: Malar., Staphyl., Tub.

Rubeola (See Measles): Tub.

Ruined (See Catastrophy, Calamity): Paratyph., Syph.

Rumbling/Grunting/Gurgling/Grumbling/Splashing: Malar.

S

Saburrale (Sordes): Paratyph.

Sacralgias: Carc.

Sacro-Sacral/Sacrum/Loin: Malar., Medo., Morg-G., Syco-Co., Tub., Var.

Sad/Morose/Melancholy/Depressed/Despondent/Low Spirited: Baci., Medo., Psor., Tub.

Said, Can not Remember What he has just: Psor.

Salads: Prot.

Salivation/Stalorrhoea/Ptyalism: B. Gaert., B. Morg., Hydroph., Malar., Morg-G., Paratyph., Psor., Syco.-Co., Syph.

Salmonella Affection (See Typhoid): Paratyph.

Salpingitis: Baci., B. Morg., Medo., Prot., Syco.-Co., Tub.

Salt/Salty: Carc., Dys.-Co., Hydroph., Medo., Morg-G., Prot., Streptococ., Syco.-Co.

Sand: Medo., Psor., Syph.

Sarcoidosis: Tub.

Sarcosis: Tub.

Satyriasis: Hydroph., Tub.

Scaly: Malan., Morb., Psor.

Scanty: Pneum., Psor., Pyro., Tub.

Sharp/Well Defined Edges: Prot.

Shell-fish: Paratyph.

Shifts (See Changes Alternates)/ Flying/Coming & Going/ Wandering: Syph.

Shining/Varnised: Medo., Pyro.

Shivering/Shuddering: Psor., Tub.

Shock/Impulse: Var.

Shooting (Pain)/Lightning like: Var.

Short: B. Morg., Carc., Diph., Hippoz., Malar., Morg-G., Pneum., Psor., Var.

Shoulder/Shoulder Blade (See Scapula): B. Morg., B. Gaert., Baci.-7., Malar., Medo., Morg-G., Psor., Syco.-Co., Tub., Var.

Sialurrhoea (See Salivation): Syco.-Co., Syph.

Sibilence: Syco.-Co.

Sick/Sickly/Sickenning/Sickly Humour: Medo., Syph., Var.

Side/Sides/Side to Side: Pyro.

Sigh/Sighing: Malar

Sight/Sightedness (See Appearance, Vision): Baci., Diph., Hydroph., Malar., Medo., Prot., Tub., Var.

Sings: Malar.

Sinusitis/Sinus: Avi., B. Morg., Hippoz., Infl., Medo., Morg-G., Osc-co., Pneum., Streptococ., Syco.-Co.

Sitting: Pneum., Psor., Syco.-Co.

Skin (See Cutano-Mucous)/ Dermo: Baci., B. Morg., B. Mut (a)., Carc., Malan., Malar., Medo., Psor., Streptococ., Syco.-Co., Syph., Tub., Var.

Skull (See Head): Medo., Pneum., Prot., Psor., Syph., Tub.

Sleep/Asleep/Somnolence/ Sleepiness/Nap (See Drowsy): Baci., B. Gaert., Carc., Dys.-Co., Malar., Medo., Morg-G., Pneum., Psor., Pyro., Streptococ., Syph., Syco.-Co., Tub., Var.

Sleeplessness (See Insomnia): Baci., Baci.-7, Carc., Malar., paratyph., Prot., Psor., Tub.

Slender (See Thin): Syph.

Slowness/Slowly (See Gradually) Sluggish: Baci.-7, Diph., Medo., Paratyph., Pert., Pyro., Syph.

Small/Little/Slight: Baci., B. Morg., Medo., Pneum., Prot., Psor., Pyro., Streptococ., Syco. Co., Tub.

Squamous: Baci., Morg-G., Tub.

Stain: Tub.

Stammering: Dys.-Co.

Stand/Standing: Malar., Pneum., Psor., Tub.

Staring: Psor.

Stare (See Frightened)/Startled: Medo., Psor.

Stasis: B. Morg., Infl.

Stenosis: Syph.

Sterility: Syph.

Sternum/Sternal/Breast Bone: B. Gaert., Psor., Syph., Var.

Stick (Wooden): **Prot., Psor.**

Sticky/Slimy/Glutty (See Adherent: Psor., Syco.-Co., Tub.

Stiffness (See Rigid): Baci.-7., Infl., Medo., Pyro., Syco.-Co., Syph., Tub., Var.

Stimylent: Medo.

Sting/Stinging: Malan.

Stomach (See Fastric): B. Gaert., B. Morg., Dys.-Co., Hydroph., Malar., Medo., Osc-co., Pneum., Pyro., Syco.-Co., Syph., Tub., Var.

Stomatitis: Medo., Paratyph.

Stools/Faeces/Manure/Fecal Matter: Anthr., Baci., B.

Gaert., Dys.-Co., Hydroph., Malar., Medo., Morg-G., Pneum., Prot., Psor., Pyro., Syco.-Co., Tub., Var.

Stops/Ceases/Arresting: Malar., Pneum.

Storm/Stormy (See Thunder Storm): B. Morg., Carc., Medo., Osc-co., Prot., Syph., Tub.

Strabismus/Squint: Syph.

Straight/Errect: Pneum., Prot.

Strain (See Urging/Tenesmus/Straining: Psor., Syph.

Strange/Stranger/Abnormal/Absurd/Unusual: Baci., Tub.

Streak: Malar., Medo.

Streptococcus: Streptococ.

Stretch/Reaching/Stretching/Stretched: Malar., Prot., Psor., Pyro., Var.

Striated: Psor.

Stricture: Syph.

Stridulous: Infl.

Strike: Tub.

Strong/Concentrated/Severe (See Abundant): B. Morg., Medo., Morg-G., Osc-co., Psor., Syco.-Co., Tub.

Psor., Syco.-Co., Syph., Tub., Var.

Sword: Syph.

Sycosis (See Mesenchymatosis): Infl., Medo., Paratyph., Pneum., Staphyl., Var.

Sympathetic: Carc.

Syndrome: Diph.

Syphilitic/Luetosic/Luetic Syphilis—Secondary & Tertiary: Hippiz., Osc.co., Syph., Var.

T

Tabes: Syph.

Tachycardia: Avi., Diph., Dys.-Co., Morb., Pert., Pneum.

Taciturn: Hydroph.

Talking (See Speaking): Carc., Malar., Medo., Pyro.

Tartar: Baci., Tub.

Taste: Dys.-Co., Malar., Medo., Morg-G., Psor., Pyro., Syco. Co., Tub.

Tear/Tearful: Streptoco.

Tear/Torn/Tearing/Rending/ Asunder: Carc., Pert., Psor., Syph., Tub., Var.

Temper: Tub.

Temperature: Prot., Pyro.

Tempest: Prot.

Temple (Head) Temporal: Psor., Pyro., Var.

Temporary: Parot., Psor., Tub.

Tendency (See Repeated) Inclination/Etiology: B. Morg., Carc., Diph., Medo., Paratyph., Pert., Psor., Pyro.

Tendon/Tendonous/Tendinitis: Infl., Syph., Var.

Tense/Tension/Tensive: B. Morg., Dys.-Co., Morg-G., Prot., Staphyl., Syco.-Co.

Testes/Testicles: Medo., Parot., Psor., Syph., Tub.

Tetani Form: Hydroph

Thick (See Viscous): Anthr., Diph., Morg-G., Prot., Pyro., Syph., Tub., Var.

Thieves/Robbers: Psor.

Thighs: Baci.-10, Carc., Malar., Medo., Syco.-Co., Syph.

Thin (See Slender): Psor.

Thinking: Carc., Hydroph., Medo., Psor.

Third: Psor.

Thirst/Thirsty: Anthr., Medo., Psor., Pyro., Var.

Thoracic (See Chest)/Thorax:
Avi., Baci.-10, Carc., Dys.-
Co., Morg-G., Prot., Syco.-
Co., Tub., Var.

Thought/Thoughtful Throat: B.
Morg., Diph., Dys.-Co.,
Hydroph., Infl., Malar.,
Medo., Morb., Morg-G.,
Pneum., Prot., Psor., Pyro.,
Syco.-Co., Tub., Var.

Throb/Throbbing: Baci-7., Dys.-
Co., Osc.co., Pyro.

Thrombosis: B. Morg., Baci.-7.

Throws: Prot.

Thumb: Baci.-7., Morg-G.

Thyroid (See Strumous): B.
Morg., Diph., Dys-co., Infl.,
Medo., Psor., Syco.-Co., Tub.

Tibia: Psor., Syco.-Co., Syph.

Tic: Dys.-Co., Syco.-Co.

Tickling/Titilation: Medo.,
Morg-G, Psor.

Tight/Tightness: Baci., Tub.,
Var.

Time: Baci.-7., Dys.-Co., Malar.,
Medo., Pneum., Pyro., Syco.-
Co., Syph., Tub.

Timid (See Fear): Baci., Dys.-
Co., Syco.-Co.

Tip (See Point): Baci.-7., Medo.,
Psor., Streptococ., Syco.-Co.

Tissues: B. Gaert.

Tobacco: Medo., Psor.

Toes/Phalanges (See Fingers):
Baci.-7., Malan., Prot.

Tongue (See Glossitis): B.
Morg., B. Gaert., Diph.,
Malar., Medo., Morg-G.,
Osc.co., Paratyph., Pert.,
Prot., Pyro., Streptococ.,
Syph., Tub., Var.

Tonsils/Tonsilitis/Quinsy: B.
Morg., Baci.-7, Diph., Dys-
Co., Medo., Morg-G., Psor.,
Streptococ., Syco.-Co., Syph.,
Tub., Var.

Too: Psor., Pyro.

Tooth/Teeth (See Molar): B.
Gaert., Carc., Malar., Medo.,
Psor., Pyro., Syph., Tub.

Toothache: Baci., Carc.,
Hydroph., Psor.

Torment/Tormented/Troubled/
Tortured/Revile: B. Morg.,
Tub.

Torpor/Torpid: Carc., Pert.

Tortion: Prot.

Tosses/Tossing: Tub.

Tottering (See Staggering): Tub.

Touch: B. Morg., Medo., Osc.co.,
Pyro., Syph.

Toximic/Toxic/Toxicosis/Intoxi-cation: Anthr., Malar., Medo., Paratyph., Pert., Psor., Pyro., Syph.

Toxico-Mania: Syph.

Traces: Malan.

Trachea/Tracheo—/Air Pas-sage: Avi., Osc.co., Pert.

Trachitis: B. Morg., Diph., Pneum.

Transverse: Medo

Travelling/Journey/Trains/Riding/Voyage/Go: Baci., B. Morg., Carc., Dys.-co., Pneum., Psor., Tub.

Trembling/Quivering/Tremu-lousness: Baci., Carc., Dys-co., Pneum., Psor., Syco.-Co., Syph., Tub., Var.

Tribadism (Sexual Relation be-tween two females or Lesbi-anism): Tub.

Trigeminal: Syph.

Trismus: Syph.

Trisomia (See Mongolism): Carc.

Troublesome/Perturbations/Bothered/Manifestation/Distressing: Baci., B. Morg., Diph., Pert., Psor., Streptococ., Syco-co., Tub.

Tuberculosis (Tubercular Con-

dition)/Tuberculinic: Avi., Baci., Baci.-7, Carc., Diph., Dys-co., Hippoz., Malar., Morb., Osc.co., Pert., Pneum., Psor., Pyro., Syco.-Co., Tub., Var.

Tumefaction (See Swelling): Parot.

Tumors/Mass (See Lump)/Growth: Medo.

Turbid/Cloudy: Malan., Osc.co., Prot., Tub.

Turns/Turning/Twisting/Tilting/Rotation/Whirling: Psor., Pyro., Tub.

Tympanum: Osc.co.

Tympanism (See Flatulence) Tympanites: Var.

Typhlitis (See Appendicitis): Tub.

Typhoid/Typhoidal: Paratyph., Psor., Pyro., Var.

Typhus (Angio Hematic]: Paratyph.

Ulceration/Ulcers (See Sores)/Cancer: Anthr., B. Morg., Dys.-Co., Hippoz., Infl., Medo., Morg-G., Pert., Prot., Psor., Pyro., Staphyl., Syco-co., Syph., Tub.

Unconscious (See Collapse & Epilepsy): Medo.

Vascular: Syph., Tub.

Vasco-Motor: Syco.-Co.

Vault: B. Gaert., Streptococ.

Vegetation/Vegetables: Psor., Syco.-Co.

Vein/Venous (See Phlebitis): B. Morg., Baci.-7, Infl., Paratyph., Prot., Tub.

Vertebra/Vertebral (Column): Baci., Medo., Paratyph., Psor., Streptococ., Syph.

Vertex/Top of the Head: B. Morg., Dys.-Co.

Vertical: Syph.

Vertigo/Giddiness/Dizziness: B. Morg., Malar., Medo., Paratyph., Pneum., Prot., Psor., Streptococ., Syph., Tub., Var.

Vesicle (See Boil)/Vesiculo/Vesicular: Anthr., B. Gaert., B. Morg., Dys.-Co., Morg-G., Prot., Psor., Pyro., Staphyl., Streptococ., Tub., Var.

Vesperal (See Evening): Diph.

Vessels/Ducts: Prot., Syph.

Viande (Titbit Foods): Morg-G., Prot., Psor.

Vibration: Streptococ.

Vice [As if Vaught in a: Pneum.

Violent/Terrible/Brutal/Fast/ Furious (See Severe): Baci., Pneum., Prot., Psor., Streptococ., Syph., Tub., Var.

Violet (See Purple): Anthr., Tub., Var.

Viral: Morg-G., Parot., Syco.-Co., Syph.

Viscera: Medo., Syph.

Viscous (See Thick/Stringy/ Tough/Ropy/Viscid/Tenacious: Hydroph., Medo., Pert., Prot., Pyro., Syco.-Co., Tub., Var.

Vision (See Sight): Dys.-Co., Medo., Streptococ., Tub., Var.

Vitality: Diph.

Vitrious: Psor.

Vocal Chords: Diph., Syph., Tub.

Voice: Diph., Hippoz., Infl., Morb., Osc.-Co., Psor., Tub.

Voluntary: Medo.

Vomit/Vomitus: B. Gaert., Baci.-10, Carc., Diph., Dys.-Co., Hydroph., Infl., Medo., Morg-G, Osc.co., Paratyph., Pert., Prot., Psor., Pyro., Streptococ., Syph., Tub., Var.

Voracious/Ravenous/Greedy/ Canine: Psor.

Winter: B. Gaert., Diph., Prot., Psor.

Without: Paratyph., Pneum., Psor., Streptococ., Syco.-Co., Tub.

Work/Function: Psor., Tub.

Worn out/Weariness: Psor.

Worry/Care, full of: Psor.

Wound/Lesion/Injury/Hurt: Hydroph., Malan., Psor.

Wrinkles/Shrivelled: Syph.

Wrist/Carpus/Carpal: B. Morg., Baci.-7, Morg-G., Pert., Prot.,

Psor., Streptococ., Syco.-Co., Var.

Writing/Writer: Medo., Prot.

Y

Yawning: Malar., Psor., Var.

Yellow: B. Morg., Dys.-Co., Malar., Medo., Osc.-Co., Prot., Psor., Pyro., Syco.-Co., Syph., Tub., Var.

Young: Carc., Tub.

Z

Zona: Morg-G., Staphyl., Var.

Zoster (Herpes) Zosterian: Var.